Neoplastic Lesions of the Skin

Demos Surgical Pathology Guides

Neoplastic Lesions of the Skin

JOSE A. PLAZA, MD
Director of Dermatopathology
Medical College of Wisconsin
Milwaukee, Wisconsin

VICTOR G. PRIETO, MD, PhD
Director of Dermatopathology
University of Texas–MD Anderson Cancer Center
Houston, Texas

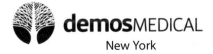
New York

ISBN: 978-1-933864-86-0
e-book ISBN: 9781935281979

Acquisitions Editor: Rich Winters
Compositor: diacriTech

Visit our website at www.demosmedpub.com

Library of Congress Cataloging-in-Publication Data

Plaza, Jose A.
  Neoplastic lesions of the skin / Jose A. Plaza, MD Medical College of Wisconsin, Milwaukee, Wisconsin, Victor G. Prieto, MD, PhD, MD Anderson Cancer Center, Houston, Texas.
      pages cm—(Demos surgical pathology guides)
  Includes bibliographical references and index.
  ISBN 978-1-933864-86-0
  1. Skin—Cancer—Diagnosis. 2. Skin—Diseases—Diagnosis. I. Prieto, Victor G. II. Title.
  RC280.S5P57 2014
  616.99′477—dc23

                                                    2013028151

Special discounts on bulk quantities of Demos Medical Publishing books are available to corporations, professional associations, pharmaceutical companies, health care organizations, and other qualifying groups. For details, please contact:

Special Sales Department
Demos Medical Publishing, LLC
11 West 42nd Street, 15th Floor
New York, NY 10036
Phone: 800-532-8663 or 212-683-0072
Fax: 212-941-7842
E-mail: specialsales@demosmedpub.com

Printed in the United States of America by Bradford & Bigelow.
13 14 15 16 17 / 5 4 3 2 1

Contents

Series Foreword

The field of surgical pathology has gained increasing relevance and importance over the years as pathologists have become more and more integrated into the health care team. To the need for precise histopathologic diagnoses has now been added the burden of providing our clinical colleagues with information that will allow them to assess the prognosis of the disease and predict the response to therapy. Pathologists now serve as key consultants in the patient management team and are responsible for providing critical information that will guide their therapy. With the progress gained due to the insights obtained from the application of newer diagnostic techniques, surgical pathology has become progressively more complex. As a result, diagnoses need to be more detailed and specific and the number of data elements required in the generation of a surgical pathology report have increased exponentially, making management of the information required for diagnosis cumbersome and sometimes difficult.

The past 15 years have witnessed an explosion of information in the field of pathology with a massive proliferation of specialized textbooks appearing in print. For the most part, such texts provide in-depth and detailed coverage of the various areas in surgical pathology. The purpose of this series is to bridge the gap between the major subspecialty texts and the large, double-volume general surgical pathology textbooks, by providing compact, single-volume monographs that will succinctly address the most salient and important points required for the diagnosis of the most common conditions. The series is organized following an organ-system format, with single volumes dedicated to individual organs. The volumes are divided on the basis of disease groups, including benign reactive, inflammatory, infectious or systemic conditions, benign neoplastic conditions, and malignant neoplasms. Each chapter consists of a bulleted list of the most pertinent clinical data related to the condition, followed by the most important histopathologic criteria for diagnosis, pertinent use of immunohistochemical stains and other ancillary techniques, and relevant molecular tests when available. This is followed by a section on differential diagnosis. References appear at the back of the volume. Each entity is illustrated with key, high-quality histological images that highlight the most salient and distinctive features that need to be recognized for the correct diagnosis.

These books are intended for the busy practicing pathologist, and for pathology residents and fellows in training who require an easy and simple overview of major diagnostic criteria and key points during the course of routine daily practice. The authors have been carefully chosen for their experience in the field and clarity of exposition in the various topics. It is hoped that this series will fulfill its purpose of providing quick and easy access to critical information for the busy practitioner or trainee, and that it will assist pathologists in their routine practice of the specialty.

Saul Suster, MD
Professor and Chairman
Department of Pathology
Medical College of Wisconsin
Milwaukee, Wisconsin

Preface

Skin neoplasms are a diverse group of diseases that may be derived from any part of the body. Their classification is quite extensive and in this book we provide a comprehensive review of the most common neoplasms encountered in clinical practice. The coverage in the book includes both benign and malignant lesions along with an update of the current diagnostic modalities. Our hope is that this book will be a concise, useful resource for pathologists, dermatopathologists and residents to become familiar with the most common cutaneous tumors and in particular with their immunohistochemical profile. The book also includes presentation of the clinical aspects of some of the common benign and malignant cutaneous lesions along with the most common differential diagnosis.

Demos Surgical Pathology Guides

Neoplastic Lesions of the Skin

Epithelial/Epidermal Lesions

1

Epidermal Nevi

Epidermal nevi are benign lesions that result from overgrowth of the epidermis. They can occur in a localized area of skin or be more extensive, covering large areas. The majority appear at birth or within the first year of life; however, they may also develop later during childhood or adulthood. They may be skin-colored or brown in color and often have a linear appearance (1).

VARIANTS

- Nevus unius lateralis: Epidermal nevus on the trunk and limbs, usually just on one side of the body.
- Ichthyosis hystrix: It is a genodermatosis (see non neoplastic diseases). Some authors use this term to describe cases of epidermal nevus that show extensive bilateral or generalized distribution.
- Inflammatory linear verrucous epidermal nevus (ILVEN): linear, persistent, pruritic plaque, usually first noted on a limb in early childhood.
- Epidermal nevus syndrome: This syndrome refers to the association of an epidermal nevus and extracutaneous abnormalities, most often affecting the brain, eye, and skeletal system (1, 2).
- Linear nevus sebaceus syndrome: Usually on head and neck. Schimmelpenning syndrome links a linear nevus sebaceus with cerebral anomalies, coloboma, and conjunctival lipodermoid lesion.
- CHILD syndrome: Congenital hypoplasia with ichthyosiform nevus and limb defects (CHILD) is inherited as an X-linked dominant disorder, and is lethal in males. It is due to mutations in the *NSDHL* gene. The CHILD nevus is either strictly on one side of the body (most often the right) with clear-cut midline demarcation, may follow Blaschko lines, or both. Other findings include hypoplasia or aplasia of limbs, chondrodysplasia punctate, etc. Histologically, the skin lesions show epidermal hyperplasia and foamy histiocytes in the dermal papillae mimicking a verruciform xanthoma (3).

PATHOLOGY (FIGURE 1-1)

■ Hyperkeratosis, papillomatosis, acanthosis, and elongation of rete ridges

■ Rarely epidermolytic hyperkeratosis, focal acantholytic dyskeratosis (FAD), and cornoid lamellae

■ In CHILD nevus, in addition to the above features there is parakeratosis admixed with hyperorthokeratosis. Also characteristic are the presence of intraepidermal neutrophils and dermal papillae filled with foamy histiocytes (mimicking verruciform xanthoma).

■ Note: The changes in epidermal nevus sometimes are subtle and may resemble acanthosis nigricans or seborrheic keratosis.

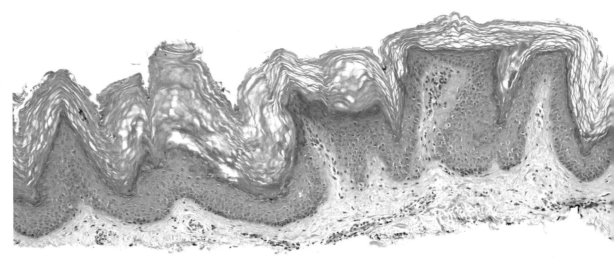

FIGURE 1-1

FIGURE 1-1   Epidermal nevus. The epidermis is papillomatous with hyperkeratosis reminiscent of a seborrheic keratosis.

Nevus Comedonicus

Nevus comedonicus is a rare disorder of pilosebaceous development. The lesions are typically present at birth or develop in early childhood. Clinically, it presents as a collection of dilated follicular ostia plugged with pigmented keratinaceous debris. It is usually unilateral, and typically found on the face, trunk, neck, and upper extremities. Nevus comedonicus syndrome is the association of nevus comedonicus with abnormalities in the central nervous system, skeletal system, and skin (4, 5).

PATHOLOGY (FIGURE 1-2)
- Dilated follicular infundibula that are closely positioned with prominent orthokeratotic plugging
- Sebaceous elements are decreased in number
- The follicular walls are lined by epithelium that often appears atrophic and is composed of a few layers of keratinocytes

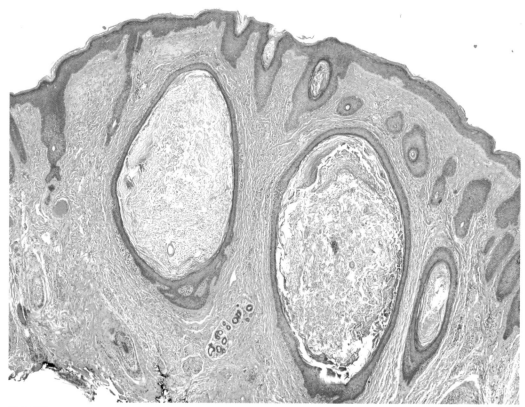

FIGURE 1-2

FIGURE 1-2   Nevus comedonicus. Dilated keratin-filled follicular invaginations. Note the absence of sebaceous glands.

Seborrheic Keratosis

Seborrheic keratosis is the most common benign tumors in older patients. Clinically, it presents as one or more, light brown, flat lesions with a velvety verrucous surface (stuck-on appearance). They can be seen almost anywhere in the body (except palms and soles), but are most common on the face, neck, and chest. The Lesser-Trélat sign is the association of multiple eruptive seborrheic keratoses with internal malignancy, most commonly adenocarcinoma of the stomach; however, it may be associated with lymphoma, leukemia, pancreatic cancer, etc. Also, multiple seborrheic keratoses may develop after inflammatory dermatoses (6).

PATHOLOGY (FIGURE 1-3A–F)
- Epidermal changes including hyperkeratosis, papillomatosis, and acanthosis
- Population of basaloid keratinocytes
- Horn pseudocysts (keratin-containing invaginations of the epidermis resembling follicular cysts)
- Commonly pigmented keratinocytes in the basal layer

VARIANTS
- Acanthotic seborrheic keratosis: It is the most common type. The surface is hyperkeratotic with a thick layer of basaloid cells interspersed with horn pseudocysts. Some of these cells typically contain melanin pigment. This variant can be confused with eccrine poroma, but there is no ductal differentiation.
- Papillomatous seborrheic keratosis: Pronounced hyperkeratosis and papillomatosis with less acanthosis and fewer horn pseudocysts.
- Stucco keratosis: Usually on lower legs of older patients. Histologically, shows church-spire rete ridges with minimal to no pseudocysts.
- Reticulated seborrheic keratosis: Numerous thin tracts of basaloid epidermal cells that are branched and interwoven. It has minimal acanthosis and horn pseudocysts are usually absent.
- Macular seborrheic keratosis: It presents as a brown macule in sun-exposed areas. It can be associated with solar lentigo. Histologically, shows a flat surface with compact stratum corneum, bridged rete ridges, and rare horn pseudocysts.

(text continued on page 6)

Seborrheic Keratosis *(continued)*

- ◼ "Clonal" (Borst–Jadassohn phenomenon) seborrheic keratosis: Well-demarcated intraepithelial nests of basaloid or larger squamous cells. These nests can mimic squamous cell carcinoma. This variant is related to irritated seborrheic keratosis in which the nests are larger and may contain spindle-shaped keratinocytes and acantholysis.
- ◼ Inverted follicular keratosis (IFK): A seborrheic keratosis that is characterized by an endophytic growth along a hair follicle. Keratinocytes characteristically show whorls/ squamous eddies of maturing squamous epithelium. There is prominent hypergranulosis suggesting possible HPV infection.
- ◼ Benign lichenoid keratosis (BLK; lichen-planus-like keratosis): Since a number of these lesions are associated with seborrheic keratosis, BLK is discussed here. BLK shows hyperkeratosis (ortho and para), hypergranulosis, irregular acanthosis, and a dense lichenoid infiltrate of lymphocytes (and scattered neutrophils, eosinophils, and plasma cells) with dyskeratotic keratinocytes (interface damage). BLK can also be associated with lentigo and actinic keratosis (AK). Due to the damage to basal keratinocytes resulting in dyskeratosis and pigment incontinence, the clinical diagnosis may include a melanocytic lesion and basal cell carcinoma (7).

FIGURE 1-3   (A) Seborrheic keratosis. Verrucous epidermis with marked acanthosis and multiple horn cysts. (B) Higher magnification of horn cysts and the basaloid cell population. (C) Acanthotic seborrheic keratosis. Smooth surface with marked acanthosis. Note the horn cysts. (D) Reticulated/adenoid seborrheic keratosis. There are irregular, interlacing narrow downgrowths of basaloid cells. (E) Macular seborrheic keratosis. Note the flat acanthotic epidermis with pigmentation of keratinocytes. (F) Inverted follicular keratosis (IFK). Endophytic growth of the epithelium with keratinocytes arranged in whorls/squamous eddies.

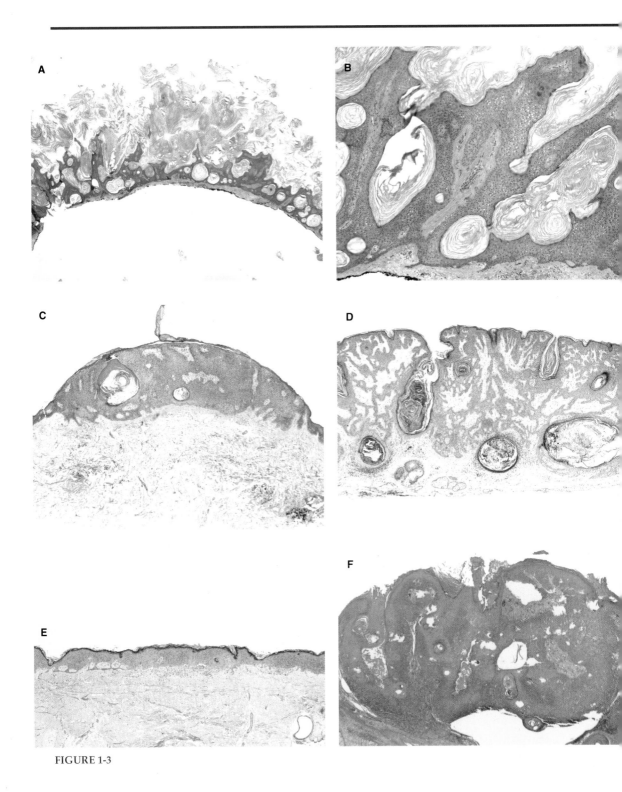

FIGURE 1-3

Warty Dyskeratoma

Warty dyskeratoma is an uncommon neoplasm that presents as whitish solitary hyperkeratotic papule with an umbilicated or pore-like center. It is more commonly located on the head and neck or back of middle-aged and elderly individuals (8).

PATHOLOGY (FIGURE 1-4)
- Cup-shaped epithelial proliferation of benign squamous cells
- The central depression is filled with a plug of keratinous material
- The epidermal component shows suprabasilar clefting with suprabasilar acantholysis and dyskeratotic cells within the lacuna
- Protruding into the lacuna are dermal papillae covered by a layer of basal cells (villi)
- Sometimes it can be seen originating from a hair follicle or sebaceous gland

DIFFERENTIAL DIAGNOSIS
Many other dermatoses (including Darier and Grover diseases) may show similar findings including the suprabasal clefting with acantholysis and dyskeratotic cells; however, the presence of deep penetrating, crateriform shape (cup-shape) in a solitary lesion is characteristic of warty dyskeratomas.

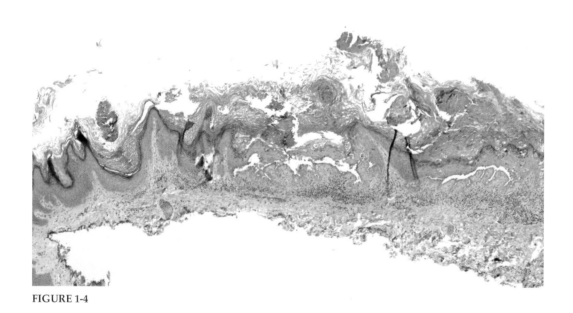

FIGURE 1-4

FIGURE 1-4   Warty dyskeratoma. A dilated cup-shaped lesion containing a keratinous plug with areas of suprabasal clefting.

Epidermolytic Acanthoma

Epidermolytic acanthoma is an acquired lesion that presents as a verrucous papule or nodule, most commonly seen on the scrotum, head and neck, and legs. This lesion develops due to a gene mutation on keratin 1 and 10 (9).

PATHOLOGY (FIGURE 1-5)
- Papillomatous and verrucous epidermis
- Hyperkeratosis and parakeratosis
- Upper epidermis and granular layer show marked vacuolation with eosinophilic keratin inclusions (epidermolytic hyperkeratosis)
- Note: Epidermolytic hyperkeratosis can be seen in many conditions including linear epidermal nevus, palmoplantar keratoderma, and in congenital bullous ichthyosiform erythroderma

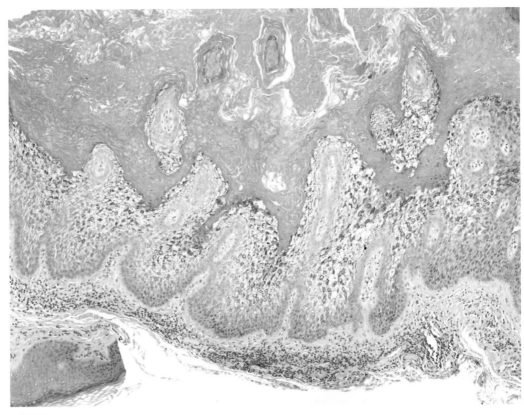

FIGURE 1-5

FIGURE 1-5   Epidermolytic acanthoma. Papillomatous epidermis with massive hyperkeratosis. Note the marked vacuolation of keratinocytes.

Acantholytic Acanthoma

Acantholytic acanthoma is a solitary lesion that presents as a keratotic papule most commonly in elderly male patients on the trunk, neck, or extremities (10).

PATHOLOGY (FIGURE 1-6)
- Papillomatous acanthotic epidermis
- Hyperkeratosis
- Acantholysis usually above basal layer (but it can affect the entire epidermis)
- Focal dyskeratosis
- In the dermis there is a superficial perivascular lymphocytic infiltrate admixed with eosinophils

DIFFERENTIAL DIAGNOSIS
Other conditions such as focal acantholytic dyskeratosis (FAD), Darier disease, or Hailey-Hailey disease may show identical histologic features but all three present with multiple lesions.

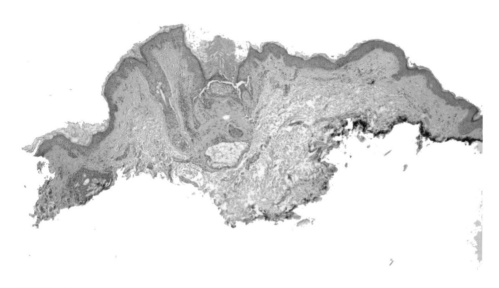

FIGURE 1-6

FIGURE 1-6   Acantholytic acanthoma. This is a solitary lesion with papillomatous architecture and acantholysis in the suprabasal layer.

Focal Acantholytic Dyskeratosis

Focal acantholytic dyskeratosis (FAD) is a common distinctive histologic pattern characterized by suprabasilar clefts around preserved papillae, acantholysis, and dyskeratotic cells. These histologic changes have been observed as an incidental finding, particularly on the trunk and many times in the re-excision specimen in a variety of skin lesions including basal cell carcinomas, nevi, dermatofibromas, epidermal nevus, pityriasis rubra pilaris, etc. (11).

PATHOLOGY (FIGURE 1-7)
- Hyperkeratosis and parakeratosis
- Focal acantholysis (intraepidermal or suprabasal) with cleft formation and dyskeratosis
- Occasional "dilapidated brick" appearance (marked intraepidermal similar to Hailey-Hailey disease)
- Occasional corps ronds and grains (similar to Darier disease)
- A diagnostic clue to FAD is the observation of multiple patterns within the same biopsy, e.g., corps ronds, next to marked intraepidermal acantholysis and next to focal suprabasal acantholysis

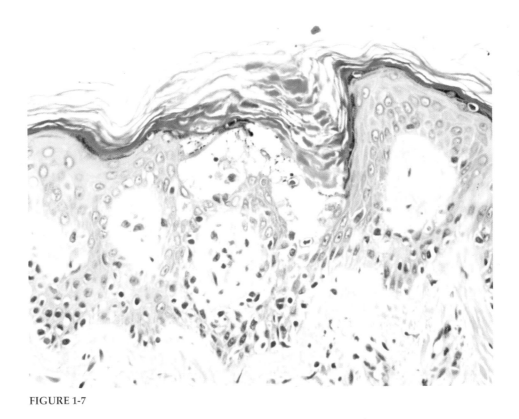

FIGURE 1-7

FIGURE 1-7   Focal acantholytic dyskeratosis (FAD). Note the focal acantholysis and dyskeratosis.

Clear Cell Acanthoma

Clear cell acanthoma is a benign solitary epidermal papule or nodule most commonly located on the lower extremities of the middle-aged and elderly. Clinically, it presents as a red nodule that can mimic a vascular neoplasms (12).

PATHOLOGY (FIGURE 1-8A, B)
- Psoriasiform hyperplasia of the epidermis with acanthosis
- Intracorneal and epidermal neutrophilic abscesses
- Dilated blood vessels
- Demarcated lateral border
- Slightly enlarged keratinocytes with pale-staining cytoplasm (glycogen-rich, highlighted by PAS)
- Mild spongiosis
- Epidermal ridges are fused
- Classically, the intraepidermal adnexal structures are spared

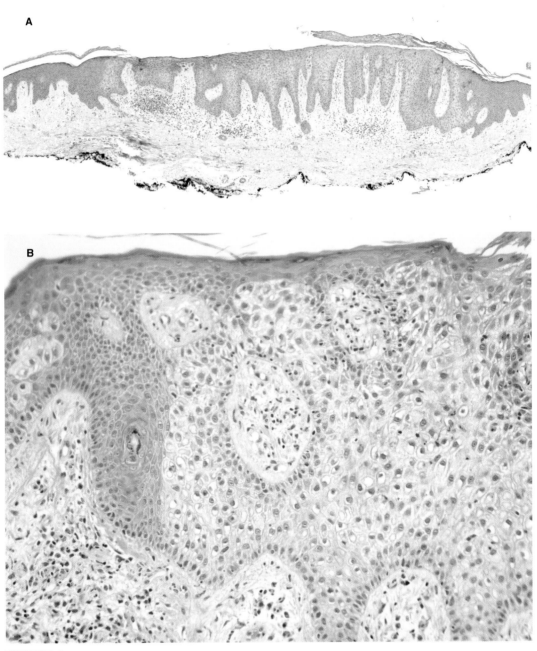

FIGURE 1-8

FIGURE 1-8   (A) Clear cell acanthoma. Circumscribed lesion with acanthotic epidermis containing pale keratinocytes. (B) Marked transition between normal epidermis and the pale staining keratinocytes at the lateral border of the lesion. The lesion has a very thin granular layer.

Actinic Keratosis

Actinic keratosis (AK) is a common, mostly sun-induced, lesion seen in White, middle-aged, or elderly patients. AK arises mostly on sun-exposed areas, such as the face, ears, bald scalp, forearms, and backs of the hands. It presents as small, red, and scaly area. AK may follow different pathways; it may regress, it may persist without major changes, or it may progress to squamous cell carcinoma. The actual percentage of lesions that progress to invasive squamous cell carcinoma remains unknown; estimates have varied from as low as 0.1% to as high as 10% (13, 14). Patients with arsenic exposure and immunosuppressed individuals may develop multiple AK.

PATHOLOGY (FIGURE 1-9A–C)
■ Epidermis exhibits hyperkeratosis and parakeratosis. There may be either irregular acanthosis or atrophy with some blunt and thick rete ridges ("Bernie's buddies")
■ Basal layer keratinocytes are cytologically atypical (hyperchromatic, irregular nuclei) and vary in size and shape (from mild to severe atypia)
■ Underlying dermis shows solar elastosis

VARIANTS
■ Atrophic AK: There is cytologic atypia of keratinocytes but only minimal acanthosis.
■ Hyperplastic AK: Atypical keratinocytes tend to bud into the papillary dermis. The dysplastic changes are seen primarily within the basal layer.
■ Acantholytic AK: Acantholysis along with dysplastic changes at the basal layer of epidermis. Sometimes this pattern can be confused with acantholytic disorders such as Darier disease. Acantholytic AK is considered to be more likely to progress to frank squamous cell carcinoma.
■ Bowenoid AK: This lesion has full-thickness keratinocytic atypia resembling that seen in Bowen disease. A distinction with a squamous cell carcinoma in situ is an artificial one, since both conditions represent part of a spectrum.
■ Pigmented AK: There is increased melanin pigment in the basal keratinocytes. Characteristically this lesion shows very little parakeratosis. Some authors (as we do) consider this lesion to be indistinguishable from large cell acanthoma.
■ Lichenoid AK: There is a band-like lymphohistiocytic infiltrate in the superficial dermis, sometimes with interface vacuolar damage of the dermal-epidermal junction.

FIGURE 1-9   (A) Actinic keratosis. Note the mounds of parakeratosis and the marked cytologic atypia of the basal cell layer of the epidermis. (B) Atrophic actinic keratosis. There are parakeratosis, epidermal atrophy, and marked basal nuclear atypia. Note the prominent solar elastosis in the dermis. (C) Hyperplastic actinic keratosis. Note the marked elongation of the rete ridges.

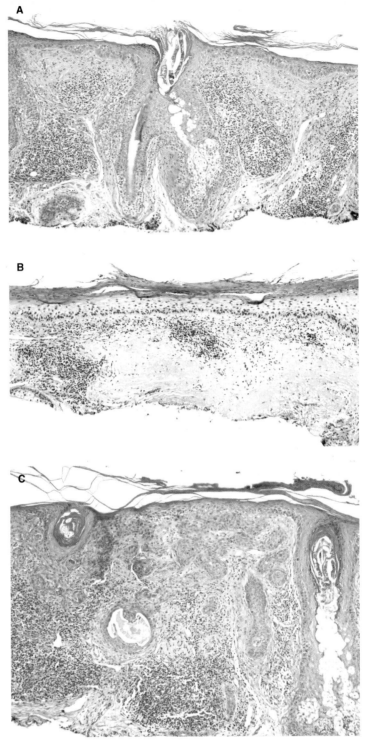

FIGURE 1-9

Squamous Cell Carcinoma

When dysplastic keratinocytic involves the entire epidermis, such lesions are then designated squamous cell carcinoma in situ (SCCis). SCCis manifests predominantly in White patients and is most common in adulthood, with the highest incidence in patients older than 60 years. It may involve any area of the body but most frequently occurs on sun-exposed areas such as the face, neck, arms, and lower legs. Clinically, it presents as slowly enlarging, irregular reddish patches. Approximately 5% of cases develop an invasive component and of these up to 30% have metastatic potential (particularly larger lesions with deep tissue and perineural invasion; see invasive SCC). Immunocompromised patients have an increased risk of developing SCCis and it tends to have a more aggressive behavior and higher recurrence rates when compared to immunocompetent patients. The etiology is possibly multifactorial including particularly solar radiation, arsenic exposure, and HPV infection (15–17).

PATHOLOGY (FIGURE 1-10A–E)
■ Epidermis shows full-thickness atypia, involving the entire epidermis including the intraepidermal areas of the cutaneous adnexa
■ Characteristic marked acanthosis with complete squamous cell dismaturation and lack of polarity
■ Keratinocytes are large and contain prominent irregular, hyperchromatic nuclei with conspicuous nucleoli and abundant cytoplasm
■ Keratinocytes may be vacuolated due to glycogen deposition resulting in clear cell change
■ Common mitotic figures and dyskeratotic cells

VARIANTS
■ Atrophic: There is thinning of the epidermis while still showing full-thickness atypia and disorganization.
■ Acantholytic: There is acantholysis. When prominent these lesions have been described as "adenoid" and may resemble both adenocarcinoma and angiosarcoma.
■ Pagetoid: There are singled and nested keratinocytes with large, pale cytoplasm alternating with strands of relatively normal intervening keratinocytes, thus resembling Paget disease or melanoma in situ. This entity is typically seen in markedly sun-damaged individuals and in Texas we sometimes refer to it as "Texas pagetoid SCC." The atypical cells of this pagetoid SCC display keratohyaline granules, thus confirming its keratinocytic differentiation (epidermal cells are the only ones in the body that contain such granules). IHC may also be helpful. Extramammary Paget and pagetoid SCCis can rarely show overlapping immunophenotypic profile (CK7, EMA, CEA); however, cases of pagetoid SCCis are positive for p63 and extramammary Paget is negative, making p63 a useful marker for such distinction. Melanoma in situ cells will express melanocytic markers (S100, MART1, HMB45 antigen) (Figure 1-10D).

FIGURE 1-10   (A) Squamous cell carcinoma in situ. Note the full thickness atypia with abnormal maturation of ketainocytes. (B) High power showing the abnormal maturation of the keratinocytes lacking polarity and showing large nuclei at all levels of the epidermis. (C) Another example showing the loss of maturation, suprabasal mitotic figures, and vacuolation. Note the markedly diminished granular cell layer. (D) Pagetoid squamous cell carcinoma in situ. Atypical keratinocytes forming single nests with pagetoid appearance. (E) Squamous cell carcinoma in situ with clear cell features. Many of the atypical cells display clear cell cytoplasm.

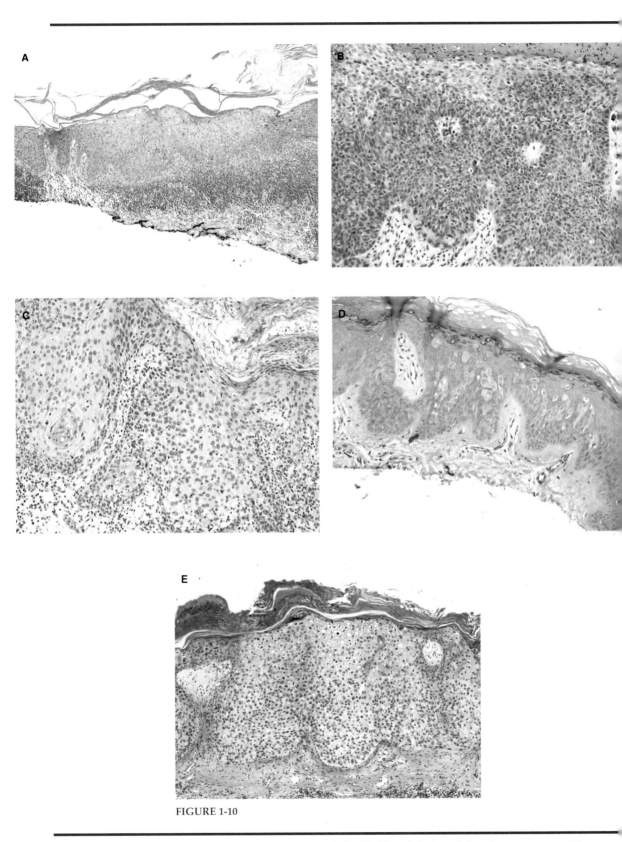

FIGURE 1-10

Invasive Squamous Cell Carcinoma

It is more common in White older males. Indeed, SCC is the second most common form of cutaneous cancer after basal cell carcinoma. The etiology of SCC is multifactorial but the likely most important factor is chronic actinic damage. Other factors include immunosuppression, radiation, HPV infection, chronic inflammation (burns, osteomyelitis), etc. The recurrence and metastasis rates are variable, with an overall recurrence rate of 3.7% to 10%. SCC after burns, radiation, and scarring are high-risk tumors with high risk of metastasis. Also related to worse prognosis are large size, invasion of deep structures, and perineural invasion (17).

PATHOLOGY (FIGURE 1-11A–G)
There is differentiation of the neoplastic cells neoplasm toward keratinization. The lesions are classified into well-differentiated, moderately differentiated, and poorly differentiated variants.

- Well-differentiated: Squamous cells shows recognizable and often abundant keratinization. It shows intercellular bridges with minimal pleomorphism. Mitotic figures are mainly seen at the base.
- Moderately differentiated: Squamous epithelial differentiation is less clear. Nuclear and cytoplasmic pleomorphism is pronounced and mitotic figures are conspicuous. Formation of keratin is less pronounced, and sometimes is limited to the formation of occasional keratin pearls and horn pseudocysts.
- Poorly differentiated: These tumors do not show clear squamous cell differentiation and it may be difficult to establish the true nature of the tumor unless intercellular bridges or an in situ component are identified.

(text continued on page 20)

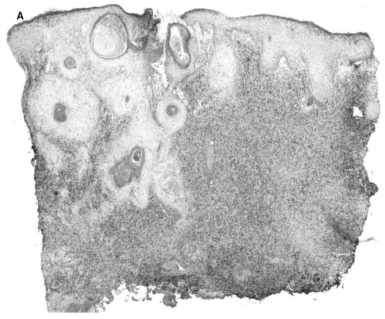

FIGURE 1-11

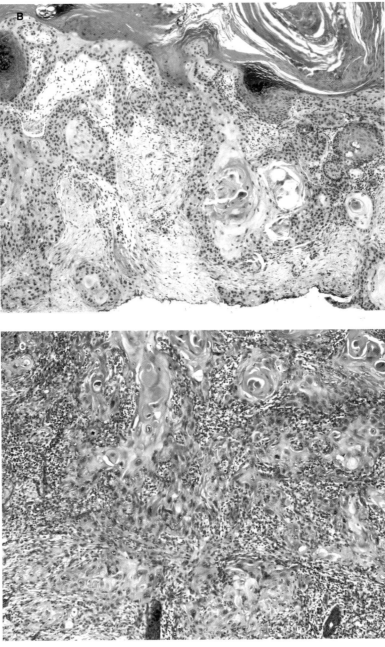

FIGURE 1-11

FIGURE 1-11   (A) Invasive squamous cell carcinoma. Nests of atypical squamous cells invade into reticular dermis. (B) Clear tumor arising from the dysplastic epidermis. Nests of atypical squamous cells invading the dermis. (C) Invading atypical squamous cells with prominent keratinization.

(continued)

Invasive Squamous Cell Carcinoma *(continued)*

HISTOLOGIC VARIANTS

Spindle cell squamous cell carcinoma (sarcomatoid carcinoma): These tumors consist of pleomorphic, spindled cells with no to minimal evidence of epithelial or squamous cell differentiation. Sometimes there is evidence of continuity with the epidermis and/ or direct transition from epithelial to spindled cell morphology. Thus, careful search for dyskeratosis or intercellular bridges may assist in making the diagnosis. Other tumors (melanoma, atypical fibroxanthoma, leiomyosarcoma) may show similar histologic findings, and the diagnosis may rely upon careful interpretation of immunohistochemical studies. Immunohistochemical studies usually show keratin expression, especially high molecular weight cytokeratins such as CK5/6, 34betaE12. p63 is also usually positive. However, sometimes these tumors may lose labeling by one or more cytokeratin antibodies and therefore it may be necessary to use a panel with several anticytokeratin antibodies. Focal positivity for muscle-specific actin (MSA) and vimentin expression is sometimes seen, suggesting a possible change toward mesenchymal phenotype (18–20) (Figure 1-11D–G).

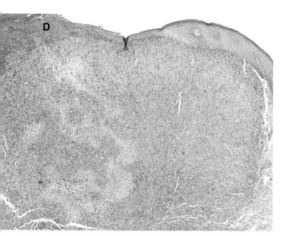 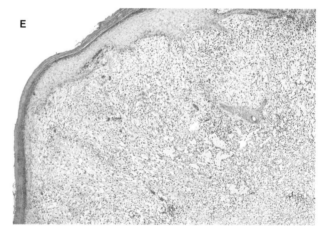

FIGURE 1-11

FIGURE 1-11 (D) Sarcomatoid squamous cell carcinoma. Malignant nodular neoplasm in the dermis with overlying ulcerated epithelium. Note the fasciculated growth pattern along with the pleomorphic spindle cells. (E) Malignant nodular neoplasm with more myxoid and pseudoglandular spaces. Note the absence of carcinoma in situ in the overlying epidermis. (F) The tumor cells strongly express p63 confirming the epithelial origin of the tumor. (G) Focal expression of CK5/6.

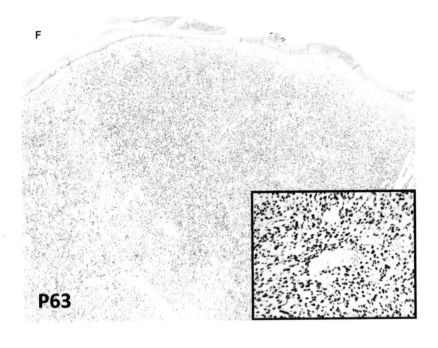

P63

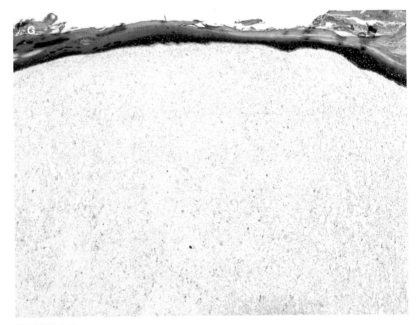

FIGURE 1-11

Verrucous Carcinoma

Verrucous carcinoma was initially described as a variant of well-differentiated squamous carcinoma arising in the oral cavity, but now this type of squamous cell carcinoma has been described on the larynx, esophagus, and multiple skin areas. They are most commonly seen in middle-aged men and usually evolve over a long period of time. The most common locations on the skin are the sole of the foot and the genital area, but lesions can affect other anatomic sites. Clinically, they present as isolated hyperkeratotic warty growths associated with the development of keratin-filled sinuses. Many cutaneous lesions can be confused both clinically and microscopically with viral warts and it is likely that some lesions have evolved within a pre-existent wart. HPV has been found in some cases (HPV types 6 and 11 are most often implicated in genital lesions) (21, 22). Verrucous carcinoma may invade adjacent structures but will only extremely rarely metastasize.

PATHOLOGY (FIGURE 1-12A, B)
- Lesions have both exophytic and endophytic components.
- The exophytic component is papillomatous with hyperkeratosis and parakeratosis.
- The endophytic component shows rete ridges that have a bulbous appearance and are composed of large well-differentiated squamous epithelial cells with a benign appearance.
- These down growths sometimes may extend into the deep dermis and the subcutaneous tissue.
- Keratinization is extensive and when accompanied by necrosis gives rise to sinuses, which are quite characteristic of this tumor.
- A diagnostic clue in many cases is the presence of increased intracellular edema (glassy appearance).
- Intraepidermal neutrophilic abscesses are common.
- Note: It is very important to render the diagnosis of verrucous carcinoma to tumors that are entirely well-differentiated and lack cellular pleomorphism. Otherwise, such tumors should be considered to be standard SCC.

DIFFERENTIAL DIAGNOSIS
- Distinguishing between viral warts and verrucous carcinoma can sometimes be challenging, especially when only the superficial portion of the specimens are available for inspection.
- Infiltration of the underlying tissue is quite characteristic of verrucous carcinomas; in contrast, warts and condylomata have an exophytic growth pattern.
- Note: In order to be able to detect the characteristic bulbous pattern of growth, specimens should contain the entire thickness of the lesion. That will allow the evaluation of the interface between the tumor and the dermis.

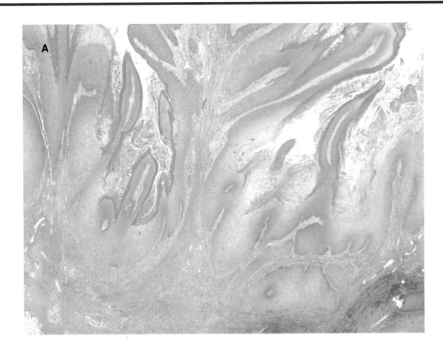

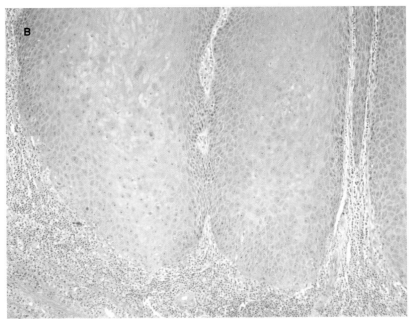

FIGURE 1-12

FIGURE 1-12   (A) Verrucous carcinoma. Large exophytic lesion with marked verrucous epidermis
with well-differentiated nests of squamous epithelium extending into dermis.
(B) Note the deceptively benign appearing, well-differentiated keratinocytes in
epidermis. The epidermal downgrowths have apparently intact basement
membrane.

Lymphoepithelioma-Like Carcinoma

This is a rare neoplasm of the skin that mimics a poorly differentiated nasopharyngeal carcinoma (lymphoepithelioma). Clinically, it presents as a solitary nodule in the head and neck area. In contrast with its nasopharyngeal counterpart, Epstein–Barr virus (EBV) has not been detected in the tumor cells. The lack of consistent epidermal involvement as well as the occasional observation of differentiation toward adnexal structures suggest the possibility of an adnexal origin (23–25).

PATHOLOGY
- The tumor may arise in the dermis or subcutis.
- Tumor cells are arranged in nests, lobules or cords of large epithelioid cells surrounded by a dense lymphoplasmacytic infiltrate.
- Tumor cells are epithelioid with an eosinophilic cytoplasm with vesicular nucleus and a large nucleoli.
- Mitosis figures are frequent.
- There is no obvious squamous cell differentiation.
- Adnexal differentiation has been sometimes reported in the epithelial nests, including ducts and sebaceous cells.
- Overlying epidermis may show obvious SCC.
- Tumor cells express cytokeratin and epithelial membrane antigen, and are negative for EBV.

DIFFERENTIAL DIAGNOSIS
- The main differential diagnosis includes metastatic disease from an undifferentiated nasopharyngeal carcinoma or lymphoepithelioma-like carcinoma from other anatomic sites.
- In such cases, clinical correlation for a primary carcinoma at other sites as well as detection of EBV are helpful in differentiating primary cutaneous tumors from metastases.

Keratoacanthoma

Keratoacanthoma is a relatively common epithelial, low-grade neoplasm of follicular origin. Clinically, it grows rapidly over few weeks followed by spontaneous resolution; however, some rare cases can progress to frank invasive or metastatic carcinoma; thus, surgical treatment often is necessary. Most keratoacanthomas present as a single discrete, flesh-colored, umbilicated nodule with a central, keratin-filled crater. These tumors arise predominantly on the exposed surfaces of the body. Sun exposure and chemical carcinogens have been implicated as etiologic factors; other cases appear to be associated with trauma, HPV infection, genetic factors, and immunocompromised status. Keratoacanthoma may rarely develop within a pre-existent nevus sebaceus. When appearing as multiple lesions, or when showing sebaceous differentiation, keratoacanthomas may be associated with Muir–Torre syndrome (26–28).

Activating mutations in BRAF are present in approximately 40 to 60 percent of advanced melanomas. In 80 to 90 percent of cases, this activating mutation consists of the substitution of glutamic acid for valine at amino acid 600 (V600E mutation) with most of the remainder consisting of an alternate substitution (lysine for valine) at the V600 locus (V to K). Inhibitors of BRAF (vemurafenib), have demonstrated antitumor activity in patients with advanced disease whose tumors have characteristic mutations in BRAF. However, the use of this drug has been implicated in the development of SCC and keratoacanthomas.

PATHOLOGY (FIGURE 1-13A–D)

- Most tumors have both an exophytic and endophytic component with crateriform architecture
- Large central keratin plug with marked squamous epithelial proliferation (the adjacent epidermis may show a collarette)
- The tumor cells are well-differentiated, often with pale-staining, eosinophilic, glassy cytoplasm with squamous keratinization
- Frequent neutrophilic microabscesses
- There are mitotic figures at the periphery of the tumor lobules
- The stroma surrounding the tumor is frequently accompanied by vascular proliferation and an inflammatory infiltrate composed of lymphocytes, histiocytes, plasma cells, neutrophils, and eosinophils
- Involution/regression: With progression, the keratin plug is lost and the proliferating epithelium tends to flatten out with underlying chronic inflammation (often lichenoid) and fibrosis. There may be also foreign body, giant-cell reaction to released keratin.

(continued)

Keratoacanthoma *(continued)*

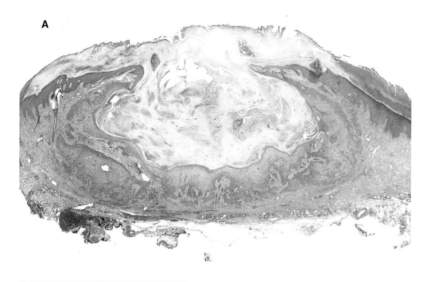

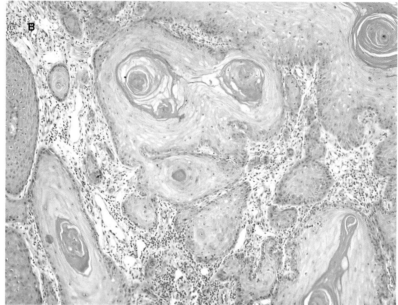

FIGURE 1-13

FIGURE 1-13   (A) Keratoacanthoma. Low power shows an endophytic lesion with lateral collarette, keratin plug, and underlying well-differentiated squamous epithelium with a smooth border. (B) Note the large keratinocytes with ample eosinophilic cytoplasm. (C) The lateral borders and the base of the tumor are commonly associated with a mixed chronic inflammatory infiltrate. (D) Characteristic neutrophilic microabscesses within epidermis.

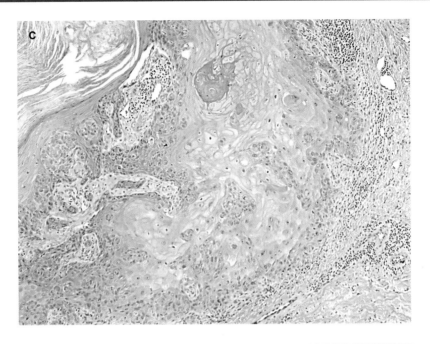

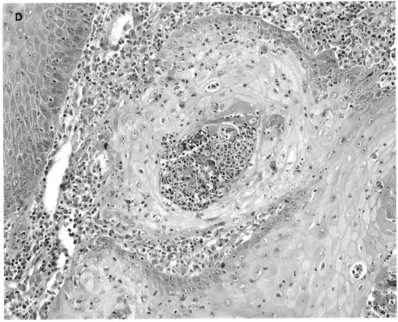

FIGURE 1-13

Bowenoid Papulosis

Bowenoid papulosis presents as a solitary or multiple verruca-like papules on the genital areas. This disease has a predilection for sexually active young adults. In males, lesions more commonly involve the glans penis and the foreskin, whereas in females the vulva is the most common location. Bowenoid papulosis is induced by HPV infection, mostly high-risk HPV-16. Prognosis is variable, as younger patients tend to have a self-limiting course, whereas older or immunocompromised patients can have a protracted course lasting years and rarely may have metastatic potential (29, 30).

PATHOLOGY (FIGURE 1-14A, B)
- Close histological resemblance to Bowen disease
- Epidermal acanthosis forming a raised plaque or papule
- Full-thickness atypia of epidermis and loss of architecture
- Keratinocytes have a hyperchromatic and pleomorphic nuclei
- Mitotic figures are frequent, sometimes of atypical forms
- Common dyskeratotic cells
- True koilocytes are rare; however, there may be vacuolated cells

DIFFERENTIAL DIAGNOSIS
Bowenoid papulosis shows histologic features reminiscent of Bowen disease as both lesions will show full-thickness atypia, numerous mitotic figures, and lack of polarization. The distinction of these two lesions rests mostly on the small size, the presence of multiple lesions, and the young age of the patient of bowenoid papulosis.

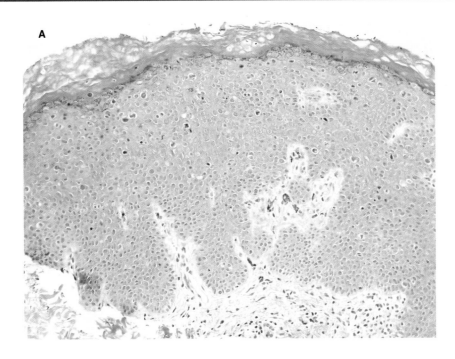

A

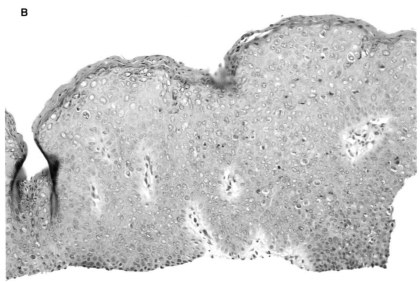

B

FIGURE 1-14

FIGURE 1-14   (A) Bowenoid papulosis. Acanthotic epidermis with hyperkeratosis and keratinocytes showing lack of maturation and pleomorphism. (B) Note the characteristic dyskeratosis, mitotic figures, and atypical keratinocytes filling the entire epidermis.

Merkel Cell Carcinoma (Neuroendocrine Carcinoma of the Skin)

Merkel cell carcinoma (MCC) is a rare tumor of neuroendocrine origin. The histogenesis of this tumor is still a matter of controversy and the most commonly accepted hypothesis is the one postulated by Tang and Toker who found dense core neurosecretory granules in the tumor cells by electron microscopy and suggested a neural crest derivation, most likely from Merkel cells. This tumor occurs primarily in elderly White patients with a slight male predilection. Clinically, it presents as a rapidly growing, solitary, purple dome-shaped papule or plaque on sun-exposed skin frequently localized in the head and neck region, followed by the extremities and trunk. MCC is a high-grade, aggressive cutaneous malignancy with a propensity for local recurrence and regional lymph node metastasis (up to 75% of cases). Sentinel lymph node biopsy is currently a frequently performed procedure in the staging of this tumor, and the finding of positive sentinel lymph nodes is a strong predictor of short-term risk of recurrence and/or metastasis. Regional spread occurs in 55% of patients and distant metastases in about 35% (skin, liver, lungs, bones, and brain). Newer studies have shown an association with polyomavirus (31–35).

PATHOLOGY (FIGURE 1-15A–G)
- Primarily a dermal tumor (sometimes invasion into the subcutis)
- Rare epidermal involvement (epidermotropism such as in Paget disease)
- Tumor cells are arranged as sheets and solid nests, rarely in a trabecular pattern
- Tumor cells are small, round to oval, of uniform size, with vesicular nucleus and multiple small nucleoli
- Frequent mitotic figures and apoptotic bodies
- Tumor cells have a scant cytoplasm, amphophilic, with poorly defined cell borders
- Frequent dense lymphoid infiltrate with formation of lymphoid follicles
- Common lymphatic and vascular invasion (important prognostic factors)
- Histological features associated with a poor outcome: Tumor size greater than 5 mm, lymphovascular invasion, invasion into subcutis (or subjacent structures), increased vascular density, increased number of mast cells, small cell size, and a high mitotic rate
- Immunohistochemistry: The majority of these tumors are positive for EMA, pancytokeratin, and CK20 (dot-like staining; although rarely it can show a cytoplasmic/membranous staining) and negative for CK7 and TTF-1 (helpful in distinguishing primary lesions from cutaneous metastases of small cell carcinoma of the lung). Also express neuroendocrine markers including chromogranin A, synaptophysin, NCAM/CD56, and NSE. MCCs can rarely be CK20–/CK7+ , CK20-/CK7- or CK20+/CK7+. Note: Dot-like staining can be seen with other epithelial markers (not only with CK20).

(text continued on page 32)

FIGURE 1-15   (A) Merkel cell carcinoma. Characteristic malignant round blue cell tumor in the dermis arranged in solid sheets and nodules. (B) Solid sheets of round blue cell tumor in the dermis. (C) The tumor cells are small, with indistinct cytoplasmic borders and a hyperchromatic nucleus. Note the numerous mitotic figures and apoptotic bodies.

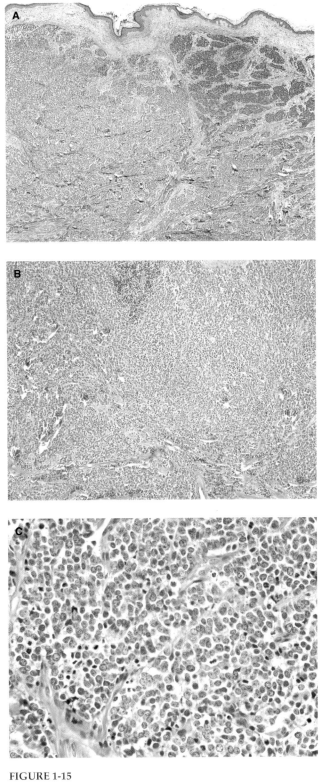

FIGURE 1-15

Merkel Cell Carcinoma (Neuroendocrine Carcinoma of the Skin) (*continued*)

DIFFERENTIAL DIAGNOSIS

■ MCC can easily be confused with other small round blue cell tumors, especially metastatic small cell carcinoma of the lung.

■ Cytokeratin 7 and TTF-1 are typically negative in MCC, in contrast with metastases from small cell carcinoma of the lung.

■ Rare cases of small cell carcinoma of the lung or from other locations (e.g., salivary glands) may express CK20, but it is usually of a weak intensity and without a dot-like pattern.

■ MCC can also be confused with lymphoma and small cell melanoma. However, the latter express lymphocytic (CD45, CD3, or CD20) and the former melanocytic markers (S-100 protein, MART1, HMB45 antigen).

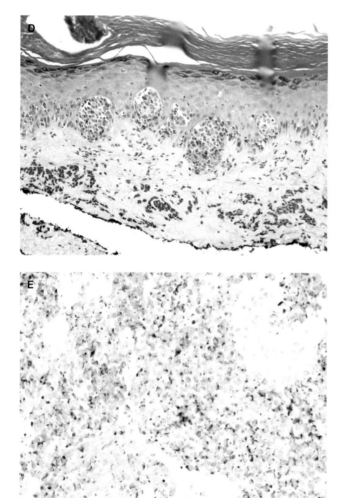

FIGURE 1-15

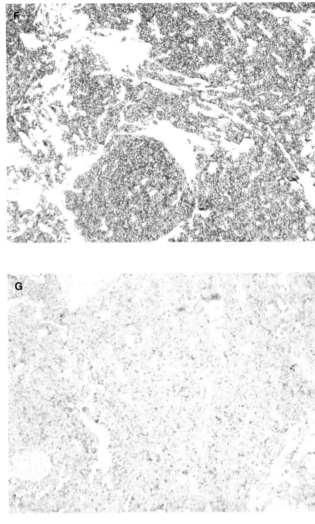

FIGURE 1-15

FIGURE 1-15   (D) Merkel cell carcinoma. Rare cases show involvement of the overlying epidermis (epidermotropism). (E) CK20 showing the classic paranuclear dot-like pattern. (F) EMA is strongly positive. (G) Strong synapthophysin expression.

Mammary and Extramammary Paget Disease

Mammary Paget disease of the breast is almost always associated with an underlying ductal carcinoma in situ or an invasive ductal carcinoma. It is predominantly a disease of females in their fifth or sixth decade, although rarely it affects males. Patients with Paget disease frequently present with a chronic eruption on the nipple and adjacent areolar skin (sometimes very similar to chronic eczema) (36, 37).

Extramammary Paget disease (EMPD) is a rare form of carcinoma in situ most commonly seen in areas rich in apocrine sweat glands, particularly the vulva and the perianal region, but it can also arise in the penis, scrotum, abdomen, axilla, etc. In most cases EMPD represents an in situ malignancy most likely derived from the intraepidermal sweat duct (apocrine glands); however, it may present as an epidermotropic metastasis (rectum, prostate, bladder, cervix, etc.). Although the prognosis is generally good, local recurrence of EMPD is common. In those cases associated with an underlying adnexal or visceral carcinoma mortality may reach 50% (38–40).

PATHOLOGY (FIGURE 1-16A–D)

■ Mammary and EMPD show similar histologic features.

■ The epidermis is acanthotic and shows a diffuse infiltration of large cells with abundant clear cytoplasm containing prominent vesicular nuclei.

■ The cells are present singly or in clusters throughout all layers of the epidermis (pagetoid spread).

■ There is focal glandular formation with signet ring cells containing intracytoplasmic mucin.

■ Pigmentation may be seen in both Paget and EMPD thus mimicking melanoma. This pigmentation is due to either prominent dendritic morphology of intraepidermal melanocytes or of transfer of melanin to keratinocytes.

■ Special stains: Tumor cells are usually positive with PAS and mucin stains (mucicarmine).

■ Immunohistochemistry: Tumor cells are usually positive for keratin AE1/AE3, EMA, and low-molecular-weight cytokeratins (CAM 5.2, CK7). There is variable expression of CEA. Negative for p63.

■ GCDFP-15 has been reported in primary EMPD (apocrine) but it is negative in secondary lesions.

■ Some cases may express Her-2/neu. This finding might indicate a possible therapeutic target.

■ S-100 protein may be expressed in some cases of mammary Paget disease but HMB-45 and anti-MART-1 are negative; thus, they can be helpful in differentiating pigmented Paget disease from melanoma.

(text continued on page 36)

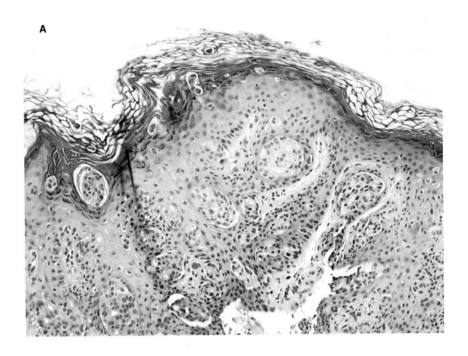

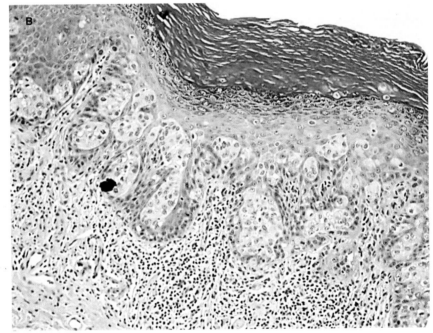

FIGURE 1-16

FIGURE 1-16   (A) Extramammary Paget disease. Acanthotic epidermis with scattered nests of atypical large cells with ample cytoplasm scattered through all layers. (B) Note that the atypical cells within epidermis characteristically lack keratohyaline granules.

Mammary and Extramammary Paget
Disease (*continued*)

DIFFERENTIAL DIAGNOSIS

Mammary Paget disease and EMPD may be confused with melanoma or with SCC in situ. Melanocytic markers, including HMB-45 antigen and Melan-A, are negative in Paget cells (up to 15% of Paget cells may express S-100). Cases of pigmented Paget disease require careful histomorphologic inspection in order to correctly interpret the immunohistochemically labeled dendritic processes of the intraepidermal melanocytes, rather than labeling of the malignant (Paget) cells. Tumor cells in SCC in situ are positive for p63 and lack mucin. While CK7 expression is useful in confirming a diagnosis of Paget disease, it is important to keep in mind that SCC may express this marker.

FIGURE 1-16   (C) Extramammary Paget disease. CK7 is strongly expressed. (D) Note the absence of p63 staining in the neoplastic cells (the adjacent normal keratinocytes are strongly positive).

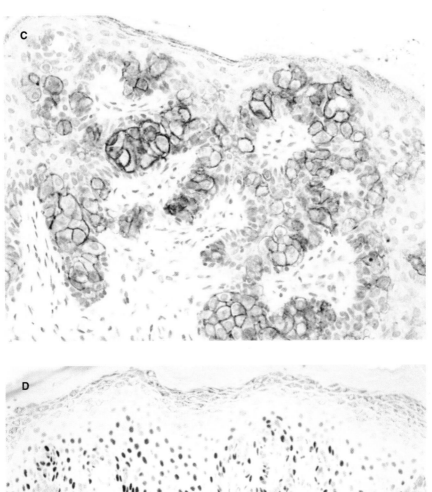

FIGURE 1-16

Adnexal Neoplasms

2

FOLLICULAR TUMORS

TRICHOADENOMA

TRICHOFOLLICULOMA

SEBACEOUS TRICHOFOLLICULOMA

TRICHOEPITHELIOMA

DESMOPLASTIC TRICHOEPITHELIOMA

TRICHILEMMOMA

DESMOPLASTIC TRICHILEMMOMA

TRICHILEMMAL CARCINOMA

TRICHOBLASTOMA

BASAL CELL CARCINOMA

NEVOID BASAL CELL CARCINOMA SYNDROME
(GORLIN–GOLTZ)

FIBROEPITHELIOMA OF PINKUS

CUTANEOUS LYMPHADENOMA

TUMOR OF THE FOLLICULAR INFUNDIBULUM

DILATED PORE OF WINER

PILAR SHEATH ACANTHOMA

PERIFOLLICULAR FIBROMA

FIBROFOLLICULOMA

TRICHODISCOMA

PILOMATRICOMA

PILOMATRICAL CARCINOMA

SEBACEOUS LESIONS

ECTOPIC SEBACEOUS GLANDS (FORDYCE SPOTS AND MONTGOMERY TUBERCLES)

SEBACEOUS HYPERPLASIA

FOLLICULOSEBACEOUS CYSTIC HAMARTOMA

NEVUS SEBACEUS

SEBACEOUS ADENOMA

SEBACEOMA/SEBACEOUS EPITHELIOMA

SEBACEOUS CARCINOMA

MUIR–TORRE SYNDROME

SWEAT GLAND (ECCRINE AND APOCRINE) NEOPLASMS

HIDRADENOMA PAPILLIFERUM

SYRINGOCYSTADENOMA PAPILLIFERUM

TUBULAR APOCRINE ADENOMA

NIPPLE ADENOMA

CERUMINOMA (CERUMINOUS GLAND TUMOR)

MYOEPITHELIOMA

SYRINGOMA

HIDRADENOMA (CLEAR-CELL HIDRADENOMA)

HIDRADENOCARCINOMAS

HIDROACANTHOMA SIMPLEX

POROMA

DERMAL DUCT TUMOR

POROCARCINOMA

SPIRADENOMA

SPIRADENOCARCINOMA

CYLINDROMA

MALIGNANT CYLINDROMA

CHONDROID SYRINGOMA (MIXED TUMOR)

MALIGNANT CHONDROID SYRINGOMA (MALIGNANT MIXED TUMOR)

PRIMARY MUCINOUS CARCINOMA

ECCRINE DUCTAL CARCINOMA

MICROCYSTIC ADNEXAL CARCINOMA

PAPILLARY ECCRINE ADENOMA

AGGRESSIVE DIGITAL PAPILLARY ADENOCARCINOMA

FOLLICULAR TUMORS

Trichoadenoma

Trichoadenoma is a follicular neoplasm that most commonly presents on the face and buttocks and less likely on the neck, upper arm, and thigh. Clinically, it presents as a solitary, skin-colored nodule that can measure up to 3 cm in maximum diameter (average 1 cm) (41, 42).

PATHOLOGY (FIGURE 2-1)
- Well-defined dermal tumor composed of epithelial islands that have a central cystic cavity containing keratinous material (infundibulocystic structures).
- Cyst wall is composed of squamous epithelium, which shows infundibular keratinization (with preserved granular cell layer).
- There are no hair shafts.
- There is a conspicuous fibrovascular stroma.
- Common foreign body granulomatous reaction.

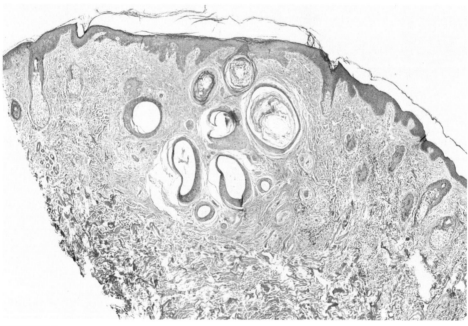

FIGURE 2-1

FIGURE 2-1 Trichoadenoma. Multiple small-to-medium cystic cavities surrounded by a fibrous stroma.

Trichofolliculoma

Trichofolliculoma is an uncommon pilar tumor. Clinically, it presents as a solitary nodule (0.5 cm) on the face (nose and earlobe), scalp, and neck. This tumor usually shows a tuft of thread-like hairs protruding from a central opening (43, 44).

PATHOLOGY (FIGURE 2-2)
- Dilated hair follicle opening to the surface
- Cystic structure lined by stratified squamous epithelium (preserved granular cell layer)
- The cystic cavity contains keratinous debris and hair shaft fragments
- Arising from the cystic wall there are numerous hair follicles (secondary and sometimes tertiary hair follicles)
- There may be abortive pilar differentiation (papillary mesenchymal bodies)

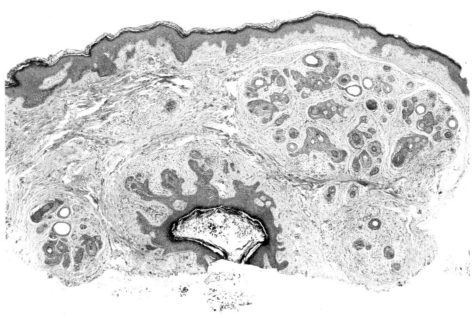

FIGURE 2-2

FIGURE 2-2   Trichofolliculoma. Dilated hair follicle with keratinous debris. Note the multiple hair follicles arising from the cystic cavity.

Sebaceous Trichofolliculoma

Sebaceous trichofolliculoma is a variant of trichofolliculoma. Clinically it presents as a depressed lesion usually on the nose, associated with one or more fistulous openings with protruding terminal hairs and vellus hairs (45, 46).

PATHOLOGY (FIGURE 2-3)
- Hamartomatous growth, with a large central cavity or sinus and with secondary branches
- Central cystic space lined by stratified squamous epithelium with granular layer
- The cavity is filled with hairs and loose epidermoid/trichilemmal-like cellular debris
- Many large sebaceous follicles
- Terminal hair follicles and vellus hair follicles are found in various stages of the hair growth cycle

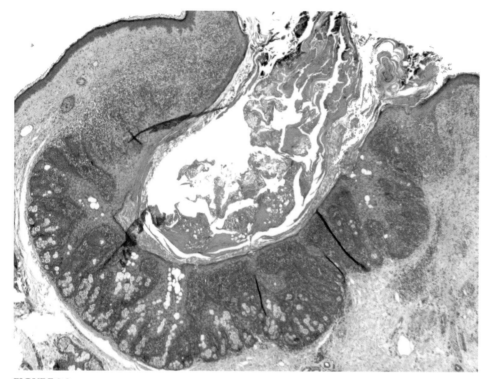

FIGURE 2-3

FIGURE 2-3   Sebaceous trichofolliculoma. Dilated follicle lined by squamous epithelium with infundibular keratinization. Note the sebaceous lobules.

Trichoepithelioma

Trichoepithelioma (TE) is a benign adnexal tumor. Although there is still controversy about their origin, many authors consider TE as a variant, more differentiated and superficial, of trichoblastoma (see also below). There are three variants of TE: solitary, multiple, and desmoplastic (see below). Solitary TEs are found as skin-colored papules, most commonly located on the nose, upper lip, and cheek (47).

Multiple, familial TE: Clinically, they present with multiple, small, skin-colored papules predominantly located on the face (most commonly on the nasolabial folds, eyebrows, eyelids, and cheeks). Familial TEs have an autosomal dominant mode of inheritance, due to a mutation in the *CYLD* (cylindromatosis) gene on chromosome 16q12–q13 (48).

Brooke–Spiegler syndrome: Associated with mutation in the *CYLD* gene. It is characterized by multiple TE, cylindromas (Turban tumor), spiradenomas, and milia (49).

Rombo syndrome: It is characterized by multiple TE, milia, vermiculate atrophy, basal cell carcinoma (BCC) and vellus-hair cysts. It is a rare condition, with a possible autosomal dominant mode of inheritance.

PATHOLOGY (FIGURE 2-4A–E)

- ◼ Identical histological features of the solitary and familial TE
- ◼ TEs are dermal tumors with continuity with the epidermis in up to 1/3 of cases
- ◼ In the dermis, there are numerous, free lining horn cysts (lined by stratified squamous epithelium) and islands of uniform basaloid cells (sometimes showing peripheral palisading)
- ◼ Characteristic branching nests of basaloid cell (frond-like appearance)
- ◼ Perilobular connective tissue sheath conspicuous and loosely arranged
- ◼ Characteristic aggregations of spindle cell fibroblasts, papillary-mesenchymal bodies
- ◼ Rupture of these horn cysts results in small foreign-body granuloma
- ◼ Frequent areas of calcification

(text continued on page 46)

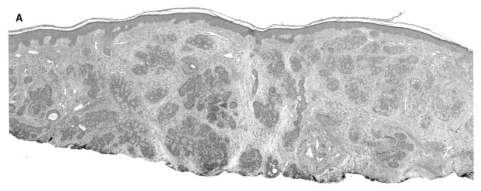

FIGURE 2-4

FIGURE 2-4   (A) Trichoepithelioma. Numerous islands of basaloid cells with frond-like appearance. Note the characteristic fibrous stroma with only minimal myxoid areas.

Trichoepithelioma *(continued)*

DIFFERENTIAL DIAGNOSIS

The main differential diagnosis is with BCC. The presence of ulceration, melanophages, marked tumor–stroma retraction artifact, and mucin deposition in the stroma favors BCC. The presence of marked epithelial frond-like structures and papillary mesenchymal body is highly indicative of TE. Mitotic figures and apoptotic cells may be present in both neoplasms but are much more common in BCC (50). When you have limited tissue to evaluate the distinction of these two neoplasms can be quite challenging. Immunohistochemical studies may be useful in the differential diagnosis but not always helpful. TE resembles the pattern in the outer root sheath, with strong reactions for keratins CK5/6 and CK8. Expression of bcl-2 is diffuse in BCC while it is predominantly peripheral in TE. CK15 is expressed in most TE and only in a subset of BCC. CK20 is expressed in Merkel cells, which are much more common in TE than in BCC. PCNA and Ki-67 (proliferative index) are increased in BCC compared to TE. Androgen receptor (AR) expression is more commonly seen in BCC than TE. The stroma of TE contains CD34+ cells but this marker is largely absent in BCC. The vast majority of TE expresses D240, and BCC are mostly negative. PHLDA-1 appears to be a promising marker as is expressed in TE and negative in BCC (426). In our experience CD10 may be most helpful since it labels the stromal cells of TE and some epithelial cells in hamartomatous/infundibulocystic BCC.

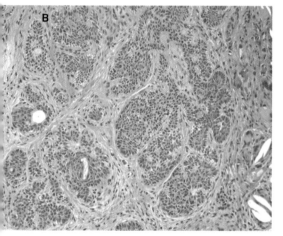 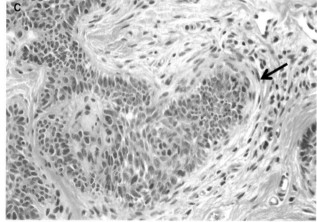

FIGURE 2-4

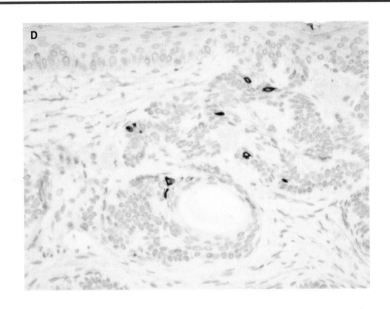

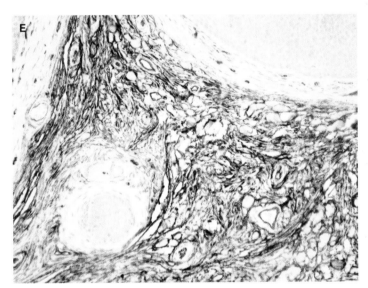

FIGURE 2-4

FIGURE 2-4 (B) Characteristic frond-like appearance. (C) Papillary mesenchymal body differentiation (arrow). (D) CK20 highlights the scattered Merkel cells within the tumor. (E) CD34 is strongly positive in the stroma.

Desmoplastic Trichoepithelioma

Desmoplastic TE is a variant that presents on the face or neck of young adults. There is a predilection for females (4:1). Clinically, it presents as an asymptomatic, solitary, annular lesion with raised borders and a depressed center, varying from 3 to 8 mm in diameter. This variant is exceptional in patients with familial TE syndromes (51, 52).

PATHOLOGY (FIGURE 2-5A, B)
- Well-circumscribed, it usually occupies the upper and mid dermis
- Central depression
- Cords and small nests of basaloid cells
- Many keratinous cysts (peripheral border of small cuboidal basal cells with prominent nuclei and scant cytoplasm)
- Tumor cords may be attached to the epidermis
- Tadpole-shaped epithelial projections extend from the peripheral layer of some of the horn cysts
- Dense and hypocellular stroma (albeit not truly desmoplastic)
- Common foreign-body giant cell reaction and calcification

DIFFERENTIAL DIAGNOSIS
The differential diagnosis of desmoplastic TE mainly includes BCC (infiltrative/morpheaform type). Desmoplastic TE is well-circumscribed and symmetric and lacks peripheral palisading, mitotic figures, apoptotic cells, mucin, necrosis, and tumor–stroma retraction artifact. BCC is not characteristically associated with keratinous-cyst formation and ruptured keratinous cysts with foreign-body granulomas. However, in small biopsies both neoplasms may show similar features and can be quite difficult to separate from each other. As mentioned above, immunohistochemistry sometimes plays a role; desmoplastic TE usually shows CK20+ Merkel cells, while such finding is only rarely seen in BCC. Up to 80% of BCC express ARs, while TE is are typically negative. Bcl-2 is expressed in a diffuse manner by the majority of BCC, but it is expressed only in the peripheral cell layer of TE. Ber-EP4 is strongly positive in BCC and is focally positive in most TE. CD10 is expressed in the stroma of TE; in contrast, BCC usually show CD10 expression in some basaloid cells but not in the stroma. PHLDA-1 is positive in desmoplastic TE and negative in BCC. P75 can also be helpful as it is mostly positive in desmoplastic TE and only rarely positive in BCC.

Desmoplastic TE may be confused histologically, especially in small biopsies, with syringoma and microcystic adnexal carcinoma (MAC). The presence of obvious duct formation rules out a tumor of follicular differentiation.

FIGURE 2-5 (A) Desmoplastic trichoepithelioma. Linear and branched epithelial strands admixed with keratinizing cysts embedded in a dense fibrous stroma. (B) The epithelial strands are composed of small cuboidal basaloid cells. Note the hypocellular stroma.

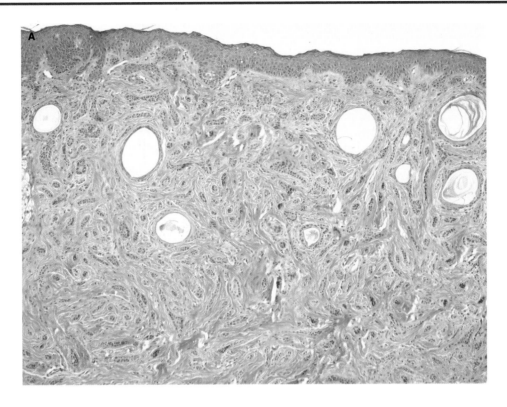

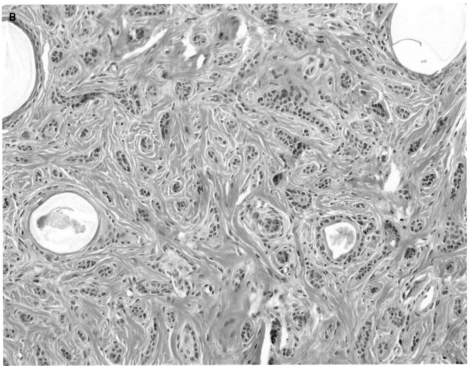

FIGURE 2-5

Trichilemmoma

Trichilemmoma is a small solitary asymptomatic warty, skin-colored papule, found almost exclusively on the face. Rarely, it can develop within a pre-existent nevus sebaceus. The presence of multiple trichilemmomas is characteristic of Cowden disease (53, 54).

Cowden disease (multiple hamartoma syndrome) is a rare disorder with autosomal dominant inheritance that is characterized by multiple, hamartomatous neoplasms of the skin and mucosa, GI tract, bones, etc. Mucocutaneous lesions include trichilemmomas, oral mucosal papillomatosis, acral keratoses, and palmoplantar keratoses. Other manifestations include thyroid adenomas and goiter, fibrocystic disease of the breast, ovarian cysts and dysgerminoma, uterine fibroids, and colonic polyps. Also, Cowden disease is associated with the development of several types of malignancies, including breast (25%–50% risk) and thyroid carcinoma (10% risk). Other associated carcinomas are colon and renal cell. Cowden disease involves a mutation in the *PTEN* gene, a tumor suppressor gene, on chromosome 10q23.31 (55, 56).

PATHOLOGY (FIGURE 2-6A, B)
- Trichilemmoma is a proliferation of the follicular outer root sheath
- It shows a sharply demarcated, symmetric neoplasm composed of one or more lobules in continuity with the epidermis and that extend into the upper dermis
- The tumor is composed of squamous cells showing variable glycogen vacuolation (clear-cell cytoplasm)
- Centrally within the lobule there may be foci of epidermal keratinization and sometimes squamous eddies
- The lobules show peripheral nuclear palisading and are composed of uniform small cells with round vesicular nuclei
- Absent pleomorphism and mitotic figures
- A thick, dense eosinophilic basement membrane surrounds the tumor (diastase-resistant, PAS-positive hyaline mantle)
- The epidermis is hyperkeratotic, sometimes verrucous and with a cutaneous horn

FIGURE 2-6 (A) Trichilemmoma. Verrucous lesion composed of squamoid cells with clear cytoplasm. Note the basaloid peripheral palisading around the lobules. (B) Uniform squamoid epithelial cells with clear cytoplasm. Note the peripheral basaloid palisading.

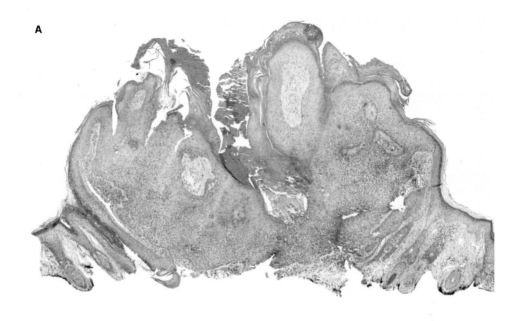

A

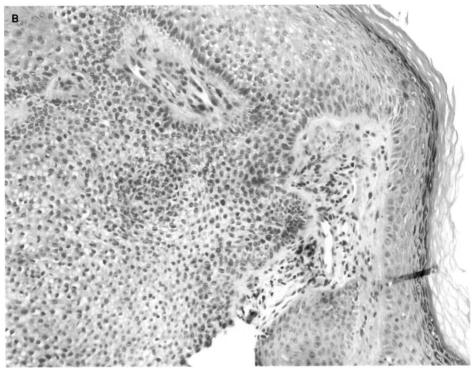

B

FIGURE 2-6

Desmoplastic Trichilemmoma

Desmoplastic trichilemmoma is a rare variant that arises from the outer root sheath or infundibular epithelium. Clinically, it most commonly presents on the face as a slow-growing, solitary, dome-shaped papule and appears to be more common in males. Rarely, it can be associated with a pre-existent nevus sebaceus. There is no association with Cowden disease (57).

PATHOLOGY (FIGURE 2-7A, B)

- The tumor shows typical areas of conventional trichilemmoma, especially at the periphery of the lesion
- In the center of the lesion, there are narrow, irregular cords of smaller epithelial cells admixed with a densely hyalinized, hypocellular stroma
- In the dermis there is a lymphocytic infiltrate

FIGURE 2-7 (A) Desmoplastic trichilemmoma. Similar to a trichilemmoma; however, the center of the lesion shows narrow irregular cords set in a hyalinized stroma. (B) Note the epithelial strands set in a hyalinized and collagenous stroma.

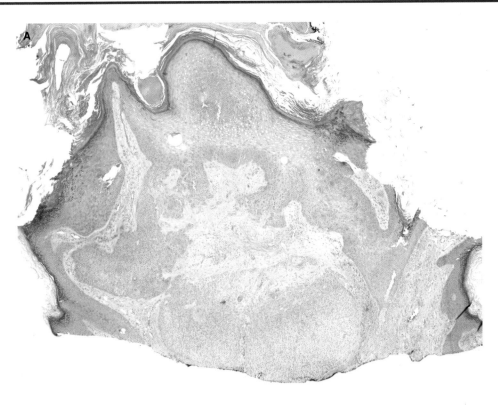

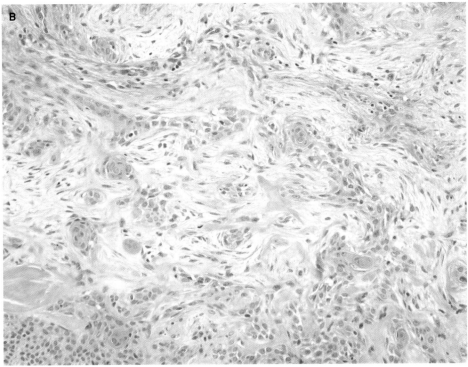

FIGURE 2-7

Trichilemmal Carcinoma

Trichilemmal carcinoma is a rare neoplasm predominantly located on sun-exposed skin of the face and extremities of elderly patients. Clinically, the lesions present as a single papule or nodule, frequently ulcerated. This tumor has an indolent clinical course and recurrences are exceedingly rare. Some authors have proposed that it may represent a clear-cell variant of SCC (58).

PATHOLOGY (FIGURE 2-8A, B)

■ Often multilobulated with infiltrative growth
■ Predominantly dermal tumor with connection to epidermis and hair follicles. The tumor cells are large with clear cytoplasm (PAS positive, diastase sensitive).
■ Tumor lobules show peripheral palisading and hyaline basement membrane
■ Frequent trichilemmal keratinization (abrupt, without keratohyaline granules)
■ Nuclear pleomorphism ranges from mild to severe
■ Mitotic figures are conspicuous, occasionally with atypical forms

DIFFERENTIAL DIAGNOSIS

The differential diagnosis includes other malignant neoplasms with clear-cell differentiation, i.e., clear-cell SCC, clear-cell porocarcinoma, and clear-cell hidradenocarcinoma. Clear-cell SCC has an infiltrative growth pattern and lacks the peripheral palisading and hyaline basement membrane seen in trichilemmal carcinoma. Also, when pilar keratinization is identified this will favor the diagnosis of trichilemmal carcinoma. Clear-cell porocarcinoma and clear-cell hidradenocarcinoma usually show ductal differentiation and intracytoplasmic lumina, which can often be highlighted by immunohistochemical studies including epithelial membrane antigen (EMA) or carcinoembryonic antigen (CEA).

FIGURE 2-8 (A) Trichilemmal carcinoma. Lobulated tumor with epidermal origin. Note the marked clear-cell differentiation. (B) High power of the epithelial cells with marked nuclear pleomorphism.

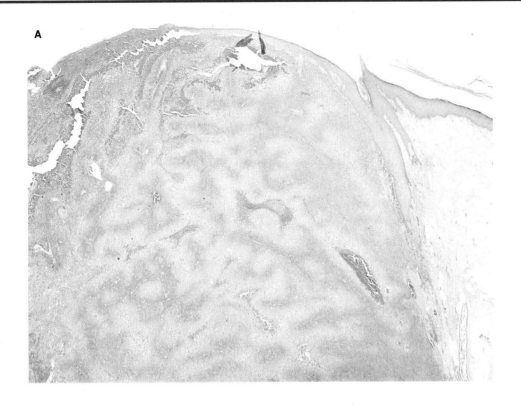

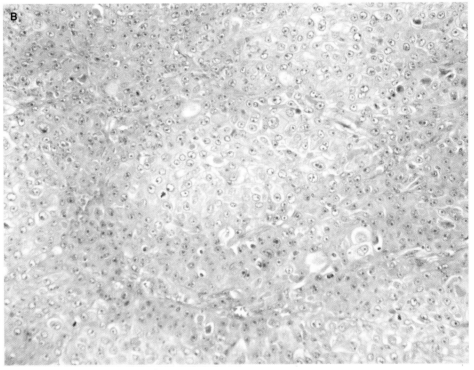

FIGURE 2-8

Trichoblastoma

Trichoblastomas are rare benign neoplasms of the hair germ, considered by some authors as deep, less differentiated TE. Clinically, they present as slow-growing solitary nodules located predominantly in the head and neck area with predilection for the scalp. Trichoblastoma most commonly presents in patients in their fifth to seventh decades of life with equal sex incidence. Trichoblastomas are present for many years, usually grow to a size of 3 cm or more in diameter and involve the deep dermis and subcutis. Trichoblastoma and syringocystadenoma papilliferum are the most common neoplasms to arise in nevus sebaceus (59).

PATHOLOGY (FIGURE 2-9A, B)
■ Large, well-circumscribed, basaloid tumor in the mid and deep dermis with focal extension into the subcutis (without epidermal connection)
■ Irregular nests of basaloid cells with peripheral palisading that mimic BCC but with variable stromal condensation and pilar differentiation
■ Fibromyxoid stroma composed of stellate and spindle fibroblasts that are associated with primitive hair-papilla formation (papillary mesenchymal bodies)
■ Stromal amyloid and Merkel cells

VARIANTS
■ Trichoblastic fibroma: This variant is composed of nests, strands, and fronds of cytologically bland, basaloid cells, often with peripheral palisading and a conspicuous fibromyxoid stroma. Larger lobules and their stroma are often arranged in a mosaic pattern, and the smaller islands of tumor cells form close clusters with little intervening stroma. This variant commonly has keratin cysts and papillary mesenchymal bodies.
■ Trichogerminoma: It is composed of lobules of basaloid cells resembling hair bulbs, with minimal intervening stroma.
■ Pigmented trichoblastoma (melanotrichoblastoma): As with other neoplasms that recapitulate hair follicle differentiation, in addition to the epithelial cells, trichoblastoma may have numerous, dendritic melanocytes. Some authors refer to these melanocytes as "passenger" cells. The presence of such dendritic melanocytes may raise the possibility of melanoma (see below).
■ Cutaneous lymphadenoma: see below.

DIFFERENTIAL DIAGNOSIS
The differential diagnosis is mainly with TE and BCC. Trichoblastomas are larger than TE and occupy deep dermis and subcutaneous tissue while TE are centered in the mid dermis. Trichoblastomas show less keratinization and lack epidermal or follicular origin. Both trichoblastomas and TE are characterized by papillary mesenchymal bodies. BCC shows retraction artifact, epidermal origin, mucin, and lack papillary mesenchymal bodies. As with pigmented Paget disease, caution should be exercised in order to determine if the pigmentation comes from the "passenger" melanocytes.

FIGURE 2-9   (A) Trichoblastoma. Multiple basaloid nodules in the dermis set in a conspicuous stroma. Note the lack of retraction artifact and mucin deposition commonly seen in BCC. (B) Note the primitive hair papilla formation.

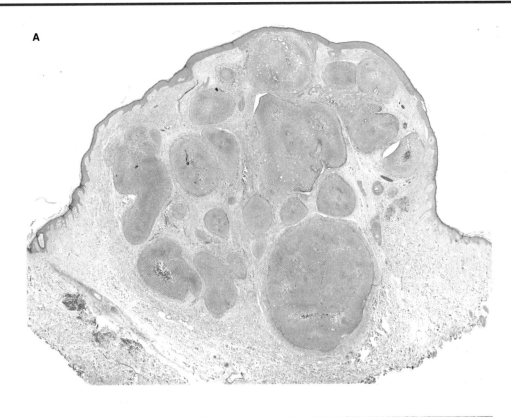

A

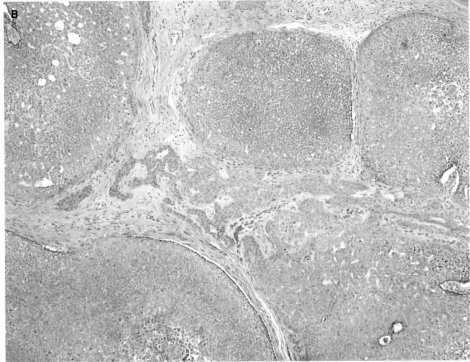

B

FIGURE 2-9

Basal Cell Carcinoma

BCC is the most common skin cancer in humans. BCCs are more commonly seen in elderly males, typically on sun-exposed skin (face is the most common site). BCCs have been reported in children and young adults, and in children there is often a clinical association with basal cell nevus syndrome and xeroderma pigmentosum. Clinically, it presents as a papulonodular tumor with a pearly, translucent edge with visible telangiectasia. Most BCCs are slow-growing, relatively nonaggressive neoplasms; however, a subset of them may have a frankly aggressive behavior with local destruction and, rarely, metastatic potential. The patched/hedgehog intracellular signaling pathway (*PTCH1*) plays an important role in both sporadic BCCs and nevoid BCC syndrome (Gorlin syndrome). *PTCH1* mutations have been found in 30% to 40% of sporadic BCCs (29–32).

PATHOLOGY (FIGURE 2-10A–H)
- The majority of BCCs show connection to the overlying epidermis
- Islands or nests of basaloid cells with peripheral palisading of the cells and haphazard arrangement of those cells in the centers of the islands
- Small tumor cells with uniform, round or oval, darkly staining nuclei and minimal cytoplasm
- Common mitotic figures and apoptosis
- Clefting at the stromal–tumor interface
- Tumor stroma contains variable amounts of acid mucopolysaccharides
- Calcification may be present in the center of the keratin cysts

VARIANTS
- Superficial: The clusters of basaloid cells are attached to the epidermis and only involve the papillary dermis.
- Nodular: This variant represents approximately 70% of all cases. It is composed of nests of basaloid cells with peripheral palisading. Retraction artifact is common. The stroma surrounding these lobules is usually loose and rich in mucin (hyaluronic acid). There may be ulceration.
- Micronodular: The nests are smaller and the peripheral palisading is not always prominent. It usually has minimal or no fibro-inflammatory response. Sometimes it infiltrates quite widely throughout the dermis and extends into the subcutis; thus, it is considered to be of a relatively high local recurrence rate.

(*text continued on page 60*)

FIGURE 2-10   (A) Nodular basal cell carcinoma. Nodular basaloid neoplasm with marked retraction artifact. Note the focal epidermal origin and the dense fibromyxoid stroma. (B) Basaloid nodule with peripheral palisading. (C) The tumor cells have indistinct cytoplasmic borders and oval basophilic vesicular nuclei. (D) Basaloid nodule with comedo necrosis. (E) Superficial basal cell carcinoma. Small basaloid tumor nests are connected in the epidermis. Note the presence of dermal fibrosis and focal chronic inflammation. (F) Hamartomatous/infundibulocystic basal cell carcinoma. Tumor nodules are small in size and uniform and are arranged around a central, dilated cystic structure. Note the absence of retraction artifact (characteristic of this variant).

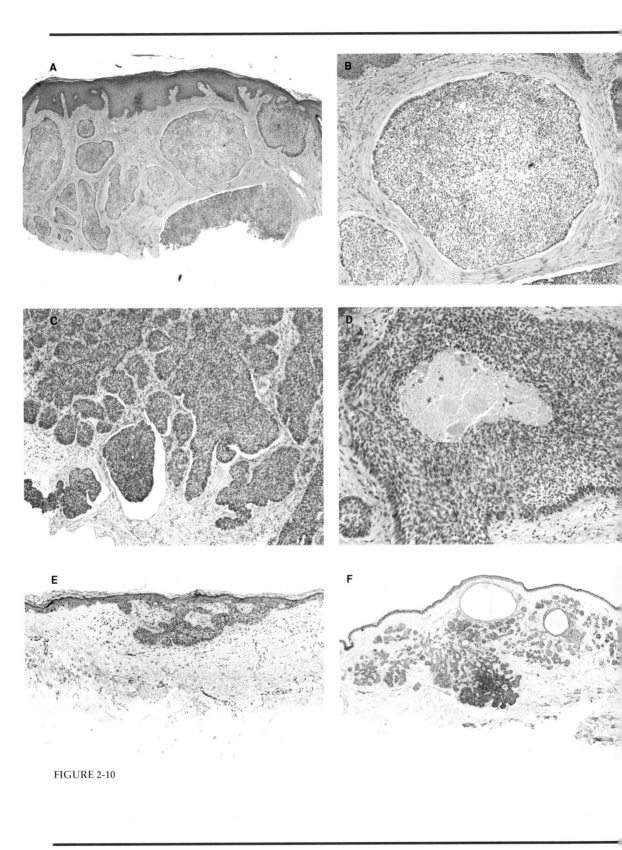

FIGURE 2-10

Basal Cell Carcinoma *(continued)*

- Infiltrating: Due to their similar pattern of growth and high local recurrence rate, we include under this term all variants with spikey contours of the tumor lobules (i.e., morpheaform, sclerodermoid, etc.). The tumor is composed of elongated strands of basaloid cells infiltrating among collagen bundles. The stroma is loose and shows an increase in fibroblasts and mucin. Often there is a nodular pattern superficially with the infiltrating nests at the periphery or base of the lesion. The tumor characteristically shows deep invasion with occasional perineural involvement. The morpheaform variant is composed of thin strands and nests of basaloid cells showing minimal peripheral palisading. The surrounding stroma is dense and sclerotic.
- The so-called keratotic variant is essentially a nodular BCC with keratotic cysts in the center of the islands.
- "Metatypical": This term is sometimes given to cases of BCC in which there are areas of typical BCC and others with extensive squamous differentiation. We prefer to diagnose such cases as BCC with squamous differentiation. Some authors suggest the term of basosquamous carcinoma, but we disagree with such practice, since the term "basosquamous" is used in gastrointestinal and genitourinary pathology for lesions with a very aggressive, even lethal course. Regardless the preferred term, these BCC with extensive squamous differentiation may be associated with a more aggressive behavior including increased risk of distant metastasis (60).

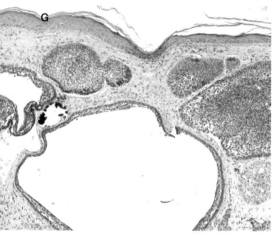
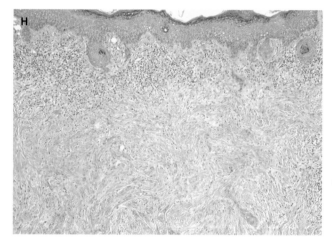

FIGURE 2-10

FIGURE 2-10   (G) Cystic basal cell carcinoma. Basaloid nodules with a cystic component. (H) Infiltrative basal cell carcinoma. The tumor cells show narrow strands of basaloid-appearing cells that are surrounded by a dense fibromyxoid stroma.

Nevoid Basal Cell Carcinoma Syndrome (Gorlin–Goltz)

Nevoid basal cell carcinoma (BCC) syndrome is characterized by multiple BCC (early age), odontogenic keratocysts of the jaw, skeletal and neurological abnormalities, ectopic calcification, cutaneous cysts, and pits of the hands and feet. It is inherited in an autosomal dominant fashion and the responsible gene, the patched homologue 1 (*PTCH1*) gene, is at chromosome 9q22.3 (33, 34).

PATHOLOGY
- Nodular and superficial variants are most common, the histologic features are identical to ordinary BCC.
- Some studies have shown that calcification, pigmentation, and osteoid metaplasia are more common in lesions occurring in the syndrome than in sporadic cases.

Fibroepithelioma of Pinkus

Fibroepithelioma of Pinkus is an uncommon neoplasm that traditionally has been regarded to be an unusual variant of BCC; however, due to its indolent behavior and often asymptomatic clinical presentation it has been suggested to be different from BCC. Fibroepithelioma of Pinkus has a predilection for females and is most commonly found on the trunk (35, 36).

PATHOLOGY (FIGURE 2-11A–C)

▪ Long, thin, branching and anastomosing basaloid epithelial strands (two to three cells thick) connected with the epidermis

▪ The basaloid strands show two types of cells: (A) lighter staining, comprising the bulk of the strand and (B) peripheral, small darker cells with a palisading pattern

▪ Loose fibrous stroma

A

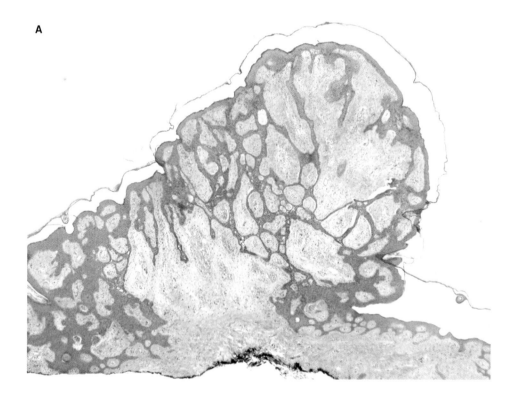

FIGURE 2-11   (A) Fibroepithelioma. Thin anastomosing and interconnecting strands of basaloid cells. Note the prominent loose stroma. (B) Higher magnification of the basaloid strands. Note the cells have a hyperchromatic cytoplasm with only minimal cytoplasm. (C) Characteristic loose fibrous stroma.

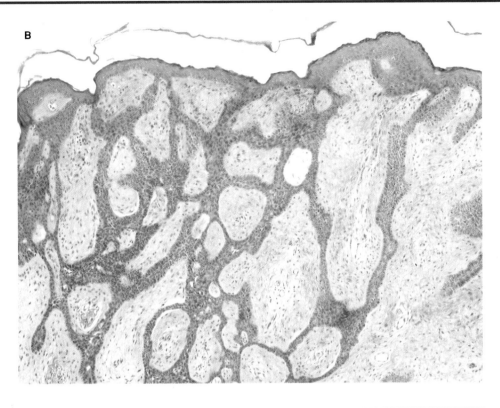

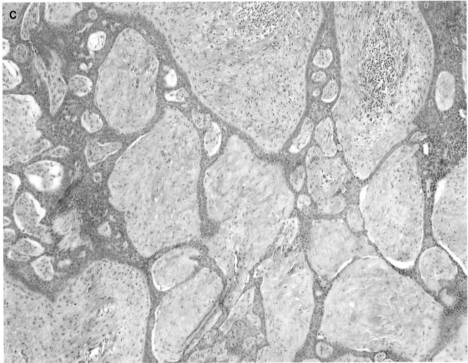

FIGURE 2-11

Cutaneous Lymphadenoma

Cutaneous lymphadenoma is a rare adnexal tumor that has recently been categorized as a variant of trichoblastoma. Clinically, the tumor presents in adults as a slow growing, small papule up to 1 cm in diameter. It is most commonly located on the face (61, 62).

PATHOLOGY (FIGURE 2-12A–C)
- Dermal location but sometimes invades the subcutaneous tissue
- Focal connection to the epidermis or a hair follicle
- Irregularly shaped lobules and trabeculae of epithelial cells embedded in a fibrous stroma
- The lobules and trabeculae have a peripheral rim of one or more layers of small basaloid cells, sometimes showing peripheral palisading, surrounding a core of large clear cells with vesicular nuclei and often containing large nucleoli (glycogen rich cytoplasm).
- Within the lobules there is an intense inflammatory infiltrate of lymphocytes, with some spillage into the stroma (there may be germinal centers).
- Follicular and sebaceous differentiation
- Small duct-like structures within the lobules
- By immunohistochemistry, the epithelial cells express keratin and sometimes EMA, while lacking CEA. CK20+ Merkel cells may be present and S-100 protein/CD1a+ dendritic cells (Langerhans cells) are often conspicuous. Within the center of the lobules there are CD30+ cells (activated lymphocytes and histiocytes).

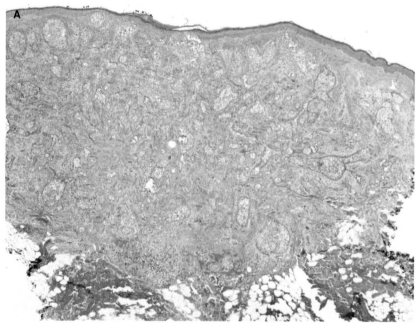

FIGURE 2-12

FIGURE 2-12   (A) Cutaneous lymphadenoma. Low magnification shows multiple irregular epithelial nodules set in a fibrous stroma. (B) The epithelial nests have a rim of basaloid cells and within the nests there are pale-stained cells. Note the sparse lymphocytic infiltrate within the nests. (C) High power of the nests with a mixture of lymphocytes and histiocytes.

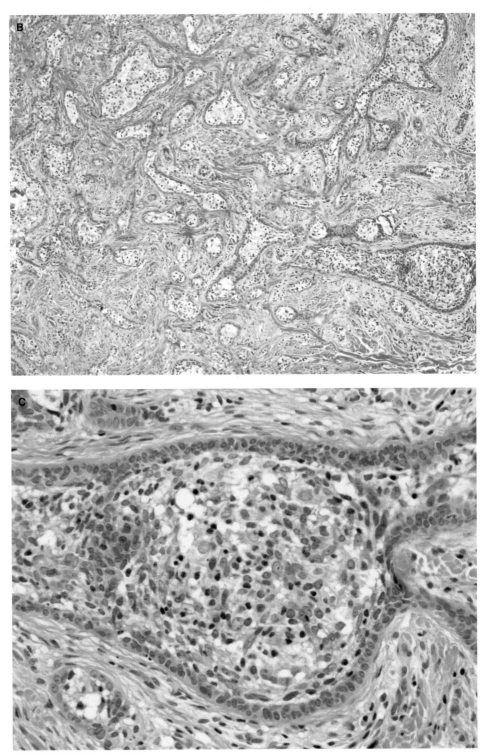

FIGURE 2-12

Tumor of the Follicular Infundibulum

This is a rare adnexal tumor that arises from or differentiates toward the follicular infundibulum. Clinically, it occurs most frequently on the head and neck, and presents as an asymptomatic solitary nodule (up to 1.5 cm in diameter). A slight female predominance is recognized and it most commonly occurs in patients older than 60 years. The eruptive form presents as a sudden onset of multiple (200 or more) hypopigmented macules and papules confined to the head, neck, and upper trunk. Tumor of follicular infundibulum may arise within a pre-existent nevus sebaceus and rarely can be associated with Cowden disease and the Schöpf–Schultz–Passarge syndrome (63).

PATHOLOGY (FIGURE 2-13)

- Plate-like fenestrated subepidermal tumor that extends horizontally under the epidermis with multiple cord-like connections to the overlying epidermis
- Pale-staining, glycogen-containing keratinocytes
- Peripheral palisading of basal cells
- Frequently with an eosinophilic basement membrane
- A dense band or brush-like network of elastic fibers is commonly demonstrated at the border of the tumor (Verhoeff stain)
- Rarely follicular bulbs, papillary mesenchymal bodies, focal sebaceous differentiation and ductal structures

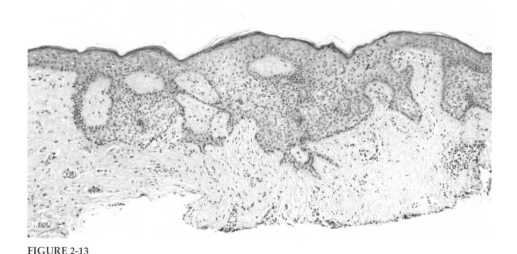

FIGURE 2-13

FIGURE 2-13   Tumor of the follicular infundibulum. Anastomosing strands of basophilic cells arising from the overlying epidermis. Note that the orientation is parallel to the epidermal surface.

Dilated Pore of Winer

Dilated pore of Winer is a relatively common adnexal tumor. Clinically, it is a solitary lesion that presents as a large comedone on the face or neck in adults and elderly patients. There is a slight male predilection (64).

PATHOLOGY (FIGURE 2-14)
- Dilated hair follicle with keratin plugging and lined by an outer root sheath epithelium in which there is infundibular keratinization (preserved granular layer)
- Acanthosis and irregular finger-like projections that radiate into the surrounding dermis, resembling the normal rete-ridge pattern of epidermis

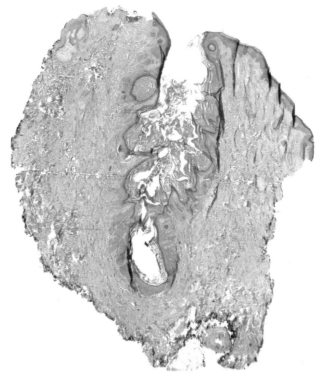

FIGURE 2-14

FIGURE 2-14   Dilated pore of Winer. Dilated hair follicle with keratin plugging. Note the small finger-like projections radiating into the surrounding dermis.

Pilar Sheath Acanthoma

Pilar sheath acanthoma is a rare follicular neoplasm usually located on the upper lip. Clinically, it presents as a solitary asymptomatic, small skin-colored nodule with a central, pore-like opening plugged with keratin. As well as other authors, we think that dilated pore of Winer and pilar sheath acanthoma are essentially the same lesion, the latter being bigger (65).

PATHOLOGY (FIGURE 2-15)
- Cystically dilated hair follicle with keratin plugging that opens onto the surface
- Many tumor lobules extend into the surrounding dermis and sometimes involve the subcutaneous fat or skeletal muscle
- Tumor lobules are composed of an outer root sheath epithelium

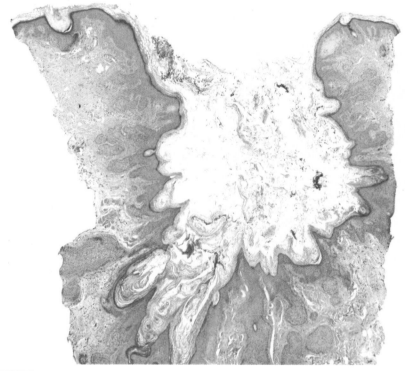

FIGURE 2-15

FIGURE 2-15   Pilar sheath acanthoma. Very similar to the dilated pore of Winer.

Perifollicular Fibroma

This rare entity is not accepted by all authors. Clinically, it may be single or multiple and presents as a flesh-colored nodule most commonly located on the face or neck. Perifollicular fibromas have been reported in association with colonic polyps and may be inherited with an autosomal dominant trait (Hornstein-Knickenberg syndrome).

PATHOLOGY (FIGURE 2-16)
■ Concentric layers of fibrous tissue ("onion skin") around hair follicles
■ Often there is a cleft that separates the fibroma from the adjacent connective tissue

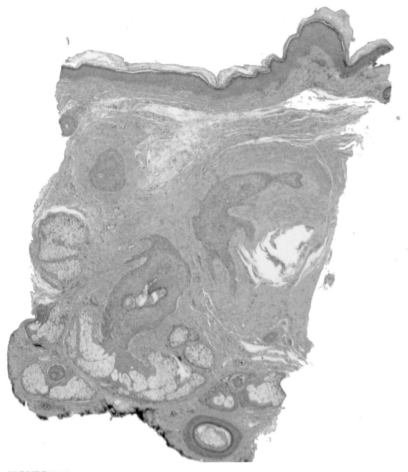

FIGURE 2-16

FIGURE 2-16   Perifollicular fibroma. Marked perifollicular concentric fibrosis.

Fibrofolliculoma

Fibrofolliculoma is a rare, benign hamartomatous condition that clinically presents as dome-shaped, yellow papules with a predilection for the scalp, face, and neck. Fibrofolliculoma can represent either an isolated condition or be part of an autosomal dominant syndrome (Birt–Hogg–Dubé syndrome) (66, 67).

PATHOLOGY (FIGURE 2-17)

- Well-formed hair follicle, with infundibular features, occasionally cystically dilated in the center
- Surrounding the infundibulum there is a well-circumscribed proliferation of loose connective tissue with some intervening mucin
- Epithelial cells, two-to-four cells thick, radiate from the infundibulum
- Often there are residual sebocytes
- Some lesions show features of both fibrofolliculoma and trichodiscoma

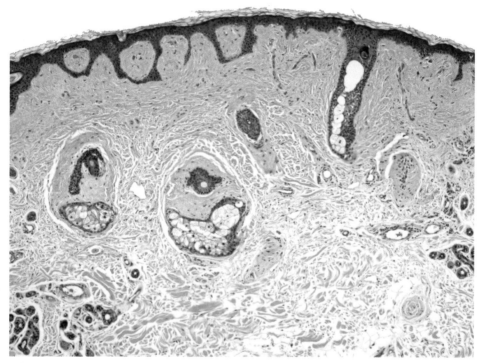

FIGURE 2-17

FIGURE 2-17   Fibrofolliculoma. Note the well-defined areas of loose connective tissue around the hair follicles.

Trichodiscoma

Trichodiscoma represents a benign proliferation of the mesodermal component of the hair disc. Clinically, there are many small, asymptomatic, round, skin-colored papules, which are distributed throughout the body. In some cases the lesions are inherited with an autosomal dominant pattern (Birt–Hogg–Dubé syndrome) (66).

The Birt–Hogg–Dubé syndrome is characterized by multiple trichodiscomas, fibrofolliculomas, and acrochorda. This autosomal dominant genodermatosis is characterized by multiple, firm papules on the face, neck, and trunk. There may be multiple or bilateral renal carcinomas, especially chromophobe renal carcinoma and renal oncocytomas. Pulmonary changes include pulmonary cysts and spontaneous pneumothorax. Other, less commonly associated conditions include parathyroid adenomas, flecked chorioretinopathy, bullous emphysema, lipomas, angiolipomas, parotid oncocytomas, neural tissue tumors, multiple facial angiofibromas, and desmoplastic melanoma (66).

PATHOLOGY
- The overlying epidermis is atrophic, and there usually is a collarette
- Dermal, nonencapsulated tumor composed of fascicles of loose, finely fibrillar connective tissue with mucin
- Fibroblasts with occasional stellate forms
- Characteristic small vessels (some with telangiectatic features)
- Peripherally to the lesion, blood vessels with a concentric arrangement of PAS-positive collagen, forming a thickened wall

Pilomatricoma

Pilomatricoma is a benign appendageal tumor with differentiation toward the hair matrix. Clinically, it usually presents as a solitary, firm nodule on the head and neck (cheek is the most common site) and upper extremities. It is most common in children, but it can be seen in adults. There is a female predominance. Patients that present with multiple lesions may have myotonic dystrophy. Recent studies have shown that there are activating mutations in beta-catenin, both in the familiar and sporadic forms. Most tumors, even if they are incompletely excised, will not recur. However there have been cases with local aggressive behavior (68, 69). Since these tumors have matrical differentiation, they may contain melanin pigment and dendritic melanocytes, similar to melanomatricomas and thus they may present clinically as pigmented lesions.

PATHOLOGY (FIGURE 2-18A, B)
■ Dermal or subcutaneous, well-demarcated multilobulated tumor surrounded by a connective tissue pseudocapsule
■ Tumor lobules are composed of a mixture of basophilic and ghost cells (these cells preserve the size and shape of the cytoplasm but lack nuclei)
■ Basophilic cells are small and uniform and usually arranged either on one side or along the periphery of the tumor islands
■ Early-stage lesions may show numerous mitotic figures, indicative of a rapid growth phase not necessarily related to a malignant potential
■ As the tumor matures, the basaloid cells evolve into ghost cells
■ Frequent multinucleated giant cells
■ As the lesion ages, the number of basophilic cells decreases
■ Melanin pigment within the basaloid keratinocytes, macrophages, or within "passenger" melanocytes
■ Calcium deposits are seen in 75% of lesions

FIGURE 2-18   (A) Pilomatricoma. Well-delineated tumor mostly composed of large areas with keratin. (B) Higher magnification showing the ghost cells and the multinucleated giant cells.

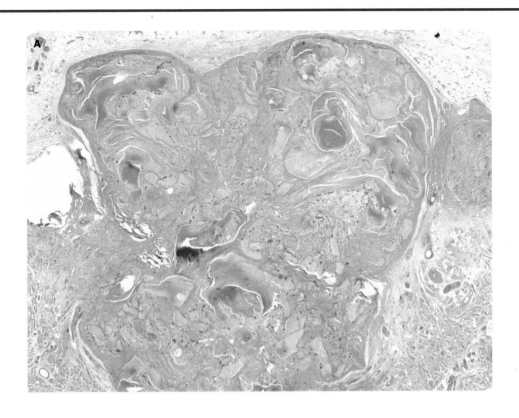

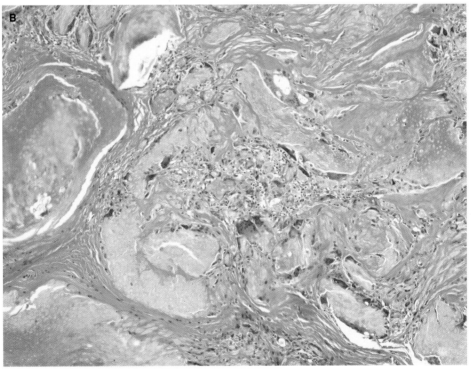

FIGURE 2-18

Pilomatrical Carcinoma

Pilomatrical carcinoma is a very rare neoplasm. In most cases the tumor arises, de novo, as a solitary lesion; however, some cases may arise in a pre-existent pilomatricoma. The tumors are usually located on the scalp and face. Pilomatrical carcinoma is most commonly seen in the elderly. These tumors have a male predominance and the tumor size ranges from 0.6 cm to up to 20 cm in diameter. Pilomatrical carcinomas are highly infiltrative neoplasms and local recurrences are common. Metastases are uncommon; however, it has been reported to spread to regional lymph nodes and to the lungs. The majority of cases show mutations in the *CTNNB1* gene (which encodes beta-catenin) (70).

PATHOLOGY (FIGURE 2-19A, B)
- Large, poorly circumscribed tumor, occasionally ulcerated
- Mainly dermal but it can infiltrate the subcutaneous fat
- Infiltrating borders with involvement of fascia or skeletal muscle
- Pleomorphic basaloid cells with prominent nucleoli
- Frequent mitotic figures (30 or more per 10 HPF) most common in early lesions
- Possible necrosis
- Keratotic material and shadow cells in the center of the basaloid islands
- Melanin pigment and intralesional melanocytes
- Possible lymphovascular or perineural invasion

FIGURE 2-19 (A) Pilomatrical carcinoma. Low power shows a poorly circumscribed tumor with infiltrating borders. (B) Note the infiltrative, irregular tumor lobules with marked pleomorphism

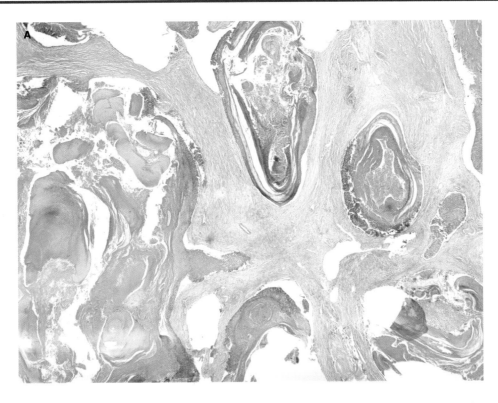

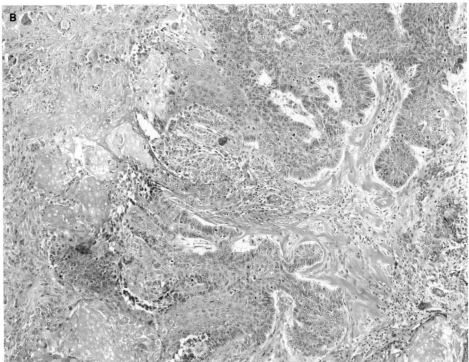

FIGURE 2-19

SEBACEOUS LESIONS

Ectopic Sebaceous Glands (Fordyce Spots and Montgomery Tubercles)

Sebaceous glands are normally found in association with a hair follicle (pilosebaceous units). Ectopic sebaceous glands without association with follicles may be found as small yellow-to-white papules (1–3 mm) near mucocutaneous junctions, especially the upper lip and in the buccal mucosa (Fordyce spots). On the vulva, Fordyce spots affect the medial aspect of the labia majora and in males the glans penis (Tyson glands). Ectopic sebaceous glands may also be found in the areolae of the breasts, where they are known as Montgomery tubercles (71).

PATHOLOGY (FIGURE 2-20)
■ Well-formed lobules or small groups of sebocytes in the lamina propria
■ Sebaceous glands open directly onto the epithelial surface

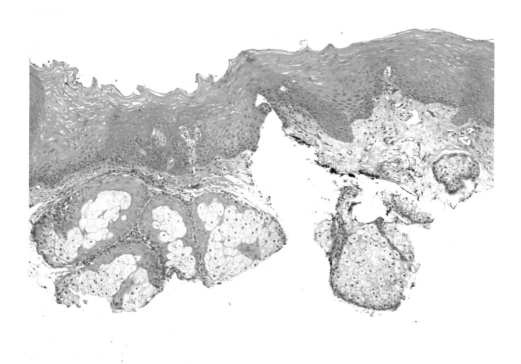

FIGURE 2-20

FIGURE 2-20   Ectopic sebaceous glands (Fordyce spots). This is a mucosal lip biopsy showing ectopic sebaceous glands in submucosal location.

Sebaceous Hyperplasia

Sebaceous hyperplasia is a common benign condition frequently clinically misdiagnosed as BCC. Lesions can be single or multiple and manifest as yellowish, soft, small papules (1–2 mm) on the face (particularly nose, cheeks, and forehead). Other less common sites of involvement include the ocular caruncle, chest, vulva, penis, and scrotum.

PATHOLOGY (FIGURE 2-21)

- Discrete, enlarged, mature sebaceous glands located around a dilated central sebaceous duct and within the papillary dermis (higher in the dermis than normal glands)
- The lobules have one or more basal cell layers at their periphery, with undifferentiated sebocytes that contain large nuclei and scant cytoplasmic lipid

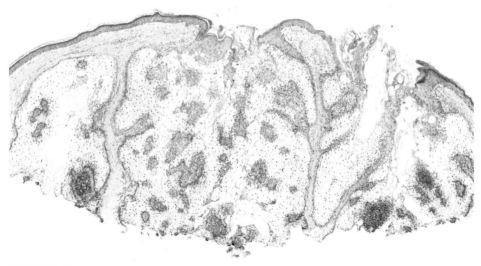

FIGURE 2-21

FIGURE 2-21   Sebaceous hyperplasia. Lobules of mature sebaceous glands around a central hair follicle.

Folliculosebaceous Cystic Hamartoma

Folliculosebaceous cystic hamartoma is a rare cutaneous hamartomatous lesion with follicular, sebaceous, and mesenchymal elements. Clinically, it presents as a small solitary symmetrical papule with a predilection for the face (characteristically on the nose). These tumors typically arise in adulthood, but the age distribution is wide and some lesions present at birth. This lesion likely represents a trichofolliculoma at its very late stage (72, 73).

PATHOLOGY (FIGURE 2-22)
- Large cystic structure lined by squamous epithelium and with many radiating sebaceous lobules
- Hair follicles at various stages in the follicular cycle
- The epithelial component is surrounded by laminated collagen and the fibroepithelial unit is separated from the adjacent stroma by cleft-like spaces
- The pilosebaceous units are embedded in a distinctive mesenchymal stroma that has variable amounts of fibrous, adipose, and vascular tissue
- The stroma shows spindled cells with eosinophilic cytoplasm and tapered nuclei (these cells can be positive for CD34 or factor XIIIa)
- Mucin may be abundant, with a perivascular disposition
- Neural and smooth muscle component

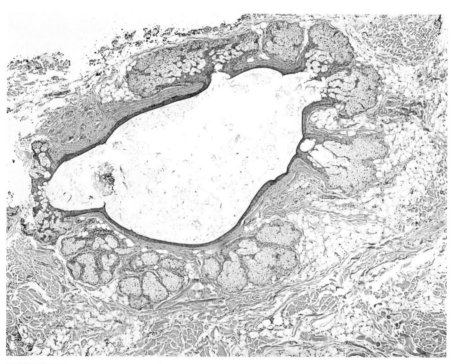

FIGURE 2-22

FIGURE 2-22   Folliculosebaceous cystic hamartoma. Cystic cavity with sebaceous glands embedded in a dense stroma. Note the mature adipose tissue.

Nevus Sebaceus

Nevus sebaceus of Jadassohn (organoid nevus) is a common hamartoma. Clinically, it presents, often at birth or early in childhood, as a solitary, hairless patch usually on the scalp. Other sites of involvement include the forehead, temples, central face, and postauricular areas. In adolescence, the lesion becomes verrucous and nodular, likely due to hormonal effect. Later in life some lesions may develop various types of adnexal tumors, including trichoblastomas (most common overall lesion), syringocystadenoma papilliferum, BCC (most common malignant tumor), and less commonly other tumors (hidradenomas, leiomyomas, sebaceous epitheliomas, apocrine cystadenomas, eccrine carcinomas, squamous cell carcinomas, sebaceous carcinomas, and keratoacanthomas) (74).

The linear sebaceus nevus syndrome is characterized by nevus sebaceus, often on the face, abnormalities of the central nervous system (seizures and mental retardation) and eyes, oral lesions, and skeletal defects (75).

PATHOLOGY (FIGURE 2-23)
- In early infancy, the sebaceous glands show a transient increase in size due to the effect of maternal hormones. When reaching adolescence they undergo marked proliferation. Afterward, the sebaceous glands tend to involute with increasing age.
- Asymmetric distribution of sebaceous glands (they are located abnormally high in the dermis, sometimes communicating directly with the surface of the epidermis)
- Absence or great reduction in the number of mature hair follicles, especially in scalp lesions
- Hairs are usually vellus type
- Ectopic apocrine glands in up to 50% of the cases.
- Papillomatous and acanthotic epidermis (especially in and after puberty).

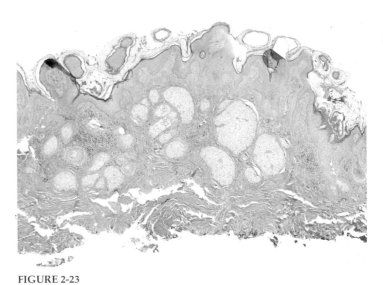

FIGURE 2-23

FIGURE 2-23   Nevus sebaceus. There is marked epidermal papillomatosis. Note the distribution of sebaceous glands and the absence of hair follicles.

Sebaceous Adenoma

Sebaceous adenoma is a rare, benign adnexal neoplasm. Clinically, it presents as a yellow, smooth-surfaced, circumscribed papule or nodule (1 cm to up to 5 cm) most often in older people. The most common locations include the face (especially the nose and cheek) and the scalp. Sebaceous adenomas, either solitary or multiple, may be associated with Muir–Torre syndrome, particularly those lesions occurring outside the head and neck region (76, 77).

PATHOLOGY (FIGURE 2-24A, B)

- Multilobulated neoplasm composed of well-defined sebaceous lobules
- The individual sebaceous lobules have a peripheral germinative layer of small basaloid cells (germinative cells) (this increased number of basaloid cells is an important characteristic in separating this lesion from sebaceous hyperplasia)
- Centrally, there are mature sebaceous cells with larger and pale staining, vacuolated cytoplasm and scalloped nuclei
- Mitotic activity is usually sparse; however, it can be prominent (as with other basaloid cutaneous neoplasms, such as pilomatricoma)
- Mature sebaceous cells outnumber the darker germinative cells. By definition greater than 50% of the tumor is composed of mature sebaceous cells.
- Lesions with less than 50% of sebocytes are termed sebaceous epitheliomas (sebaceomas).
- Cystic degeneration, germinative cells with mild nuclear pleomorphism, and moderate mitotic activity in some cases may be associated with the mismatch repair (MMR)-deficient subtype of Muir–Torre syndrome.
- Lesions with features of both keratoacanthoma and sebaceous differentiation are very commonly associated with the Muir–Torre syndrome.

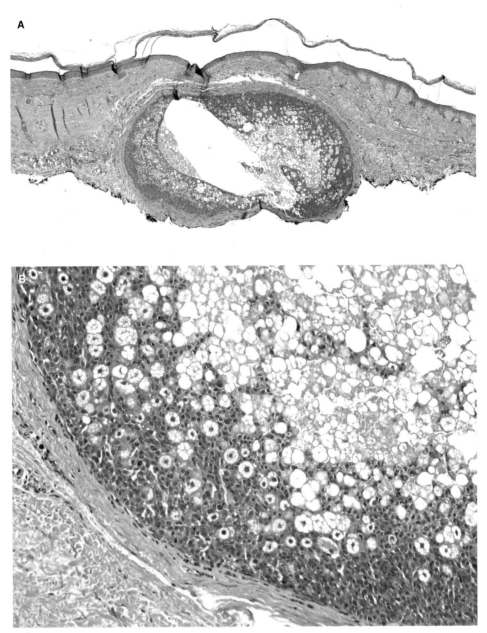

FIGURE 2-24

FIGURE 2-24   (A) Sebaceous adenoma. Well-defined sebaceous lobule in the dermis with a peripheral layer of basaloid/primitive cells. (B) The periphery of the tumor is composed of basaloid cells and inner sebocytes (note the characteristic scalloped nuclei).

Sebaceoma/Sebaceous Epithelioma

These two terms have been used to describe lesions with basaloid cells and focal sebaceous differentiation (i.e., <50% of the tumor). Furthermore, some authors have suggested that sebaceous epithelioma should be left for those BCC lesions with sebaceous differentiation. We prefer to designate those lesions with obvious characteristics of BCC (i.e., peripheral cleft and mucinous stroma) and sebocytes as BCC with sebaceous differentiation and leave the term of sebaceous epithelioma (sebaceoma) for lesions showing the architecture of sebaceous adenoma but with a minority of sebocytes (Figure 2-25A–D).

DIFFERENTIAL DIAGNOSIS
■ BCCs with sebaceous differentiation show peripheral palisading, clefting artifact, mucin deposition, and a loose fibromyxoid stroma. Mature sebaceous cells express EMA and D2-40, and this expression is uncommon in BCCs. BCCs express Ber-EP4, whereas sebaceous neoplasms do not. Adipophilin will detect sebocytes but will not allow differentiating BCC with sebaceous differentiation from sebaceous neoplasms.

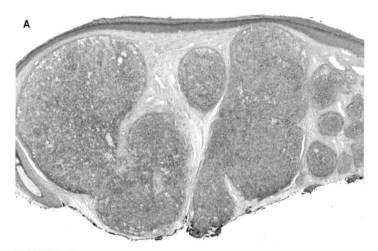

FIGURE 2-25

FIGURE 2-25   (A) Sebaceous epithelioma. Multinodular tumor separated by connective tissue septa. (B) Higher magnification showing the basaloid cells randomly admixed with small sebocytes. (C) Sebaceous epithelioma (rippled variant). Note the rippled-pattern on low magnification. (D) Higher magnification showing the palisading basaloid cells. The sebocytes are only focally seen in this variant.

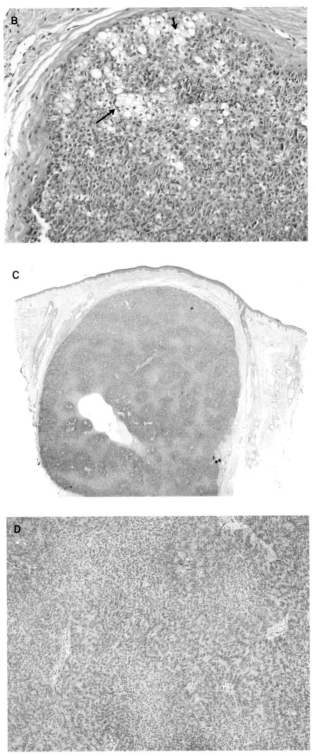

FIGURE 2-25

Sebaceous Carcinoma

Sebaceous carcinomas are rare and have been historically divided in two groups: the periocular and extraocular variants.

The periocular variant is more common (>75% of cases) and arises from the Meibomian glands and glands of Zeiss. They have a slight female predominance and more commonly involve the upper eyelid. Clinically, they sometimes may present as a chalazion, and thus the diagnosis may be delayed. One-third of cases develop lymph node metastases, more commonly to the preauricular and cervical nodes, with subsequent involvement of lung, liver, brain, and bone. The 5-year mortality rate is about 20% (metastatic cases show 50% 5-year mortality).

The extraocular variant involves particularly the head and neck of elderly patients; however, rare sites include the leg, trunk, foot, labia, penis, etc. The prognosis is probably similar to that of the periocular tumors.

Extraocular lesions are more likely to be associated with Muir–Torre syndrome, and such carcinomas appear at a younger age (78–80).

PATHOLOGY (FIGURE 2-26A–E)

- The tumor cells are arranged in lobules or sheets of cells separated by a dense fibrous stroma.
- The tumor lobules are composed of an admixture of basophilic germinative sebaceous cells with large nuclei, usually with multiple eosinophilic nucleoli, and more mature cells with finely vacuolated cytoplasm.
- There usually is central necrosis (comedo type).
- There are variable numbers of mitotic figures.
- The tumor may extend deeply and often involves the subcutaneous tissue and even the underlying muscle.
- The periocular variant often shows intraepithelial pagetoid upward migration or, less commonly, a carcinoma in situ change (up to 1/3 of all cases). These changes are rare in extraocular cases.
- In poorly differentiated carcinomas, the tumor cells are more pleomorphic and hyperchromatic and may contain only rare sebocytes.
- Poor prognostic features include: large tumor size (>1 cm), multicentricity, lymphovascular invasion, orbital extension, poor differentiation and extensive infiltrative growth pattern.
- Sebaceous carcinomas are strongly positive for EMA, ARs and with CAM 5.2. It is negative for CEA, S100p, and GCDFP-15. Note: In poorly differentiated carcinomas EMA can be negative or only focally positive.
- Adipophilin has recently been shown to be helpful since it labels the intracytoplasmic vacuoles of sebocytes. This vacuolar pattern should be distinguished from the granular pattern seen in macrophages and basaloid cells.

(*text continued on page 86*)

FIGURE 2-26   (A) Intraepithelial sebaceous carcinoma. Intraepithelial atypical cells with marked Bowenoid features. (B) Higher magnification showing focal cytoplasmic vacuolation (diagnostic clue). (C) An example of poorly differentiated sebaceous carcinoma. The tumor is composed of irregular lobules composed of dark-staining germinative cells. Note the comedo-like necrosis. In this particular case sebaceous differentiation was difficult to appreciate on H&E.

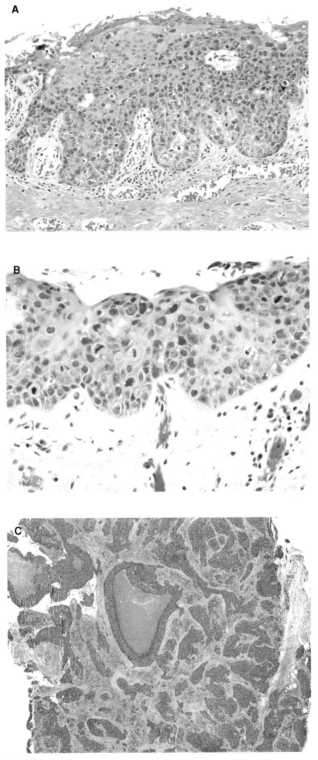

FIGURE 2-26

Sebaceous Carcinoma (continued)

DIFFERENTIAL DIAGNOSIS

■ Sebaceous carcinoma must be distinguished from BCC and SCC (clear-cell type and poorly differentiated).

■ Clear-cell SCC lacks lipid staining and is positive with Alcian blue, PAS, or mucicarmine (glycogen). Also, adipophilin would be negative. However, there is a group of purely intraepidermal carcinomas with obvious squamous differentiation (keratohyaline granules) that also contains intracytoplasmic vacuoles with scalloped nuclei, thus identical to sebocytes. These lesions have been designated as SCC with sebaceous differentiation or sebaceous carcinoma in situ.

■ Sometimes sebaceous carcinomas can be difficult to distinguish from BCC. A recent immunohistochemical study showed that an EMA+/Ber-EP4+ immunophenotype favors sebaceous carcinoma; an EMA+/Ber-EP4- phenotype favors SCC; and an EMA-/Ber-EP4+ favors BCC. In addition, roughly 60% of BCC show focal expression of AR. Adipophilin is a useful marker to separate these two neoplasms.

FIGURE 2-26   (D) Sebaceous carcinoma. In this example many of the atypical cells have a subtle vacuolated cytoplasm (diagnostic clue). (E) Expression of adipophilin by immunohistochemistry. Note the vacuolated staining in the cytoplasm of these atypical cells.

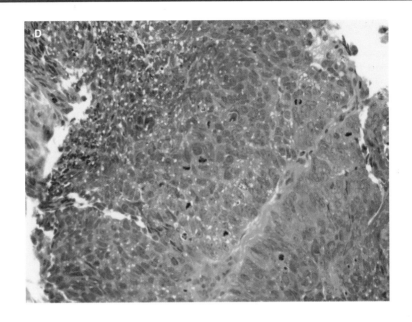

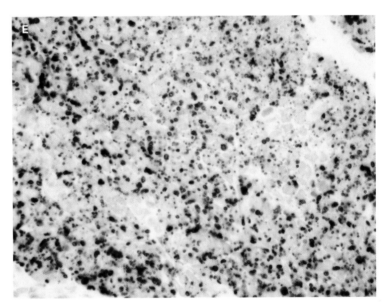

FIGURE 2-26

Muir–Torre Syndrome

Muir–Torre syndrome (MTS) is considered a subtype of the more common hereditary nonpolyposis colorectal cancer (HNPCC) syndrome. This condition is associated with an inherited defect in a DNA *MMR* gene, which eventually leads to microsatellite instability (MSI). MTS is characterized by the presence of sebaceous tumors (often multiple and outside the head and neck) in association with visceral neoplasms, usually gastrointestinal carcinomas. Keratoacanthomas, epidermal cysts, and colonic polyps are other common findings. Multiple sebaceous tumors occurring before the age of 50 years are strong indicators of MTS. Sebaceous hyperplasia may also be seen in MTS, but it is not considered to be a marker of the disease. The skin tumors may precede or follow visceral cancer (although sebaceous neoplasms usually develop after the visceral cancer). The internal neoplasms in MTS, which can be multiple, generally behave less aggressively than the non-MSI counterparts. Common malignancies include gastrointestinal (>50%), bladder and renal pelvis, endometrium, breast, and hematological (81–83).

MTS has usually an autosomal dominant pattern of inheritance. At least 70% of tumors from these patients show MSI. The malignancies in patients with MTS associated with MSI presented at a significantly younger age. Mutations in one of the DNA *MMR* genes *MLH1*, *MSH2*, and *MSH6*, have been described in these patients. A mutation in *MSH2* represents the majority of cases (90%), followed by *MSH6* mutations. These mutations can be detected when the nuclear staining of one of these proteins is absent in the tumor cells (84, 85).

PATHOLOGY (FIGURE 2-27A–G)
■ The sebaceous tumors of MTS may have unusual histomorphological features: cystic changes and keratoacanthoma-like architecture.
■ Some tumors may mimic BCC with some sebaceous differentiation.
■ Some tumors may show significant cytologic atypia (it has been proposed by some authors that these atypical features could be predictive of malignant transformation).

FIGURE 2-27   (A) Sebaceous epithelioma with verrucous features in a patient with Muir–Torre syndrome. Note the basaloid cells admixed with many sebocytes at the base of the tumor. (B) Sebaceous epithelioma with cystic features in a patient with Muir–Torre syndrome. Note the rim of basaloid cells at the periphery. (C) Higher magnification at the periphery of the tumor shows the characteristic sebaceous differentiation.

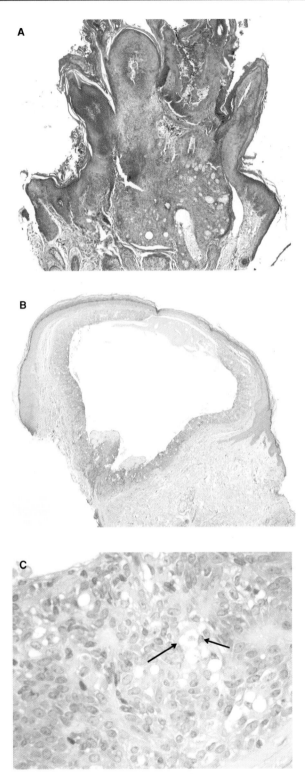

FIGURE 2-27

(continued)

Chapter 2: Adnexal Neoplasms 89

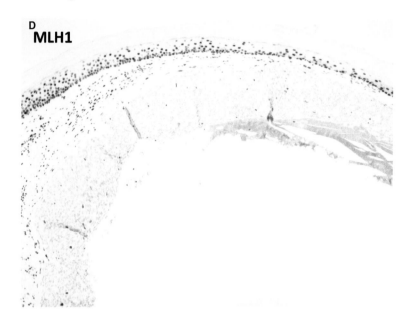

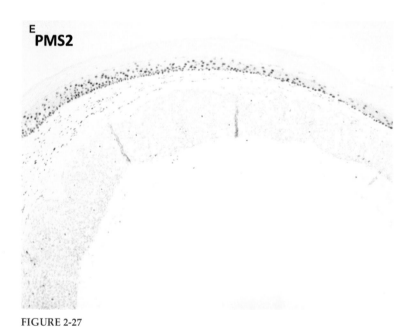

FIGURE 2-27

FIGURE 2-27   (D) Sebaceous epithelioma with cystic features in a patient with Muir–Torre syndrome. *MLH1* immunohistochemical stain showing loss of expression within the tumor cells. (E) *PMS2* immunohistochemical stain showing loss of expression within the tumor cells.

F
MSH2

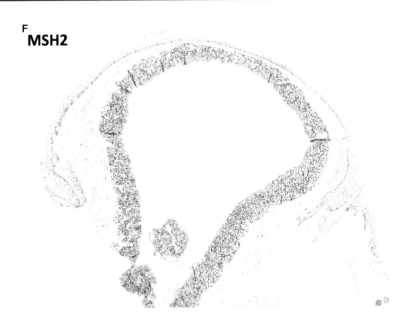

G
MSH6

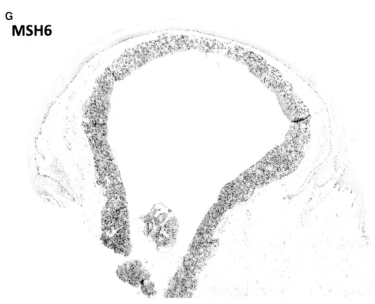

FIGURE 2-27

FIGURE 2-27   (F) Sebaceous epithelioma with cystic features in a patient with Muir–Torre syndrome. *MSH2* immunohistochemical stain showing expression within the tumor cells. (G) *MSH6* immunohistochemical stain showing expression within the tumor cells.

SWEAT GLAND (ECCRINE AND APOCRINE) NEOPLASMS

Hidradenoma Papilliferum

Hidradenoma papilliferum is a benign apocrine neoplasm that is almost always found in the vulva and perianal regions. Rare cases have been reported on the face, scalp, and chest (so-called ectopic cases). Patients are usually young or middle-aged women (rarely in males). Clinically, it presents as an asymptomatic solitary nodule, usually less than 1 cm in diameter (86, 87).

PATHOLOGY (FIGURE 2-28A, B)
- Mainly a dermal tumor that is relatively well-circumscribed and sometimes may show continuity with the overlying epidermis
- Partially cystic with papillary processes that project into cystic spaces (occasional glandular structures)
- Possible cribriform pattern
- Papillae may have arborizing trabecular pattern
- The epithelial lining is double layered in both the papillary and glandular areas. The inner layer is composed of small myoepithelial cells with round hyperchromatic nuclei; the outer layer has tall columnar cells with pale eosinophilic cytoplasm and nipple-like cytoplasmic projections on the surface (decapitation secretion).
- Although there may be visible mitotic figures, they do not predict aggressive behavior

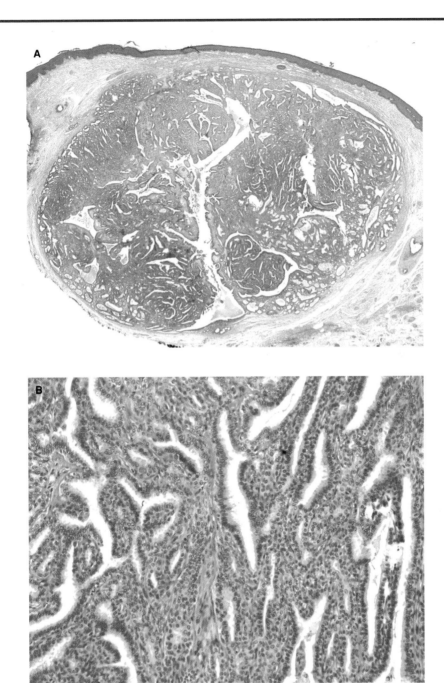

FIGURE 2-28

FIGURE 2-28   (A) Hidradenoma papilliferum. Well-defined tumor nodule in the dermis with papillary
configuration. (B) Higher magnification showing the double layer of epithelium in the
papillary areas along with conspicuous decapitation secretion.

Chapter 2: Adnexal Neoplasms   *93*

Syringocystadenoma Papilliferum

Syringocystadenoma papilliferum is a benign neoplasm of uncertain histogenesis; some authors believe it has an apocrine origin. Clinically, it presents more commonly as an isolated, raised warty plaque (1–3 cm) mostly on the scalp and forehead, but rarely in other locations including the breast, arm, thigh, eyelids, popliteal fossa, scrotum, vulva. Lesions may be present at birth or develop in childhood. Tumors on the scalp can be associated with nevus sebaceus in 1/3 of cases. BCC can be associated in approximately 10% of the cases (88, 89).

PATHOLOGY (FIGURE 2-29A, B)
- Usually invaginations arising from the overlying epidermis (the adjacent epithelium shows hyperplastic changes).
- In the middle portion of the tumor there are epithelium-lined papillae that communicate with duct-like structures in the lower portion of the tumor. In the upper portion the papillae are lined by stratified squamous epithelium with a transition into double-layered columnar epithelium. The latter is composed of an inner layer of small cells and an outer layer of tall columnar cells with abundant eosinophilic cytoplasm.
- The stroma of the papillary processes has dilated blood vessels and many plasma cells.
- Dilated ducts may form cystic spaces with internal villous projections.

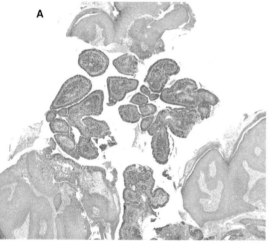
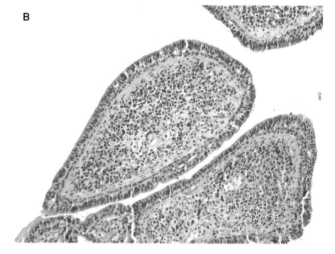

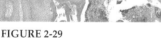
FIGURE 2-29

FIGURE 2-29 (A) Syringocystadenoma papilliferum. Low magnification showing an exophytic papillary lesion protruding into the invaginations of the surface epithelium. (B) Higher magnification showing the papillae covered by an outer layer of columnar cells. Note the conspicuous plasma cells in the stroma (diagnostic clue).

Tubular Apocrine Adenoma

Tubular apocrine adenoma (also known as apocrine adenoma) is a rare benign, adnexal tumor with female predominance. Clinically, it presents as a slow-growing nodular lesion, most common on the scalp (also eyelid, axilla, leg, and genitalia). Lesions that present on the scalp often are associated with a nevus sebaceus and syringocystadenoma papilliferum (90, 91).

PATHOLOGY (FIGURE 2-30A, B)

- Dermal lesion with circumscribed lobules of tubular structures (it may infiltrate the subcutis). Cystic changes are common.
- Occasional connection to epidermis through duct-like structures
- Well-formed tubules, lined by a double or multilayered epithelial cell layer composed of columnar cells with eosinophilic cytoplasm and uniform round nuclei
- Decapitation secretion in some tubules with glandular differentiation
- Papillae devoid of stroma project into the lumina of some tubules
- Intraluminal papillae lacking a fibrovascular core
- Possible cystic degeneration, follicular and sebaceous differentiation
- Fibrous stroma with only minimal inflammatory response

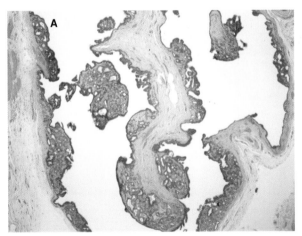
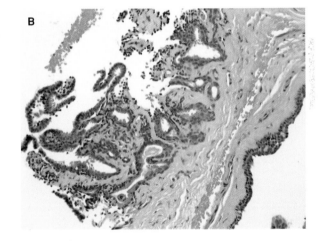

FIGURE 2-30

FIGURE 2-30   Tubular apocrine adenoma. (A) Nodular neoplasm with cystic changes and tubular structures. (B) Higher magnification showing ductal differentiation and tubules with apocrine differentiation.

Nipple Adenoma

Nipple adenoma (florid papillomatosis of nipple) is a benign adnexal tumor that more commonly presents in middle-aged females (30–50 years of age). It is believe to arise from the ducts of the nipple. Clinically, it presents as a unilateral, erythematous and sometimes eroded lesion that clinically may resemble eczematous dermatitis or Paget disease. Sometimes there is an associated nodule with serous or bloody nipple discharge (92).

PATHOLOGY (FIGURE 2-31A, B)

- Dermal tumor, nonencapsulated but well-circumscribed, with adenomatous and papillary architecture
- It may connect with the overlying epithelium but there is no pagetoid extension in the epidermis (histologic distinction with intraductal breast carcinoma)
- Glandular spaces are lined by columnar, eosinophilic cells with decapitation secretion and a myoepithelial cell layer. There are mitotic figures of normal morphology
- Some of the ducts have papillary projections into the lumen and may show cystic degeneration
- Stroma can be fibrotic or hyalinized with focal plasma cell infiltrate

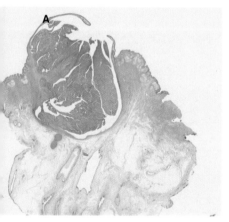 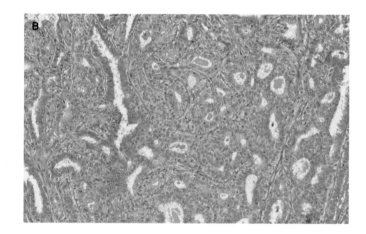

FIGURE 2-31

FIGURE 2-31   Nipple adenoma. (A) Low power showing a well defined tumor in dermis that connected to the overlying epidermis. (B) High power showing the glandular spaces with papillary projections.

Ceruminoma (Ceruminous Gland Tumor)

Ceruminoma is a rare adnexal tumor that arises from the modified apocrine glands of the external auditory canal. In the past, the term ceruminoma was used in all glandular tumors arising in the external auditory meatus. Clinically, it presents in adult patients as a pedunculated papule/nodule in the external auditory canal (hearing loss can be associated in 25% of cases). Ceruminous gland tumors are classified as benign and malignant (ceruminous gland adenocarcinoma) (93, 94).

PATHOLOGY
- Well-circumscribed nodule composed of glands lined by a double layer of epithelium (inner columnar cells with eosinophilic cytoplasm often showing decapitation secretion and outer myoepithelial cells)
- Cystic degeneration
- Rarely pleomorphism and mitotic figures
- Ceruminous gland adenocarcinoma can be exceedingly difficult to distinguish from adenoma, particularly in small biopsies, since the main feature is the infiltrative border in the former. These lesions may recur and be locally aggressive
- Note: It is advised that all these ceruminous lesions undergo full excision to rule out the possibility of malignancy.

Myoepithelioma

Myoepithelioma is a rare, benign adnexal neoplasm that arises from the peripheral myoepithelial cells in eccrine and apocrine glands. Clinically, it presents as a nodular neoplasm most commonly located in the extremities, head and neck, and trunk. The tumors range in size from 0.5 to 2.5 cm. The age range is wide but there is a predilection for male adolescents and young adults. Lesions usually behave in an indolent fashion; there may be local recurrence and rare distant metastases. Frankly malignant myoepitheliomas are rare, with an increased risk of local recurrence and metastatic potential (95, 96).

PATHOLOGY
- Nonencapsulated, well-defined dermal nodule, sometimes involving subcutaneous tissue
- Spindle, epithelioid, histiocytoid, and myoepithelial cells without evidence of ductal differentiation. When ducts are found those cases are termed mixed tumors/pleomorphic adenomas (also see below)
- Cells arranged in solid sheets or with a reticular or fascicular pattern
- Monomorphous cells devoid of pleomorphism
- Rare mitotic figures
- Myxoid or collagenous, hyalinized stroma
- Radially orientated collagenous crystalloid inclusions
- Overlying hyperplastic epidermis with peripheral collarette
- Immunohistochemistry: The tumor cells express S100p, vimentin, EMA, and GFAP, supporting their myoepithelial origin. They also express p63 and smooth muscle markers including smooth muscle actin (SMA), calponin, and muscle-specific actin (MSA). Desmin is rarely expressed. Cytokeratin expression is variable
- Malignant myoepithelioma is composed of tumor cells with marked nuclear pleomorphism, high-mitotic count, and tumor necrosis. There may be lymphovascular and perineural invasion

Syringoma

Syringomas are common benign adnexal neoplasms. Clinically, they present as asymptomatic skin-colored, small, dermal papules on the lower eyelids and upper cheeks. They appear at puberty or in early adult life and show a marked female predominance. An eruptive variant has been described in which many papules appear (mostly on the neck, chest, axillae, and upper extremities). The clear-cell variant of syringoma may be associated with diabetes mellitus. Syringomas appear to be more common in patients with Down syndrome (97, 98).

PATHOLOGY (FIGURE 2-32A–C)
- Numerous small ducts, embedded in a sclerotic stroma, in superficial dermis
- Ducts lined by two layers of cuboidal epithelial cells and with a lumen filled with eosinophilic amorphous debris (the lumen may be lined a cuticle)

(text continued on page 100)

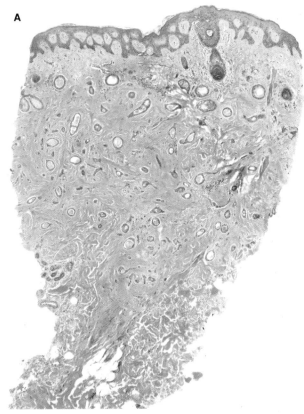

A

FIGURE 2-32

FIGURE 2-32   (A) Syringoma. Low power showing the epithelial strands and small cysts in the dermis embedded in a dense fibrous stroma.

Syringoma (*continued*)

- Some ducts have elongated tails with a characteristic comma-shaped or tadpole appearance
- Solid nests and strands of cells, sometimes having a basaloid appearance
- Clear-cell variant: The ducts are lined by cells with pale or clear cytoplasm containing glycogen. This clear-cell change may involve only part of the tumor or be limited to the cells adjacent to the duct lumina. This variant is associated with diabetes mellitus.

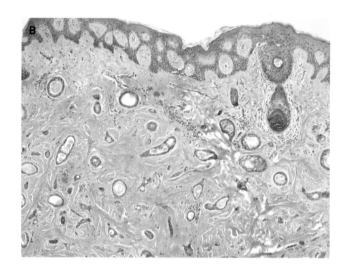

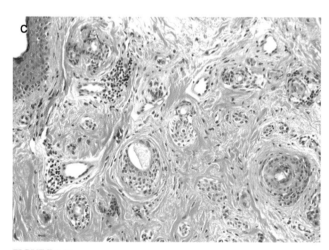

FIGURE 2-32

FIGURE 2-32   (B) Syringoma. Note the epithelial strands showing a characteristic tadpole appearance. (C) Syringoma with clear cell change. Epithelial strands with clear cytoplasm.

Hidradenoma (Clear-Cell Hidradenoma)

Hidradenoma (clear-cell hidradenoma, nodular hidradenoma, solid–cystic hidradenoma) is an adnexal tumor that arises from the distal excretory duct of eccrine sweat glands. Clinically, it presents as a slowly enlarging, solitary, solid or cystic nodule (average 0.5–2 cm in diameter). It is most commonly seen in middle-aged or elderly females anywhere on the body, but the head and neck is the most common site. A chromosomal translocation t(11;19) (q21;p13) involving the *CRTC1* and the *MAML2* genes has been reported in approximately 50% of lesions (more prevalent in tumors with clear-cell features); this translocation is shared by some salivary gland tumors including mucoepidermoid carcinoma and Warthin tumor. Although regarded as benign, hidradenomas can recur after inadequate excision. Malignant transformation is rare (99–102).

PATHOLOGY (FIGURE 2-33A–C)
- Well-circumscribed and nonencapsulated dermal tumor (it may involve the subcutaneous fat and it rarely connects with the overlying epidermis)
- Lobulated and sometimes with cystic degeneration

(text continued on page 102)

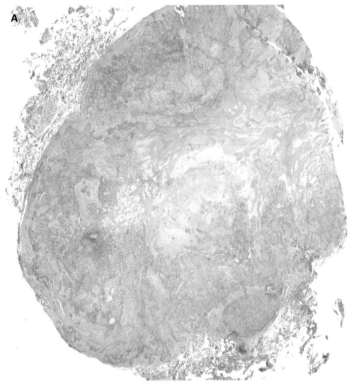

FIGURE 2-33

FIGURE 2-33   (A) Hidradenoma. Well-defined, lobulated tumor in the dermis with marked stromal hyalinization.

Hidradenoma (Clear-Cell Hidradenoma) *(continued)*

- Different proportions of two types of cells: Polyhedral with rounded vesicular nuclei with nuclear grooves and slightly basophilic cytoplasm. A second type, round, with clear cytoplasm and small dark nuclei. A predominance of clear cells (clear-cell hidradenoma) is noted in less than one-third of cases.
- The clear cells contain glycogen and PAS-positive, diastase-resistant material
- Duct-like structures are often present, some of which resemble eccrine ducts
- Focal apocrine decapitation secretion
- Tumors may show squamous differentiation, squamous eddy formation or full keratinization
- Cystic degeneration can be prominent (solid–cystic hidradenoma)
- Intervening stroma varies from delicate vascularized cords of fibrous tissue to dense hyalinized collagen
- Rare mitotic figures
- Some tumors can be highly vascular, forming perivascular pseudorosettes and hemangiopericytoma-like areas
- Note: In rare instances, circumscribed, benign-appearing tumors may show atypical features such as focal cytologic atypia (nuclear pleomorphism with prominent nucleoli and giant cell forms), and mitotic activity (two or more mitotic figures per 10 HPF). These histologic changes may correlate with an increased risk of recurrence and a possible malignant biological potential (thus the term atypical hidradenoma). Such lesions should probably be completely excised.

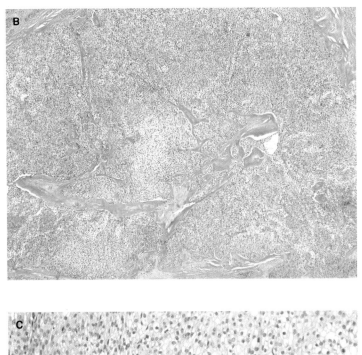

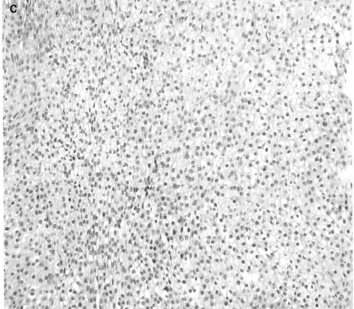

FIGURE 2-33

FIGURE 2-33 (B) Hidradenoma. Note the polyhedral cells and the cells with clear cytoplasm. (C) Higher magnification showing cells with clear cytoplasm and devoid of cytologic atypia or mitotic figures.

Hidradenocarcinomas

Hidradenocarcinomas are exceedingly rare adnexal neoplasms. Clinically, they present as an intradermal ulcerated nodule more commonly located on the face and extremities. They are most commonly seen in middle-aged to elderly patients. These tumors behave in an aggressive fashion with a high recurrence rate if incompletely excised (50%–75%). Metastatic and mortality rates are relatively high with a reported 5-year disease-free survival of only 30% (103); the lymph nodes, lungs, and bones are the most common metastatic sites. An associated benign hidradenoma can be identified in some tumors. Similar to hidradenomas, hidradenocarcinomas may rarely show the t(11;19) translocation (103–105).

PATHOLOGY (FIGURE 2-34A–C)
- Lobules and sheets of epithelial cells, with an irregular, infiltrative contour
- Focally clear cytoplasm (glycogen rich)
- Marked cytologic atypia and pleomorphism with varying degrees of mitotic activity
- Sometimes only focal clear-cell change, with a predominance of basaloid or squamous morphology (there may be extensive squamous differentiation)
- Characteristic intracytoplasmic ductal differentiation
- Focal to extensive tumor necrosis
- Note: Within the spectrum of low-grade hidradenocarcinomas, there seem to exist deceptively histologically benign tumors almost indistinguishable from hidradenomas but still capable of regional or distant metastasis. Thus, lesions with only mild cytologic atypia, but with mitotic figures (particularly abnormal forms) and a focal infiltrating growth pattern should be classified as low grade hidradenocarcinomas

FIGURE 2-34   (A) High grade hidradenocarcinoma. Infiltrative irregular tumor nodules embedded in a desmoplastic stroma. (B) Higher magnification showing epithelioid cells with squamoid features and only focal clear-cell changes. Note the ductal differentiation. (C) Prominent cytologic atypia of the tumor cells.

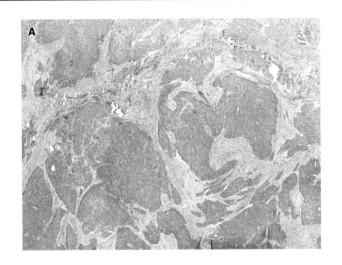

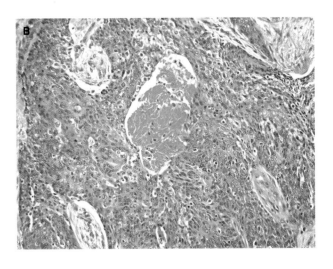

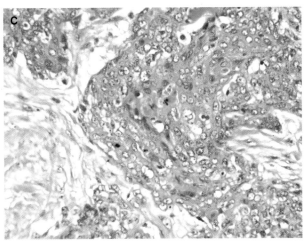

FIGURE 2-34

Hidroacanthoma Simplex

Hidroacanthoma simplex (intraepidermal poroma) is a rare benign adnexal neoplasm that likely arises from the acrosyringium. Clinically, it presents as a solitary nodular lesion that can be misdiagnosed as seborrheic keratosis or SCC in situ. It is more commonly seen on the distal extremities of elderly patients (106).

PATHOLOGY (FIGURE 2-35A, B)

■ Well-demarcated nests within an acanthotic epidermis (dermis is unaffected)
■ Tumor cells are smaller than the adjacent epidermal keratinocytes and show a cuboidal shape with vesicular nuclei containing a small nucleolus (similar to poroma cells)
■ Occasional ductal structures and intracytoplasmic lumina
■ Clear-cell change (intracytoplasmic glycogen)
■ Rare melanin pigment

FIGURE 2-35   (A) Hidroacanthoma simplex. Well-demarcated nests within epidermis. (B) Note the size of the tumor cells, which are smaller than the adjacent keratinocytes.

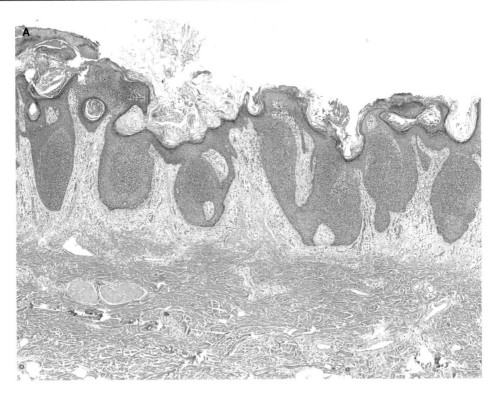

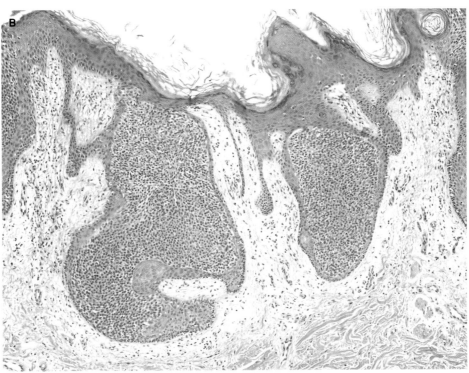

FIGURE 2-35

Poroma

Poroma (eccrine poroma) is a benign adnexal tumor that most likely arises from the cells of the outer layer of the acrosyringium and upper dermal eccrine duct; however, some cases may have apocrine origin. Clinically, it is more commonly seen in middle-aged or elderly patients, as a solitary, pedunculated, skin-colored nodule (up to 3 cm in diameter). It is most common on the sole or sides of the foot, but it can be seen in many other anatomic locations. Multiple lesions (eccrine poromatosis) are rare and may occur in the setting of chronic scarring and resemble acrosyringeal nevi (107, 108).

PATHOLOGY (FIGURE 2-36A–C)
- Cords and tongues of uniform poroid cells extending into the dermis from the undersurface of the epidermis
- Sharp demarcation between the epidermal keratinocytes and the monomorphic smaller cuboidal poroid cells
- Tumor cells are attached to each other by prominent intercellular bridges
- Ductal lumina and small cysts may also be seen within the tumor, thus confirming the diagnosis
- Intracytoplasmic lumina with cuticular borders
- Usually highly vascular stroma
- Ductal lumina can be highlighted by PAS staining or EMA and CEA by immunohistochemistry
- Occasional melanin pigment

A

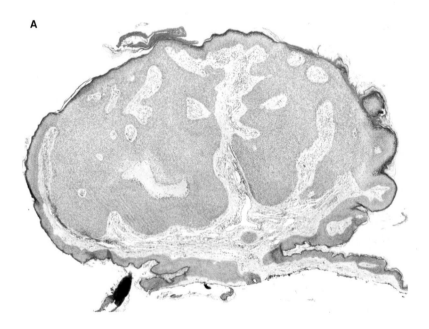

FIGURE 2-36   (A) Poroma. Tongues of epithelium arising from the epidermis. Note the clear transition between the adjacent keratinocytes and the poroid cells. (B) Higher magnification of the monomorphic cuboidal poroid cells. The presence of ductal lumina is a diagnostic clue. (C) High magnification of the characteristic monotonous epitheliod cells.

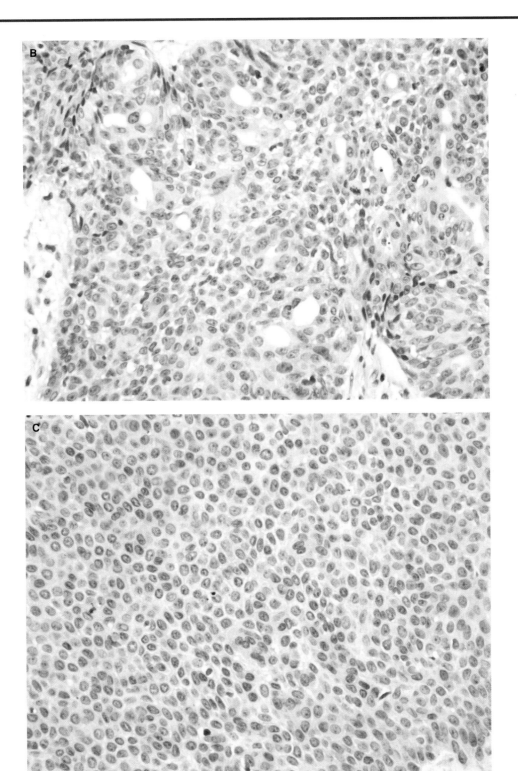

FIGURE 2-36

Dermal Duct Tumor

Dermal duct tumor is a rare benign adnexal neoplasm that likely arises from the intradermal segment of the eccrine duct. Clinically, it occurs on the head and neck or limbs and presents as a flesh-colored, firm nodule measuring up to 2 cm in diameter. It is more commonly seen in elderly females (108, 109).

PATHOLOGY (FIGURE 2-37A, B)
- Lobules of basaloid tumor cells within the dermis (epidermis is usually uninvolved)
- Small, cuboidal, uniform tumor cells showing ductal lumina. The tumor may occasionally connect with a normal-appearing eccrine duct
- Intracytoplasmic lumina, rarely also cystic spaces
- Rare mitotic figures
- Occasionally melanin pigment
- Anti-EMA and CEA highlight the ductal structures

FIGURE 2-37   (A) Dermal duct tumor. Tumor lobules of basaloid cells with prominent ductal structures. Note the lack of epidermal involvement. (B) Tumor lobules composed of small uniform cuboidal cells showing ductal lumina formation.

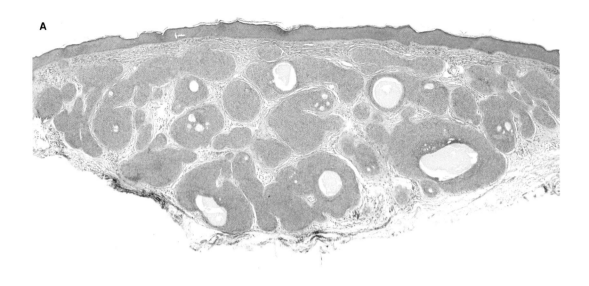

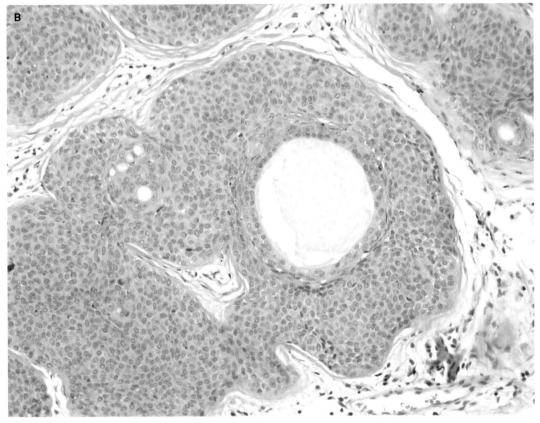

FIGURE 2-37

Porocarcinoma

Porocarcinoma is a rare, malignant adnexal neoplasm that most likely arises from the intraepidermal portion of the eccrine sweat gland duct epithelium. The tumor most often occurs in the elderly with slight predilection for females. Some porocarcinomas arise from a pre-existing benign lesion (poroma) manifesting with recent increase in size. Clinically, it presents as a dome-shaped nodule that tends to ulcerate. The tumors are most often located on the lower limb, trunk, head, and upper limb. Porocarcinoma has propensity for local recurrence and metastatic potential (propensity for epidermotropic metastases). Studies have suggested that the incidence of an aggressive clinical course is less than previously believed. However, once metastases appear the prognosis is poor with a high mortality rate (110–112).

PATHOLOGY (FIGURE 2-38A, B)
- The intraepidermal component (in situ) is composed of nests and islands of basaloid cells with ducts, associated with cytological features of malignancy including nuclear pleomorphism and mitotic activity
- The invasive component shows broad anastomosing cords and solid columns and nests of large cells extend into the dermis to varying levels
- Clear-cell areas and melanin pigment
- Focal tumor necrosis
- Occasional extensive squamous differentiation
- Ductal differentiation and intracytoplasmic lumina can be highlighted by immunohistochemical studies (EMA or CEA expression)
- Note: Some rare tumors may appear deceptively bland and are only recognized as being malignant based on their infiltrative growth

FIGURE 2-38   (A) Porocarcinoma. Note the broad anastomosing lobulated trabeculae with ductal differentiation. (B) Higher magnification showing the atypical cells with ductal differentiation. Some cells show intracytoplasmic lumina.

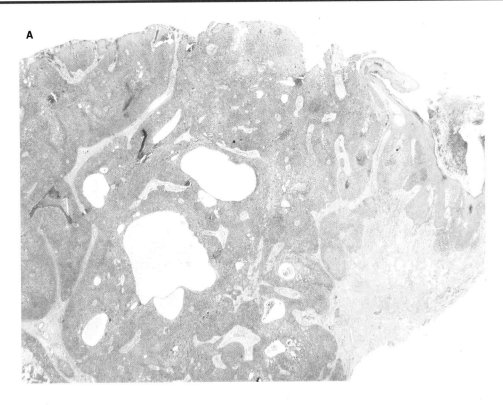

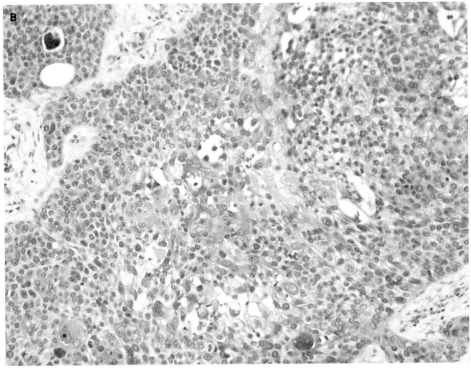

FIGURE 2-38

Spiradenoma

Spiradenoma is a benign adnexal tumor. Clinically, it presents as a painful, solitary gray-pink nodule. Tumors are commonly seen in adults and tend to arise on the head and neck, trunk, and, less commonly, arms and legs. It can be associated with nevus sebaceus. Multiple eccrine spiradenomas can be familial and inherited in an autosomal dominant pattern. Spiradenomas can be associated with multiple TEs and cylindromas as part of the morphologic spectrum of Brooke–Spiegler syndrome (113, 114).

PATHOLOGY (FIGURE 2-39A, B)

- One or more well-delineated basophilic nodules in the dermis and sometimes invading into the subcutis (no connection to the epidermis)
- Occasional small satellite lobules
- Some cases show retraction artifact between the lobule capsule from the surrounding tissues
- Tumor nodules have aggregates of cells arranged in sheets, cords, or with a trabecular arrangement
- Two cell types of tumor cells: small dark basaloid cells with hyperchromatic nuclei at the periphery of the lobule, and more frequent larger cells with a pale vesicular nucleus, toward the center of the lobules
- Hyaline droplets within the center of the lobules
- Thin bands of fibrous tissue rich in vessels within the tumor lobules
- Ductal differentiation
- Rare mitotic figures
- Occasional cystic degeneration filled with a finely granular eosinophilic material
- Focal squamous eddies and lymphocytes infiltrating the tumor lobules
- Edematous stroma among tumor lobules. Sometimes large vessels with hemorrhagic areas
- Some cases show overlapping features with cylindromas (see below)

FIGURE 2-39   (A) Spiradenoma. Circumscribed tumor nodules in the dermis composed of basophilic cells. Note the lack of epidermal involvement. (B) Note the two types of cells, the basophilic cells small cells and the larger cells. Characteristic fibrous bands of tissue within the tumor.

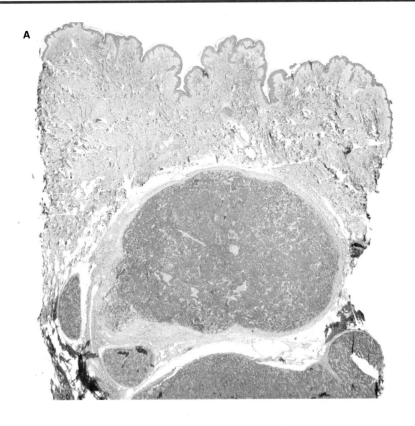

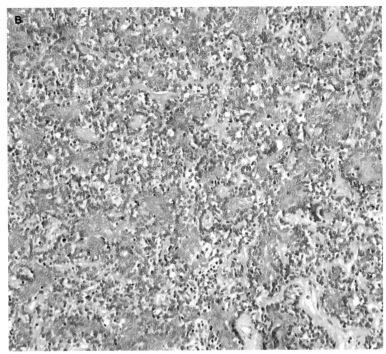

FIGURE 2-39

Spiradenocarcinoma

Spiradenocarcinoma is a very rare neoplasm believed to arise from transformation of a long-standing benign spiradenoma. Clinically, the tumors are solitary and there is a history of increase in size, change in color, or ulceration. The size ranges between 0.5 cm and 15 cm. In most cases the lesions have been present for a long time. It mainly affects middle-aged patients (mean age 55 years), most commonly in the upper extremities. Tumors are typically sporadic and solitary, but rarely can they be associated with Brooke–Spiegler syndrome. Most spiradenocarcinomas are aggressive, high-grade tumors with an approximate recurrence rate of 30%, a metastasis rate of at least 20%, and a mortality of 20%. Common metastatic sites include local regional lymph nodes and lung (115, 116).

PATHOLOGY

- Most spiradenocarcinomas contain areas of benign spiradenoma
- Malignant features include cytologic atypia (marked nuclear pleomorphism, prominent nucleoli, and brisk mitotic activity), infiltrating borders, necrosis, and hemorrhage
- Lack of the normal dual cell population normally seen in spiradenomas
- Malignant transformation change in spiradenoma shows two histomorphological patterns. (A) Abrupt transition to a carcinomatous or sarcomatous component (including leiomyosarcomatous, chondrosarcomatous, or osteosarcomatous differentiation). (B) Low-grade tumor in which the lobular architecture of spiradenoma is retained. This pattern shows a loss of the dual cell population and is composed of only basaloid cells with mild atypia and increased mitotic figures
- Immunohistochemistry with anti-EMA or CEA will highlight ductal differentiation

Cylindroma

Cylindroma is a common, benign adnexal tumor. Clinically, it present as tender, solitary red nodules (about 1 cm in diameter). There is strong predilection for middle-aged and elderly females. The majority occurs on the head, neck, and scalp. Scalp lesions can coalesce and grow to a large size ("turban tumor"). Multiple cylindromas occur in familial cylindromatosis and Brooke–Spiegler syndrome, inherited in an autosomal dominant fashion. The gene responsible for multiple cylindromas is the *CYLD* gene on chromosome 16q12–q13. Local aggressive behavior and malignant transformation are uncommon, mostly seen in long-standing turban tumors of the scalp. Studies have suggested both apocrine and eccrine differentiation (117, 118).

PATHOLOGY (FIGURE 2-40A, B)

■ Ill-defined dermal tumors composed of irregularly shaped islands and cords of basaloid cells (arranged in a jigsaw pattern)
■ No connection with the overlying epidermis
■ Occasional subcutaneous involvement
■ The tumor islands are surrounded by conspicuous eosinophilic hyaline bands (diastase-resistant, PAS-positive basement membrane; type IV and type VII collagen).
■ Tumor islands are composed of two cell types: At the periphery there are small cells with scant cytoplasm and hyperchromatic nuclei; second, central and larger cell with vesicular nuclei
■ Ducts and droplets of hyaline material in the cell nests
■ Stroma is composed of loosely arranged collagen with an increased number of fibroblasts
■ Some cases have overlapping features with spiradenoma (more solid pattern with light and dark cells)

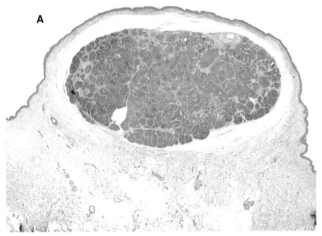 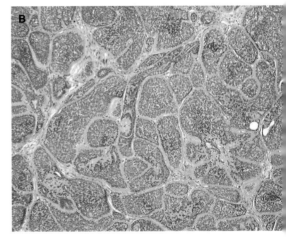

FIGURE 2-40

FIGURE 2-40 (A) Cylindroma. Dermal tumor composed of irregular islands and cords of basaloid cells (jigsaw pattern). (B) The irregular islands of basaloid cells are surrounded by eosinophilic hyaline bands.

Malignant Cylindroma

Malignant cylindroma is an extremely rare adnexal neoplasm. These tumors arise more commonly in long-standing cylindromas associated with the autosomal dominant multiple tumor variant. Malignant cylindromas are more likely located on the scalp of older females. These tumors are aggressive and have a high recurrence and metastatic rate (119–121).

PATHOLOGY
- Frequently associated with a cylindroma
- Nodules and cords of basaloid cells with infiltrating growth pattern and loss of mosaic appearance, hyaline membrane, or dual population of cells
- Nuclear pleomorphism, prominent nucleoli, and frequent atypical mitotic figures
- Some tumors may show squamous cell differentiation

Chondroid Syringoma (Mixed Tumor)

Chondroid syringoma (mixed tumor) is a rare adnexal neoplasm that is composed of both epithelial and mesenchymal components. These tumors are thought to originate from both secretory and ductal segments of the sweat gland (both eccrine and apocrine variants). Clinically, it presents as a nonulcerating solitary, slowly growing nodule on the head or neck (especially forehead and scalp) of middle-aged and elderly males (122, 123).

PATHOLOGY (FIGURE 2-41A, B)

- Well-delineated, multilobulated, and composed of mixed epithelial and mesenchymal elements
- Dermal lesion without connection to the overlying epidermis (occasional invasion of the subcutaneous fat)
- The lobules are separated by fibrous septa
- The epithelial structures are arranged singly, in cords and nests, or as irregular tubuloalveolar and ductal structures
- Stroma characteristically composed of homogeneous chondroid areas alternating with myxoid or densely collagenous, eosinophilic, and hyalinized areas
- Focal cystic degeneration, keratinous cysts, and squamous differentiation
- Clear-cell change, apocrine decapitation, and mucinous, columnar, and hobnail metaplasia
- Absence of pleomorphism or tumor necrosis; sparse mitotic figures
- Foci of follicular (infundibular, isthmic, as well as trichilemmal) and sebaceous differentiation (cells with vacuolated cytoplasm and scalloped nuclei)
- Foci of calcification, and rarely osteoid stroma or mature adipocytes

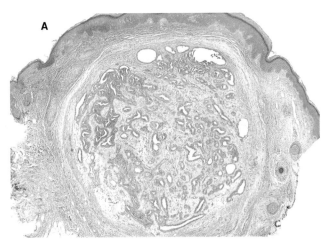
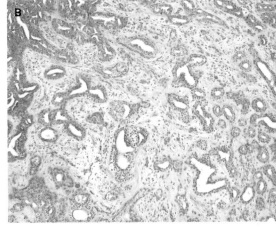

FIGURE 2-41

FIGURE 2-41   (A) Chondroid syringoma. Lobular neoplasm in the dermis composed of epithelial and mesenchymal elements. Note the light, myxoid stroma. (B) Higher magnification showing the epithelial component arranged in cords and irregular tubuloalveolar and ductal structures within a myxoid stroma.

Malignant Chondroid Syringoma (Malignant Mixed Tumor)

Malignant chondroid syringoma (malignant mixed tumor) is a rare high-grade neoplasm. Most of these tumors develop de novo, but they may appear within a pre-existent, benign chondroid syringoma. Clinically, it presents as a skin-colored nodule most commonly seen in the distal extremities (especially the foot). The tumors show a predilection for females and most often arise in the sixth decade of life. Metastatic rate is close to 60% and mortality rate is 25% (124, 125).

PATHOLOGY
- In many cases, the diagnosis will depend on the identification of a benign component (chondroid syringoma)
- Features that favor malignancy include infiltrative growth pattern, nuclear pleomorphism, atypical mitotic figures, and tumor necrosis. Also, vascular and lymphatic invasion
- Excessive mucoid matrix and extensive chondroid elements also favor malignancy
- Rare chondrosarcomatous differentiation
- Frequent satellite lesions in the dermis and subcutaneous fat, likely related to their high-risk of recurrence
- Note: In cytologically benign lesions, the presence of an infiltrative growth pattern or satellite lesions should be viewed with caution and prompt complete excision.

Primary Mucinous Carcinoma

Primary mucinous carcinoma is a rare neoplasm showing a predilection for the face (particularly the eyelids), scalp, axilla, and trunk. Clinically, it presents as a slowly growing, skin-colored, reddish nodule. The tumor is more commonly seen in middle-aged and elderly patients (median age is 62 years). These tumors are locally aggressive and commonly recur. Metastases to regional nodes and widespread dissemination occur in about 15% of cases (126–128).

PATHOLOGY (FIGURE 2-42A–D)
■ Dermal (or subcutaneous) tumor
■ Large pools of mucin separated by thin fibrovascular septa
■ Small islands of epithelial cells floating within the mucin
■ Epithelial component more pronounced at the periphery of the lesion
■ Cuboidal tumor cells, sometimes with vacuolated cytoplasm, and centrally located, round vesicular nuclei
■ Cribriform appearance alternating with areas of small glandular or tubular spaces. Rare solid pattern
■ Rare signet ring cells
■ Comedo necrosis
■ Some cases show an intraglandular (in situ) component thus supporting a diagnosis of primary rather than metastatic origin
■ Rare microcalcifications and psammoma bodies
■ Rare mitotic figures
■ Special stains: The mucin is PAS (diastase-resistant), Alcian blue (pH 2.5), mucicarmine, and colloidal iron-positive. It is hyaluronidase resistant and sialidase labile, confirming that it is a sialomucin. This feature helps in distinguishing this tumor from a metastatic mucinous carcinoma from the gastrointestinal tract.
■ Immunohistochemistry: The tumor cells are positive with CAM5.2, AE1/AE3, and for EMA and CEA. The tumor cells are CK7 positive and CK20 negative. S-100 protein expression is variable. The tumor cells express estrogen and progesterone receptors. A layer of myoepithelial cells may be focally highlighted by anti-p63, calponin, SMA, and with CK5/6. Myoepithelial cells are preserved in areas of carcinoma in situ and, when present, this a helpful feature in confirming the primary, cutaneous origin of the tumor.

DIFFERENTIAL DIAGNOSIS
Primary mucinous carcinoma is often difficult to distinguish from metastatic lesions, especially from mucinous breast cancer. Gastrointestinal and ovary neoplasms may also enter in the differential diagnosis. Primary mucinous carcinoma may be distinguished from gastrointestinal tumors by mucin stains. The former contains abundant sialomucin (Alcian blue pH 2.5) in contrast to gastrointestinal tumors, which show sulfamucins (Alcian blue pH 1.0 and 0.4). Also, primary mucinous carcinomas are CK20 negative as opposed to gastrointestinal tumors. Metastatic breast cancer is very difficult to distinguish as the histologic and immunophenotypic features are very similar; however, a helpful clue in this distinction is the presence of a myoepithelial layer in the in situ component of primary cutaneous mucinous carcinoma (highlighted by immunohistochemistry for p63, calponin, SMA, or with CK5/6). Clinical information is critical.

(continued)

Primary Mucinous Carcinoma *(continued)*

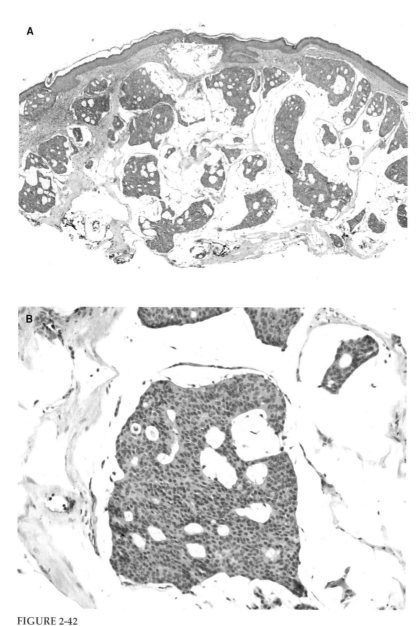

FIGURE 2-42

FIGURE 2-42   (A) Primary mucinous carcinoma. Islands of epithelial cells embedded in a mucinous stroma. (B) Islands of epithelial cells composed of cuboidal cells arranged in cribriform structures. (C) P63 immunohistochemical study showing no expression in the neoplastic component. (D) Calponin immunohistochemical study showing expression in the preserved myoepithelial cell layer confirming the presence of an in situ component.

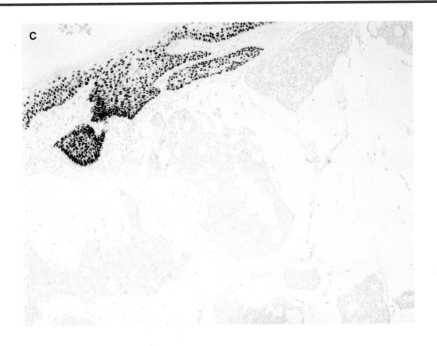

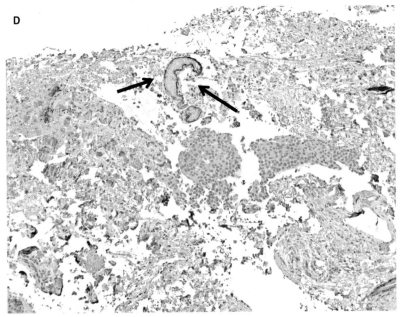

FIGURE 2-42

Eccrine Ductal Carcinoma

Eccrine ductal carcinoma is a rare adnexal neoplasm. Clinically, it presents as a slowly growing, infiltrating plaque or nodule on the scalp, the extremities or trunk in middle-aged and elderly patients. It has a propensity for local recurrence and occasional metastases. These tumors have striking similarities to infiltrating ductal carcinoma of the breast and can therefore be easily overlooked for a metastatic neoplasm (129, 130).

PATHOLOGY (FIGURE 2-43A–D)
- The tumor is situated in the lower dermis and often extends into the subcutaneous fat
- No connection with the epidermis
- Nests, cords, and tubular structures of cuboidal epithelium showing marked ductal differentiation
- Less commonly thin strands and solid nests
- Intracytoplasmic lumina
- Usually mild pleomorphism and few mitotic figures
- Dense, sometimes sclerotic, fibrous stroma
- Common perineural and lymphovascular invasion
- PAS-positive diastase-resistant material in the lumina of the tubular structures
- Immunohistochemistry: Tumor cells express cytokeratin and CEA. Some tumors may also express estrogen and progesterone receptors, S-100, and GCDFP-15. As most primary epithelial and adnexal neoplasms of the skin, the tumor cells express P63 (remember metastatic adenocarcinomas are mostly p63 negative).

DIFFERENTIAL DIAGNOSIS
The histological features of eccrine ductal carcinoma are very similar to those seen in invasive ductal breast carcinoma. Furthermore, multiple immunohistochemical markers will be positive in both types of lesion (estrogen and progesterone receptors, Her-2-neu, and even mammoblogin). Eccrine ductal carcinomas most likely are positive for P63, calretinin, or D2-40 while metastatic breast tumors are usually negative. However, careful clinical and radiological examination of the breasts is recommended before labeling such a tumor as being of primary eccrine neoplasm (131, 132).

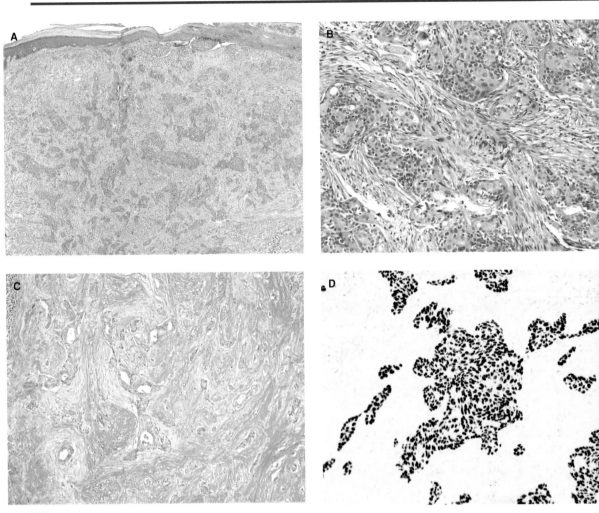

FIGURE 2-43

FIGURE 2-43   (A) Eccrine ductal carcinoma. Dermal infiltrative neoplasm composed of irregular
cords embedded in a desmoplastic stroma. (B) Higher magnification showing the
irregular epithelial cords with ductal differentiation. Note the marked desmoplastic
stroma. (C) Another case showing only scattered tubular structures that are highly
infiltrative in deep dermis. (D) Sometimes it is challenging to differentiate an eccrine
ductal carcinoma from a metastatic adenocarcinoma. In this case, P63 is strongly
positive confirming the diagnosis of a primary eccrine carcinoma.

Microcystic Adnexal Carcinoma

Microcystic adnexal carcinoma (MAC) is a rare, locally aggressive malignant adnexal neoplasm with sweat duct and follicular differentiation. Clinically, it presents as a slowly growing, indurated, plaque or nodule, usually on the upper lip and periorbital regions. There is a possible female predominance. The tumor presents in a wide age range; however, the majority of patients are in the seventh decade. The tumor is characteristically indolent with some cases having been present for years before the initial diagnosis. Local recurrence reportedly occurs in almost 50% of cases, but this is much less common if the surgical margins are free of tumor in the initial excision. Sometimes due to lack of familiarity and inadequate small biopsies, it can be initially misdiagnosed as a syringoma, with potential serious consequences for the patient (133–135).

PATHOLOGY (FIGURE 2-44A–C)
- It usually involves the entire dermis and the subcutaneous tissue, and it may extend into the underlying skeletal muscle and bone
- Ill-defined and only rarely connected with the overlying epidermis or hair follicles
- The superficial part of the tumor is composed of numerous, small keratinous cysts, merging into smaller cysts, and solid islands and strands of cells of with basaloid and squamous epithelium
- The deeper component consists of smaller nests and strands with ductal differentiation and a highly infiltrative growth pattern in a dense, hyalinized stroma
- Intracytoplasmic lumina are sometimes detected (characteristic diagnostic feature)
- In some cases, the deeply located ducts show a tadpole-like configuration similar to that seen in syringoma
- The dense fibrous stroma becomes more sclerotic in the deep infiltrative areas
- Frequent perineural invasion
- Rare cytological atypia or obvious mitotic figures
- Immunohistochemistry: Tumor cells are labeled with AE1/AE3 and EMA and also express CK7. Anti-EMA and CEA highlight the ducts and the intracytoplasmic lumina. In one study, Ber-EP4 was negative in MACs and positive in BCC.

DIFFERENTIAL DIAGNOSIS
MAC must be separated from desmoplastic TE, syringoma, and morpheaform BCC. Desmoplastic TE lacks the deep and infiltrative growth pattern, perineural infiltration, and ducts seen in MAC. Syringomas are very similar to superficial MAC especially in small limited biopsies where the deep, infiltrative component is absent. Keratocysts and mild nuclear atypia are against the diagnosis of syringoma. Morpheaform BCC lacks ductal differentiation and intracytoplasmic lumina.

FIGURE 2-44   (A) Microcystic adnexal carcinoma. Deep infiltrative neoplasm showing follicular and ductal differentiation. Note the sparse lymphocytic aggregates. (B) Higher magnification showing small nests and strands with ductal differentiation (narrow arrow) embedded in a dense, hyalinized stroma. Note the small keratinous cysts (wide arrows). (C) High power of the infiltrative strands of epithelial cells.

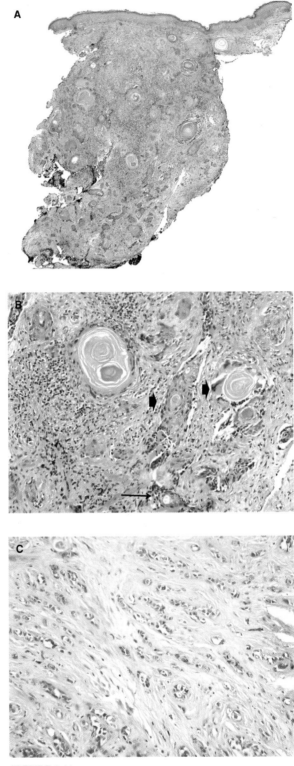

FIGURE 2-44

Papillary Eccrine Adenoma

Papillary eccrine adenoma is a rare benign adnexal tumor. It presents more commonly on the extremities and it particularly affects African American females (4:1). It is a slow-growing erythematous or brown nodule. The lesions have a tendency to recur locally. Due to the existence of aggressive digital papillary adenocarcinoma, it is important to consider all glandular lesions with focal papillary growth located on acral locations as potentially malignant (see below) (136, 137).

PATHOLOGY (FIGURE 2-45A, B)
- The tumor is composed of a well-circumscribed, unencapsulated growth of dilated branching duct-like structures in the dermis
- These ducts are lined by two or more layers of small eosinophilic cells with regular, round or oval nuclei containing small nucleoli
- Intraluminal papilla may project into the cystic spaces and may form a cribriform pattern
- Focal squamous cell differentiation
- Clear-cell change due to cytoplasmic glycogen accumulation
- Some lumina contain an amorphous eosinophilic material
- Absent decapitation secretion
- Absent nuclear pleomorphism or atypical mitotic figures
- The tumor may be associated with a subtle lymphoplasmacytic infiltrate (sometimes with lymphoid follicles)
- Dense stroma, sometimes hyalinized

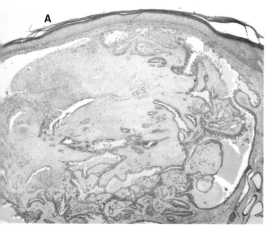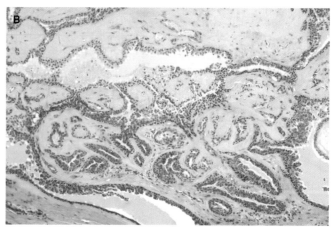

FIGURE 2-45

FIGURE 2-45   Papillary eccrine adenoma. (A) Nodular neoplasm composed of dilated branching duct-like structures. (B) Ducts are lined by two layers of cuboidal cells. Note the lumina filled with amorphous material.

Aggressive Digital Papillary Adenocarcinoma

Although originally conceived as a spectrum of benign and malignant papillary lesions in the digits, none of the histological or clinical parameters was predictive of recurrence or metastasis. Thus, all such lesions are better regarded as potentially malignant tumors and the designation of "adenocarcinoma" should be the preferred term. These tumors are rare adnexal neoplasms and occur almost exclusively on the fingers and toes and adjacent parts of the palms and soles. Clinically, it presents as a slow-growing, deep-seated, multinodular tumor. The tumor is most commonly seen in adults and males are more often affected than females (10:1). These tumors have a propensity to recur after narrow excisions (recurrent rate of roughly 50%). Metastases occur in 14% of cases and most commonly affect the lung and lymph nodes (136–138).

PATHOLOGY (FIGURE 2-46A, B)
- Multinodular and poorly circumscribed, in the deep dermis. It can extend into the subcutaneous fat and may occasionally infiltrate skeletal muscle, tendon, or bone
- No connection with the overlying epidermis
- Multiple tubuloalveolar and ductal structures with areas of papillary projections protruding into cystic lumina
- Solid growth pattern is observed in 20% of cases. Some of these cases have only very focal papillary areas
- Occasional lymphovascular invasion
- The glands are lined by one or two layers of columnar epithelium with eosinophilic cytoplasm and round vesicular nuclei. Typically these glands are fused in a back-to-back pattern.
- Common clear-cell change and squamous metaplasia
- Occasional decapitation secretion
- Most cases only show mild to moderate cytologic atypia
- Scattered mitotic figures
- Stroma varies from thin fibrous septa to areas of fairly dense, fibrous collagen

DIFFERENTIAL DIAGNOSIS
Aggressive digital papillary adenocarcinoma may mimic metastatic carcinomas with papillary features including breast, thyroid or gastrointestinal neoplasms. By immunohistochemistry, the epithelium expresses keratin, P63, S-100 protein, and ductal CEA. The majority of metastatic adenocarcinomas are negative for P63. In general, a diagnosis of aggressive digital papillary adenocarcinoma should be considered any time a papillary neoplasm is encountered in acral locations.

(continued)

Aggressive Digital Papillary Adenocarcinoma *(continued)*

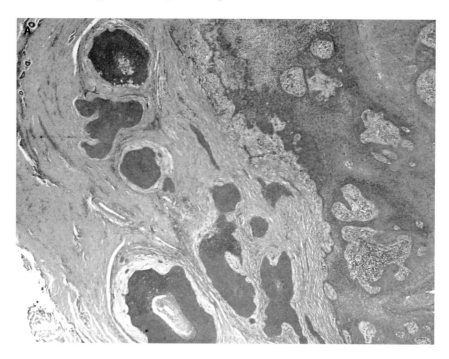

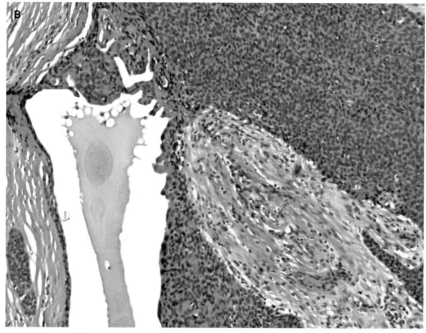

FIGURE 2-46

FIGURE 2-46   (A) Aggressive digital papillary adenocarcinoma. Infiltrative multinodular neoplasm with ductal differentiation. (B) Note the focal papillary projections into the cystic lumina.

Cutaneous Cysts

3

Follicular Infundibular Cyst

Follicular infundibular cyst (also known as epidermoid cyst) most commonly occurs in the face, neck, and trunk. These cysts are derived from the pilosebaceous follicle, specifically from the infundibular portion of the hair follicle. Clinically, they present as dome-shaped papules/nodules with a central punctum. Multiple follicular cysts may be associated with Gardner syndrome or with cyclosporine therapy in transplant patients (139).

PATHOLOGY (FIGURE 3-1A, B)
■ Unilocular cyst lined by stratified squamous epithelium showing epidermal keratinization (keratohyaline granules and loosely packed, laminated orthokeratin)

VARIANTS
■ In patients with Gardner syndrome the epithelial lining occasionally shows focal basaloid proliferation with ghost-cell changes (pilomatricoma-like changes) (140).
■ Sometimes follicular cysts may show hybrid features including trichilemmal cysts, pilomatrixomas, and/or eruptive villus hair components.
■ Malignant epidermal neoplasms may rarely arise in the wall of a follicular cysts (usually SCC or BCC) (141, 142).
■ Favre–Racouchot syndrome occurs as a clinical triad of follicular cysts, comedones, and prominent solar elastosis. This triad is seen in elderly patients around the orbit and malar areas.
■ Milia are superficial keratinous cysts. Clinically, they present as small white/yellow papules.

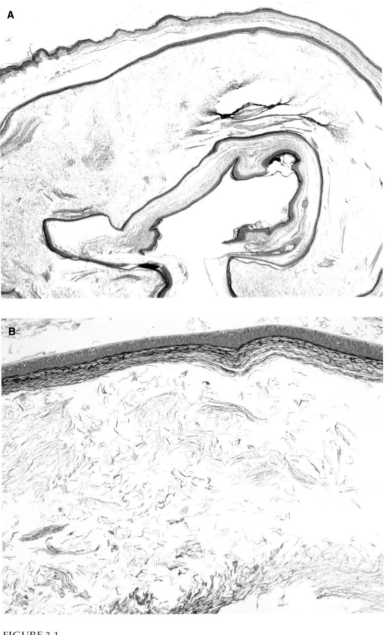

FIGURE 3-1

FIGURE 3-1   (A) Follicular infundibular cyst. Cyst lined by squamous epithelium. Note the laminated keratin. (B) Squamous epithelium with preserved granular cell layer.

Follicular Trichilemmal Cyst (Pilar Cyst)

Follicular trichilemmal cysts (pilar cyst) are believed to originate from the isthmic portion of the follicle. These cysts are found as solitary or multiple intradermal or subcutaneous papules/nodules with a predilection for the scalp (144).

PATHOLOGY (FIGURE 3-2A–C)
■ Lined by stratified squamous epithelium showing trichilemmal keratinization (compact, laminated keratin without keratohyaline granules)
■ Common cholesterol clefts and calcifications

A

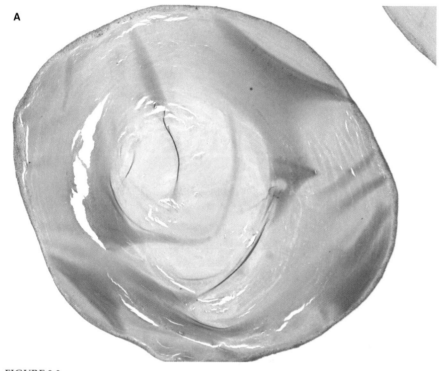

FIGURE 3-2

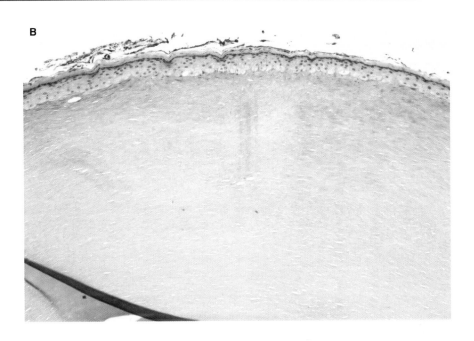

B

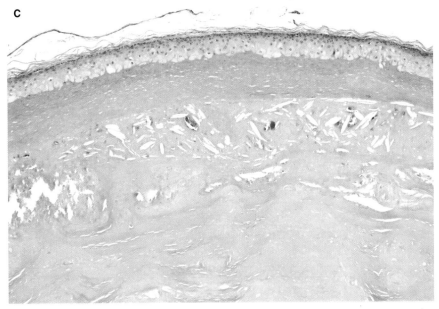

C

FIGURE 3-2

FIGURE 3-2 (A) Follicular trichilemmal cyst (pilar cyst). Cyst lined by stratified squamous epithelium with compact keratin in the lumen. (B) Higher magnification showing the stratified squamous epithelium and absence of granular layer. Note the compact eosinophilic keratin in the lumen. (C) Cholesterol clefts and calcifications within the compact keratinous lumen.

Proliferating Trichilemmal Cyst

This is a rare, benign neoplasm, apparently of external root sheath derivation. In the majority of cases it appears to be associated with a preexistent pilar cyst. The tumors are large and multinodular, measuring from 2 cm to 10 cm in diameter. These neoplasms are most commonly found on the scalp of middle-aged or elderly females (145, 146).

PATHOLOGY (FIGURE 3-3A–C)

- Lobular intradermal proliferation of squamous cells
- Sharply defined, regular lobules with noninfiltrative borders
- Trichilemmal keratinization with necrosis
- Nests of squamous cells may extend into the adjacent connective tissue (simulating squamous cell carcinoma), but the proliferation of nests is mostly inward into the cyst (squamous eddies formation)
- Focal mild cellular atypia; mitotic figures confined to the basal epithelium
- There may be focal cystic areas or remnants of a trichilemmal cyst
- Features favoring the diagnosis of proliferating trichilemmal cyst over squamous cell carcinoma include the presence of trichilemmal keratinization, cystic dilatation, hyaline basement membrane, and calcification. On the other hand, lesions with a biphenotypic pattern of growth with benign and atypical keratinocytes support the diagnosis of carcinoma arising in a proliferating trichilemmal cyst

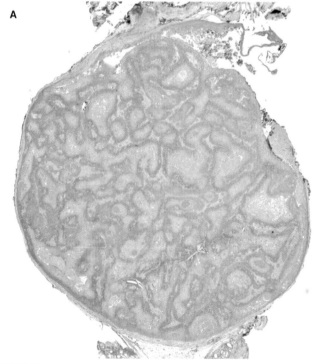

A

FIGURE 3-3

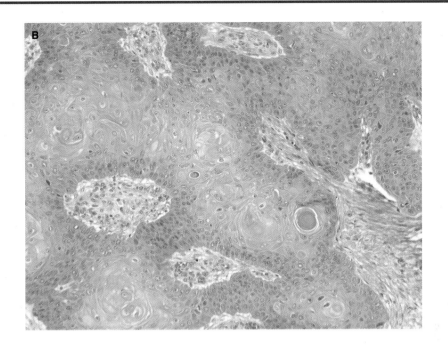

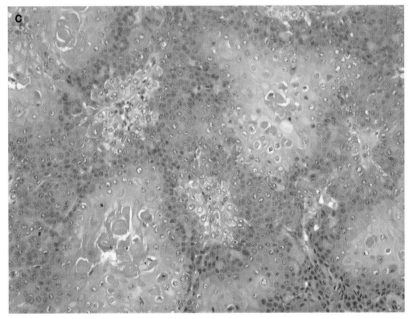

FIGURE 3-3

FIGURE 3-3   (A) Proliferating trichilemmal cyst. Well-defined lobule of squamous cells. Note the
proliferation of squamous cells is most inward into the cyst. (B) Higher magnification
of well-differentiated squamous cells with some squamous eddies. (C) Characteristic
trichilemmal keratinization.

Pilonidal Cyst

Pilonidal cyst is a common cyst, usually in White males in their second to third decade of life. Clinically, it presents as a chronic, painful, draining sinus at the base of the spine or in the intergluteal cleft (147, 148).

PATHOLOGY (FIGURE 3-4A, B)
- Cyst is lined by stratified squamous epithelium
- Due to frequent rupture frequently there is also granulation tissue with scarring and hair shaft fragments
- Common abscesses and foreign body reaction

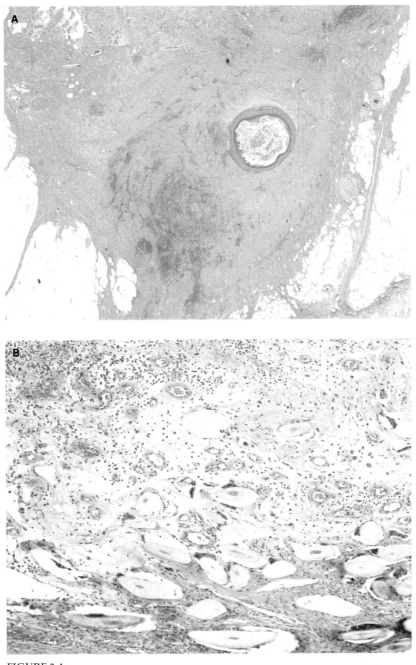

FIGURE 3-4

FIGURE 3-4   (A) Pilonidal cyst. Cystic structure lined by squamous epithelium. Note the
surrounding granulation tissue and scarring changes. (B) Higher magnification
showing the characteristic floating hair shaft fragments.

Verrucous Cyst

Verrucous cyst is a rare variant of follicular cyst that is usually associated with human papillomavirus (HPV) infection. Lesions are more commonly located on the face, back, and arms (149, 150).

PATHOLOGY (FIGURE 3-5A, B)
■ Reminiscent of a follicular infundibular cyst
■ The cyst wall is lined by papillomatous squamous epithelium with hyperkeratosis and conspicuous hypergranulosis
■ Keratohyaline granules are enlarged
■ Occasionally koilocytes
■ Laminated keratin in the cyst cavity

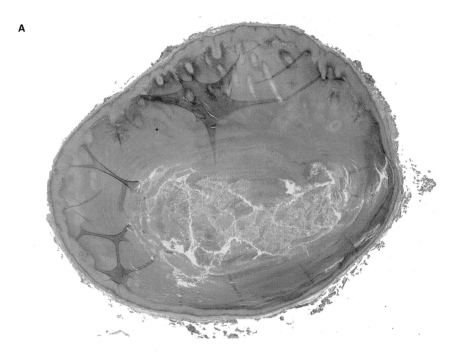

A

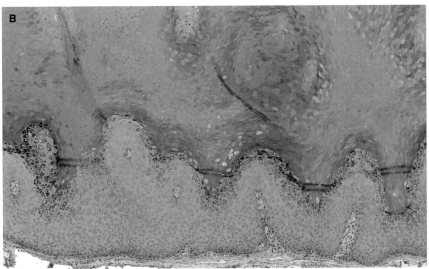

B

FIGURE 3-5

FIGURE 3-5   (A) Verrucous cyst. Cyst lined by squamous epithelium with marked hypergranulosis (enlarged keratohyaline granules). (B) Higher magnification of cyst wall with marked hypergranulosis and enlarged keratohyaline granules.

Vellus Hair Cyst

Vellus hair cysts present as multiple, small, asymptomatic papules with a predilection for the chest of children or young adults. Eruptive vellus hair cysts develop after occlusion of the infundibulum. These cysts have been reported in patients with steatocystoma, suggesting a possible relationship; however, their pattern of keratin expression is different (vellus hair cysts express keratin 17 but no keratin 10, while steatocystomas express both keratins 17 and 10). Vellus hair cysts have been related to some genodermatosis including ectodermal dysplasia and pachyonychia congenital (151–153).

PATHOLOGY (FIGURE 3-6A, B)
■ Dermal cysts are lined by stratified squamous epithelium
■ Focal trichilemmal and infundibular keratinization
■ Lumen contains laminated keratin and numerous vellus hair shaft

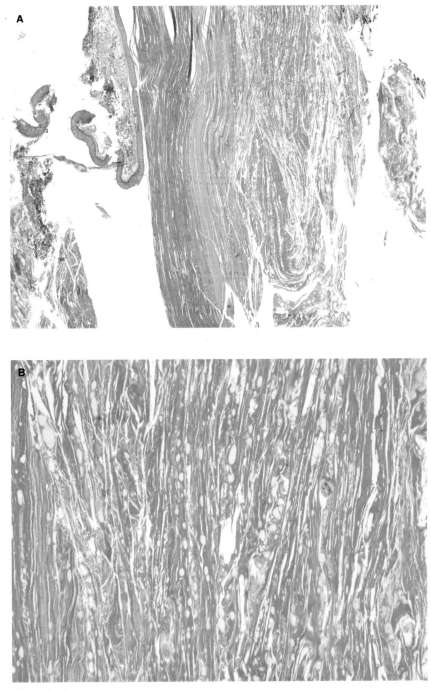

FIGURE 3-6

FIGURE 3-6   (A) Vellus hair cysts. Cyst lined by stratified squamous epithelium and dense keratin. (B) Higher magnification of the cavity showing multiple vellus hair shafts.

Steatocystoma Multiplex

This lesion usually presents as multiple, small yellowish to skin-colored papules, mostly on the chest; however, they may be found on the face, scalp, trunk, vulva, and the extremities. They are mostly sporadic, but may occur with autosomal dominant inheritance. In the familial form, mutations are localized to the keratin 17 (*K17*) gene, in areas identical to mutations found in patients with pachyonychia congenita type 2. Solitary lesions are rare and referred as steatocystoma simplex (151, 154).

PATHOLOGY (FIGURE 3-7A, B)
■ The lining of the cysts is usually undulating with stratified squamous epithelium (only a few cells thick and without a granular layer) and maturing into a eosinophilic cuticle
■ Characteristic sebaceous glands of varying size attached to the wall
■ Note: Steatocystomas multiplex and simplex have the same histologic features

FIGURE 3-7   (A) Steatocystoma. Cyst lined by undulating squamous epithelium with a eosinophilic cuticle. Note the sebaceous glands around the cyst. (B) Higher magnification showing the eosinophilic cuticle.

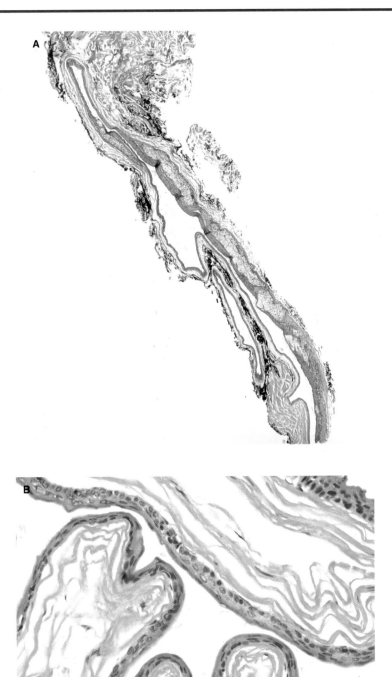

FIGURE 3-7

Dermoid Cyst

Dermoid cysts are dermal or subcutaneous cysts of ectodermal origin found along lines of embryonic fusion; predominantly on the lateral angle of the eye or the midline of the forehead or neck (155, 156).

PATHOLOGY (FIGURE 3-8A, B)
■ Cysts are lined by keratinizing squamous epithelium with attached pilosebaceous structures (these appendages are fully mature)
■ Sebaceous glands may empty directly into the cyst
■ Also eccrine and apocrine glands, as well as smooth muscle in the wall

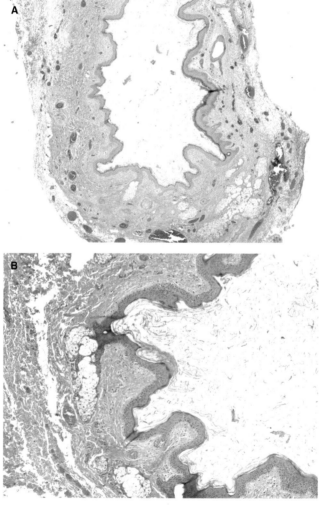

FIGURE 3-8

FIGURE 3-8   (A) Dermoid cyst. Cyst lined by squamous epithelium and with attached pilosebaceous units. Note the surrounding sebaceous glands. (B) Higher magnification of the attached sebaceous glands.

Hidrocystoma

Hidrocystomas are benign tumors of sweat gland origin. They can be eccrine or apocrine. They present as solitary lesions of the face, trunk, or popliteal fossa, with a strong predilection for the periorbital area (157).

PATHOLOGY (FIGURE 3-9A, B)

◼ Unilocular, in close proximity to eccrine glands
◼ Lined by two layers of cuboidal epithelium with eosinophilic cytoplasm
◼ Lumen may show pale eosinophilic secretions
◼ In the apocrine type, there is decapitation secretion

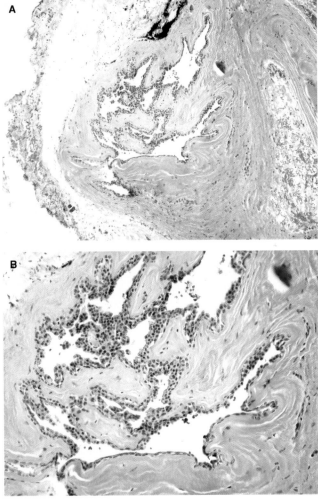

FIGURE 3-9

FIGURE 3-9   (A) Hidrocystoma. Unilocular cyst lined by an attenuated cuboidal epithelium. (B) Higher magnification of the two layers of cuboidal epithelium (eccrine type).

Cutaneous Ciliated Cyst

Cutaneous ciliated cysts occur almost exclusively in young women. Most commonly arise on the legs, buttock, and foot. These cysts are generally thought to be of paramesonephric derivation (Müllerian) (158, 159).

PATHOLOGY (FIGURE 3-10A, B)
- Unilocular or multilocular cyst with some intraluminal papillae
- Cyst lined by cuboidal or columnar ciliated epithelium
- Focal squamous metaplasia
- Note: Ciliated epithelium can also be observed in other cysts including bronchogenic, branchial, and thyroglossal

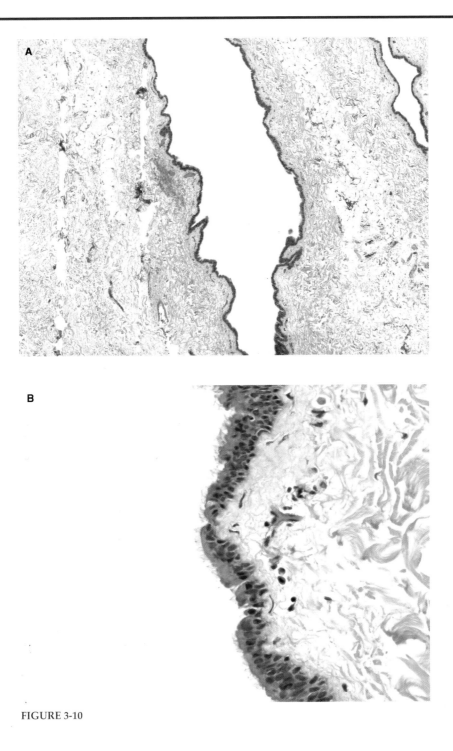

FIGURE 3-10

FIGURE 3-10   (A) Cutaneous ciliated cyst. Cyst lined by columnar epithelium. Note the papillary
projections into the lumen. (B) Higher magnification of the cyst lined by columnar
epithelium. Characteristic ciliated epithelium.

Thyroglossal Duct Cyst

Thyroglossal cysts are congenital anomalies from vestigial remnants of the tubular thyroid gland. Most commonly, they present in the first decade of life; however, they can be seen also in adults. They usually present as fluctuant swellings in the midline of the neck along the line of thyroid descent (160, 161).

PATHOLOGY (FIGURE 3-11A, B)
■ Cysts are lined by cuboidal columnar or squamous epithelium, often ciliated
■ Frequently seen in association with an epithelial-lined tract
■ Adjacent tissue shows thyroid follicles and lymphoid aggregates
■ Rarely with cutaneous adnexal structures

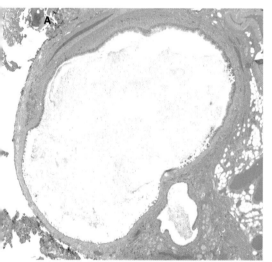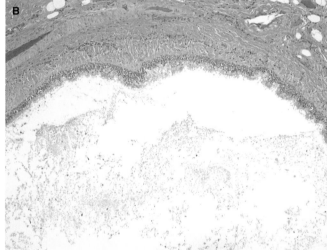

FIGURE 3-11

FIGURE 3-11   (A) Thyroglossal duct cyst. Low magnification showing the cyst lined by cuboidal epithelium. Note the thyroid glands next to the cyst. (B) Higher magnification of the cyst lined by cuboidal ciliated epithelium.

Cervical Thymic Cyst

These cysts are more commonly seen in children and characteristically present in the anterior triangle from the angle of mandible to manubrium sterni (more commonly of the left side). These cysts develop from remnants of the thymopharyngeal duct (162).

PATHOLOGY
- Cysts are unilocular or multilocular
- Lined by stratified squamous epithelium (also columnar, cuboidal or ciliated)
- Thymic remnants such as Hassall corpuscles
- Lymphoid aggregates are seen in the adjacent stroma

Branchial Cleft Cyst

Branchial cleft cysts are congenital cysts that arise on the lateral part of the neck from a failure or incomplete involution of branchial cleft structures during embryonic development. They presents as a solitary, painless mass in the neck of a young patient (160, 163).

PATHOLOGY (FIGURE 3-12A, B)

- Cyst lined by stratified squamous epithelium with keratinous debris; however, the cysts can be also lined with ciliated columnar epithelium.
- Lymphoid aggregates are seen in the adjacent stroma (germinal center formation can be prominent).

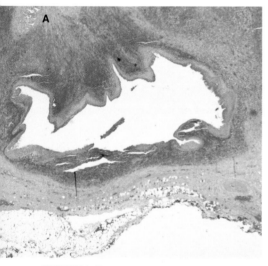 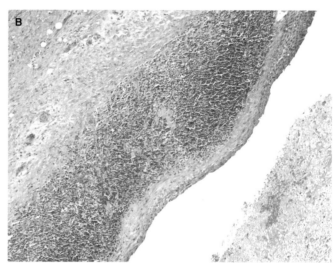

FIGURE 3-12

FIGURE 3-12   (A) Branchial cleft cyst. Cyst lined by squamous epithelium and surrounded by lymphoid aggregates. (B) Higher magnification of the squamous epithelium and lymphoid aggregates.

Bronchogenic Cyst

Bronchogenic cysts on the skin are extremely rare. This lesion is four times more common in men than in women. The most common location is the suprasternal notch, followed by the presternal area, neck, and scapula (164, 165).

PATHOLOGY (FIGURE 3-13A, B)

▪ Cyst lined by a ciliated pseudostratified columnar epithelium (it may be also nonciliated)
▪ Lymphoid follicles, smooth muscle cells, seromucinous, and goblet cells
▪ Cartilage can be present in a minority of cases

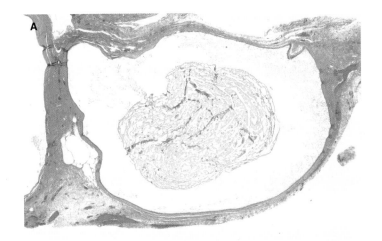

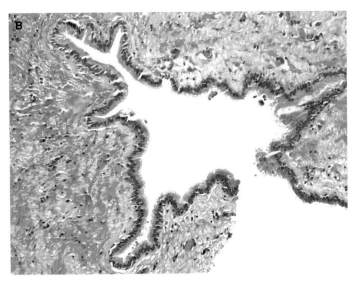

FIGURE 3-13

FIGURE 3-13   Bronchogenic cyst. (A) Low magnification of the cyst. (B) Cyst lined by ciliated columnar epithelium.

Median Raphe Cyst

Median raphe cysts are midline-developmental cysts that can occur anywhere from the anus to the urinary meatus. Most of these cysts are present from birth and remain undetectable until adolescence, occurring as a solitary freely movable nodule on the ventral aspect of the penis (glans) (160, 166).

PATHOLOGY (FIGURE 3-14A, B)

- The cyst does not communicate with the urethra
- Cyst is lined by a pseudostratified, columnar, or stratified squamous cell epithelium
- Occasionally ciliated epithelium and goblets cells

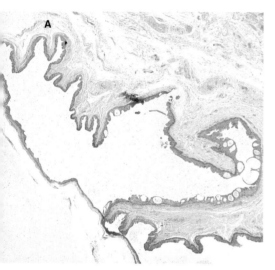
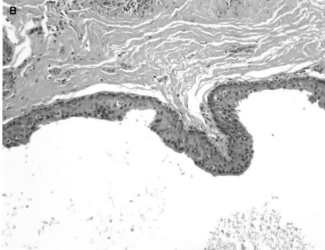

FIGURE 3-14

FIGURE 3-14   (A) Median raphe cyst. Cyst lined by squamous epithelium. Note the mucous glands within the wall. (B) Higher magnification showing the stratified squamous lining.

Pseudocyst of the Auricle

A pseudocyst of the auricle manifests as a painless swelling on the lateral or anterior surface of the pinna. A history of minor trauma may accompany the clinical history (167).

PATHOLOGY (FIGURE 3-15A, B)

■ Pseudocysts of the auricle lack pathognomonic features
■ Lesion shows an intracartilaginous cystic space devoid of an epithelial lining
■ Usually with degeneration of the adjacent cartilage
■ The epidermis and dermis overlying the pseudocyst are usually normal

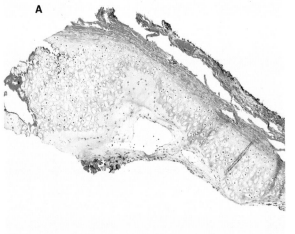 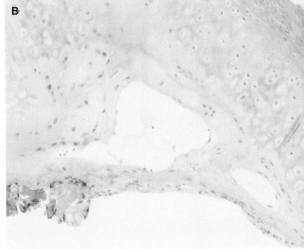

FIGURE 3-15

FIGURE 3-15   (A) Pseudocyst of the auricle. Note the intracartilaginous cyst with no epithelial lining. (B) Higher magnification of the cysts.

Connective Tissue Tumors

4

ADIPOCYTIC AND SMOOTH MUSCLE TUMORS

LIPOMA

ANGIOLIPOMA

SPINDLE CELL LIPOMA

PLEOMORPHIC LIPOMA

NEVUS LIPOMATOSUS SUPERFICIALIS/DERMATOLIPOMA

PILAR LEIOMYOMA

ANGIOLEIOMYOMA

SMOOTH MUSCLE HAMARTOMA

LEIOMYOSARCOMA

FIBROUS AND MYOFIBROBLASTIC TUMORS

KELOID

NODULAR FASCIITIS

ELASTOFIBROMA

NUCHAL FIBROMA

GARDNER FIBROMA

FIBROEPITHELIAL POLYP (ACROCHORDON)

PLEOMORPHIC FIBROMA

SCLEROTIC FIBROMA (STORIFORM COLLAGENOMA)

SUPERFICIAL ACRAL FIBROMYXOMA

SUPERFICIAL ANGIOMYXOMA

ACQUIRED DIGITAL FIBROKERATOMA

FIBROUS HAMARTOMA OF INFANCY

INFANTILE DIGITAL FIBROMATOSIS

FIBROMATOSIS

ANGIOFIBROMAS (ADENOMA SEBACEUM)

FIBROUS PAPULE OF THE NOSE

PEARLY PENILE PAPULES

FIBROHISTIOCYTIC TUMORS

MULTINUCLEATED CELL ANGIOHISTIOCYTOMA

DERMATOFIBROMA

DERMATOFIBROSARCOMA PROTUBERANS

FIBROHISTIOCYTIC LESION WITH ATYPICAL FEATURES

GIANT CELL TUMOR OF TENDON SHEATH

ANGIOMATOID FIBROUS HISTIOCYTOMA

ATYPICAL FIBROXANTHOMA

PLEXIFORM FIBROHISTIOCYTIC TUMOR

VASCULAR NEOPLASMS

INFANTILE HEMANGIOMA

VERRUCOUS HEMANGIOMA

CHERRY ANGIOMA

PYOGENIC GRANULOMA/LOBULAR CAPILLARY HEMANGIOMA

ARTERIOVENOUS HEMANGIOMA

MICROVENULAR HEMANGIOMA

HOBNAIL HEMANGIOMA

ACQUIRED ELASTOTIC HEMANGIOMA

ANGIOKERATOMA

SPINDLE CELL HEMANGIOMA
(HEMANGIOENDOTHELIOMA)

CUTANEOUS EPITHELIOID ANGIOMATOUS NODULE

EPITHELIOID HEMANGIOMA (ANGIOLYMPHOID
HYPERPLASIA WITH EOSINOPHILIA)

GLOMERULOID HEMANGIOMA

VENOUS LAKE

INTRAVASCULAR PAPILLARY ENDOTHELIAL HYPERPLASIA
(MASSON TUMOR)

LYMPHANGIOMA

ECCRINE ANGIOMATOUS HAMARTOMA

GLOMUS TUMOR

REACTIVE ANGIOENDOTHELIOMATOSIS

INTRAVASCULAR HISTIOCYTOSIS

EPITHELIOID HEMANGIOENDOTHELIOMA

CUTANEOUS ANGIOSARCOMA

ATYPICAL VASCULAR LESION

KAPOSI SARCOMA

KAPOSIFORM HEMANGIOENDOTHELIOMA

NEURAL NEOPLASMS

NEUROFIBROMA

SCHWANNOMAS

PALISADED ENCAPSULATED NEUROMA

PERINEURIOMA

GRANULAR CELL TUMOR

NERVE SHEATH MYXOMA

CELLULAR NEUROTHEKEOMA

ADIPOCYTIC AND SMOOTH MUSCLE TUMORS

Lipoma

Lipomas are common benign adipocytic neoplasms. Clinically, they present as asymptomatic slow-growing, painless, subcutaneous tumors with a predilection for the upper trunk, upper extremities, thighs, and neck. Obese patients are more commonly affected. Lipomas show clonal karyotypic abnormalities in up to 75% of cases and the most common translocations involve the long arm of chromosome 12 and chromosome 3 (168–170).

PATHOLOGY (FIGURE 4-1A, B)
- The tumor is usually encapsulated and composed of sheets of mature adipose tissue divided by thin, delicate fibrous septa containing a few blood vessels.
- Frequently with a fibrous capsule.
- Occasional degenerative changes characterized by fibrosis, fat necrosis, and/or myxoid changes (especially in old or traumatized lesions).
- Fibrolipomas variants show increased stromal fibrous tissue.
- Rarely, the lipomatous component is mildly atypical showing cells with vacuolated nuclei.
- Note: These atypical lypocytes must not be confused with lipoblasts, seen in liposarcomas, which are characterized by intracytoplasmic lipid vacuoles with scalloping of peripherally located hyperchromatic nuclei.

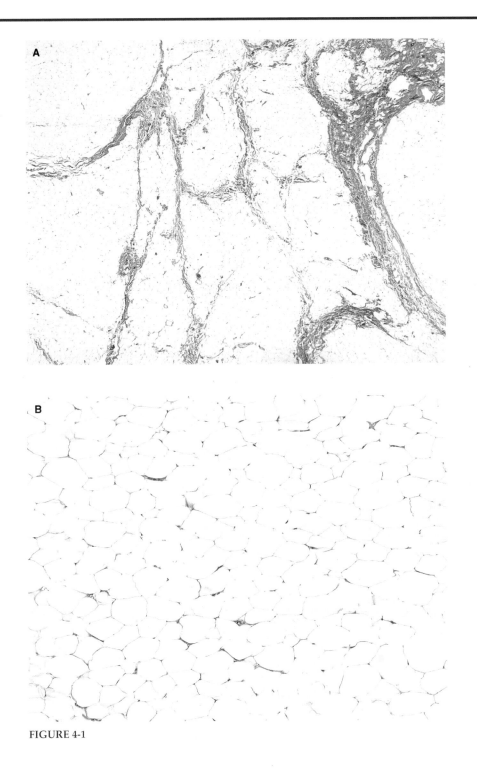

FIGURE 4-1

FIGURE 4-1 (A) Lipoma. Mature adipose tissue with thin strands of fibrous tissue. (B) Higher magnification showing benign appearing adipocytes.

Angiolipoma

Angiolipomas are benign subcutaneous tumors. These tumors are often multiple and appear after puberty. They are more commonly seen in the upper limbs, especially the forearm and are typically tender. A family history is found in about 10% of cases. Subcutaneous angiolipomas have a normal karyotype, as opposed to the majority of adipose neoplasms, including lipomas; thus, angiolipomas have been regarded as a hamartoma of blood vessels and fat, rather than a true adipose neoplasm (171).

PATHOLOGY (FIGURE 4-2A, B)
■ The tumor is usually encapsulated (thin fibrous capsule) and composed of variable proportions of mature adipocytes and anastomosing small blood vessels.
■ The vascular component consists of groups of capillaries.
■ Luminal microthrombi are a diagnostic clue.

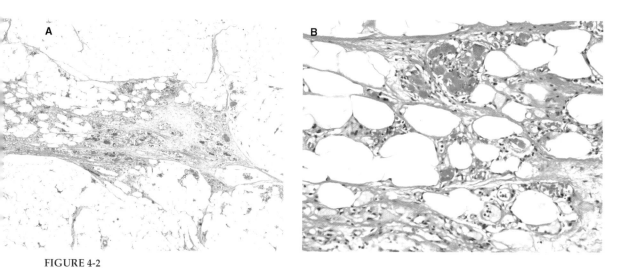

FIGURE 4-2

FIGURE 4-2   Angiolipoma. Mature adipocytes with irregular anastomosing blood vessels. Note the micro thrombi in the lumen. (B) Higher magnification showing the luminal microthrombi.

Spindle Cell Lipoma

Spindle cell lipoma is a benign adipocytic neoplasm. Clinically, it is most commonly seen in the shoulders, upper back, and back of the neck of men in the fifth to seventh decades of life. It presents as a painless, slowly growing, subcutaneous, or, less commonly, dermal lesion that usually measures less than 5 cm in diameter. Monosomy or partial loss of chromosomes 13 and 16 are the most common alterations (172, 173).

PATHOLOGY (FIGURE 4-3)

- The tumor is unencapsulated and well-circumscribed.
- Dermal spindle cell lipomas tend to be more ill-defined.
- The tumor is composed by mature univacuolated adipocytes and spindle cells.
- The spindle cells are small and elongated and arranged haphazardly. Occasionally they may show a palisaded or fascicular pattern in some areas.
- Some spindle cells may show small cytoplasmic vacuoles.
- The spindle cells are separated by variable amounts of hyaline bundles of collagen.
- Rare giant cells
- Frequent mast cells
- Sometimes the stroma shows focal myxomatous change.
- Absence of lipoblasts
- A few tumors have a prominent vascular pattern.
- Some cases contain only few or no adipocytes.
- The spindle cells are positive for CD34.

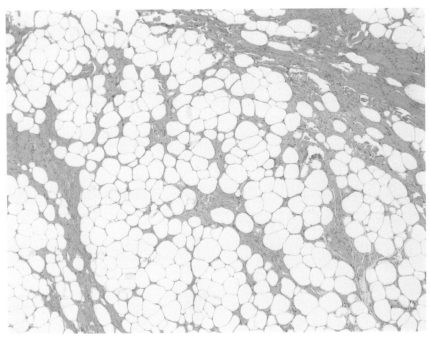

FIGURE 4-3

FIGURE 4-3   Spindle cell lipoma. Ill defined lesion composed of adipocytes, spindle cells, and epithelioid cells. Note the hyaline bundles of collagen.

Pleomorphic Lipoma

Pleomorphic lipoma is a benign tumor of adipose tissue that represents a variant of spindle cell lipoma. Clinically, it presents as a subcutaneous mass (5 cm in diameter). This tumor has a predilection for the shoulders, back of the neck, and back of middle-aged and elderly males. Cytogenetically, it shows a consistent loss of chromosome 16q, similar to spindle cell lipomas, supporting that these tumors are part of the same spectrum (174, 175).

PATHOLOGY (FIGURE 4-4A, B)

■ The tumor is circumscribed and composed of mature adipose tissue, collagen, and myxoid areas interspersed with cellular foci of varying amounts.

■ The tumor has variable number of spindle and giant cells.

■ The giant cells have marginally placed and often overlapping nuclei, the so-called "floret cells."

■ Occasional multivacuolated lipoblasts

■ Rare mitotic figures

■ Focal collections of lymphocytes and plasma cells

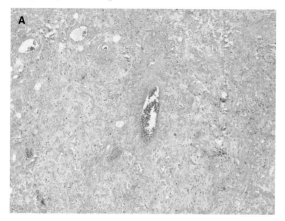

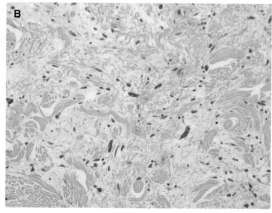

FIGURE 4-4

FIGURE 4-4   Pleomorphic lipoma. (A) The lesion is composed of adipocytes and atypical spindle cells. (B) The tumor shows many spindle cells with marked pleomorphism and "floret" cells.

Nevus Lipomatosus Superficialis/Dermatolipoma

Nevus lipomatosus superficialis (Hoffmann–Zurhelle) is a rare type of connective tissue nevus that is characterized by the presence of mature adipose tissue in the dermis. It is found as plaques or solitary unilateral lesions. The plaque type presents as multiple flesh-colored lesions that are present at birth or develop in the first two decades of life. The most common location is around the gluteal area. The solitary type presents as a solitary nodule that can be located anywhere on the body, but more commonly seen on the trunk. Usually appear around the fifth decade of life. Some authors do not believe in the existence of this solitary variant and regard them as skin tags (dermatolipomas). It is our opinion that this term should be applied only to congenital lesions and that it should not be used for acquired lesions in adults. Dr. Scott McNutt has proposed the designation of dermatolipoma for similar lesions arising in adults. Such lesions may be associated with diabetes (176, 177).

PATHOLOGY (FIGURE 4-5)
- The lesion shows lobules of mature fat in the superficial dermis.
- These fatty lobules are located particularly around small blood vessels.
- Vascular spaces are increased in number.
- There may be areas of loose fibrous tissue, diminished elastic fibers, and reduced numbers of epidermal appendages.
- Note: Nevus lipomatosus superficialis is indistinguishable from the cutaneous papules of focal dermal hypoplasia.

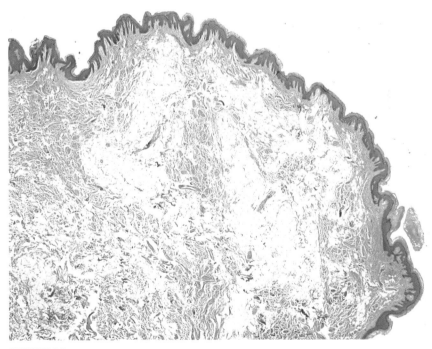

FIGURE 4-5

FIGURE 4-5   Dermatolipoma/nevus lipomatosus superficialis. Polypoid lesion with small lobules of mature fat in the dermis.

Pilar Leiomyoma

Pilar leiomyomas appear as tender, dermal papules commonly located on the face, back, and extensor surfaces of the extremities. Multiple lesions are more frequent than solitary lesions and can affect more than one area of the body. Familial occurrence has been reported occasionally. Multiple cutaneous leiomyomas have been related to uterine leiomyomas. Recently an association with papillary or collecting duct renal cell carcinoma has been identified and the syndrome is now termed "hereditary leiomyomatosis and renal cell cancer" (HLRCC). Loss of function in the gene FH (1q42.3 q43) results in fumarate hydratase deficiency (178, 179).

PATHOLOGY (FIGURE 4-6A–C)
■ These tumors are ill defined, nonencapsulated, and centered in the dermis.
■ Usually a Grenz zone
■ Bundles of smooth muscle arranged in an interlacing and sometimes a whorled pattern
■ The cells have abundant eosinophilic cytoplasm and elongated nuclei with blunt ends.
■ There may be focal areas with cytological atypia similar to that seen in symplastic leiomyomas of the uterus.
■ Long-standing tumors may have fibrous tissue in the stroma, and occasionally this shows focal hyalinization.
■ IHC: The tumor cells are positive for SMA, desmin, and h-caldesmon.
■ Most authors consider that smooth muscle lesions that infiltrate the subcutaneous tissue or show mitotic figures should be considered malignant, i.e., leiomyosarcomas.

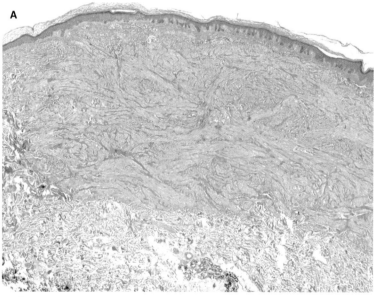

FIGURE 4-6

FIGURE 4-6   (A) Pilar leiomyoma. Irregular and interlacing bundles of smooth muscle in the dermis. (B) Higher magnification the interlacing bundles of smooth muscle devoid of cytologic atypia. (C) Cells are strongly positive for smooth muscle antigen (SMA).

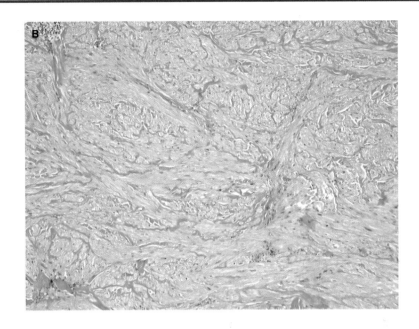

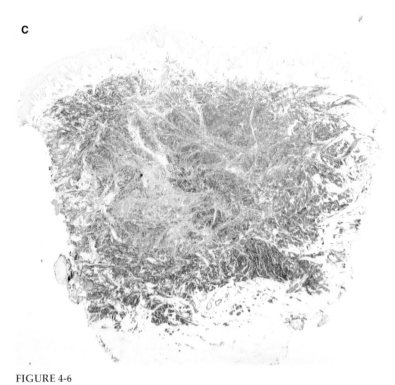

FIGURE 4-6

Angioleiomyoma

Angioleiomyomas are common benign neoplasms that originate from vascular smooth muscle. They usually present as solitary, slow-growing nodules on the lower extremities of middle-aged women. Tumors are firm, gray-white round to oval painful nodules that usually measure less than 2 cm in diameter (180, 181).

PATHOLOGY (FIGURE 4-7A, B)

- Well-circumscribed and encapsulated lesions
- Interlacing bundles of uniform smooth muscle cells between numerous small vascular channels
- Majority of vessels are thick walled, with several layers of smooth muscle in their walls.
- Calcification can be extensive (more common in acral location).
- Some cases contain collections of mature adipocytes (angiomyolipoma).
- The vascular spaces may show marked sinusoidal architecture.
- Rarely, there are cells with enlarged hyperchromatic nuclei.
- IHC: The tumor cells are positive for SMA, desmin, and h-caldesmon.
- Note: HMB-45 is negative as opposed to the renal lesions.

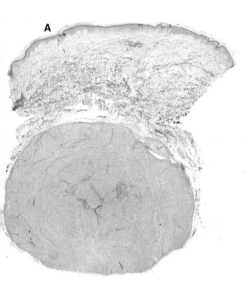
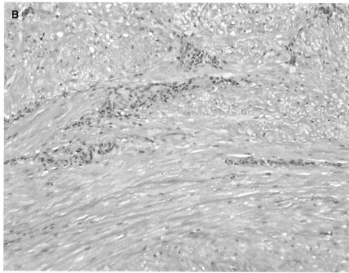

FIGURE 4-7

FIGURE 4-7   (A) Angioleiomyoma. Well-defined nodule in deep dermis composed of layers of smooth muscle and vascular spaces. (B) Higher magnification showing the layers of smooth muscle and blood vessels.

Smooth Muscle Hamartoma

Smooth muscle hamartoma (congenital smooth muscle hamartoma) is a rare cutaneous lesion that is usually congenital and typically recognized at birth or early infancy. It presents as a flesh-colored or lightly pigmented plaque up to 10 cm in diameter on the extremities or trunk (more commonly located on the lumbosacral area and the proximal extremities). Within the plaques there may be small, "gooseflesh"-like papules (182, 183).

PATHOLOGY
- Well-defined mature smooth muscle bundles in the dermis, haphazardly oriented in several directions
- Some smooth muscle bundles surround the hair follicles.
- Often there is a thin retraction space around the bundles.
- There may be bundles of nerve fibers.
- IHC: The lesion is positive for SMA and desmin.

Leiomyosarcoma

Cutaneous leiomyosarcomas are rare tumors that may arise in the dermis. Tumors usually arise from the arrector pili muscles and commonly affect the extensor surfaces of the extremities. There is male predominance, and the age of presentation ranges from 40 to 60 years. Subcutaneous extension is present in two-thirds of cases. Dermal leiomyosarcomas may recur locally in up to 30% of cases but metastases are very rare (184–186).

PATHOLOGY (FIGURE 4-8A–C)
- The dermal tumors are ill defined and the subcutaneous variant tends to be more circumscribed and nodular.
- Are composed of infiltrative interlacing fascicles of elongated spindle-shaped cells with eosinophilic cytoplasm and eccentric, blunt-ended (cigar-shaped) nuclei.
- There may be nuclear palisading.
- There is variable nuclear pleomorphism; higher degree of cytologic atypia is usually seen in the subcutaneous variant.
- There are cases with only occasional mitotic figures; however, is not uncommon to detect hot spots with a higher number of mitotic figures.
- Small lymphoid aggregates are sometimes present within the tumor.
- IHC: Tumors are strongly positive for SMA, calponin, desmin, and h-caldesmon. Occasional focal expression of keratin, CD34, or S100.

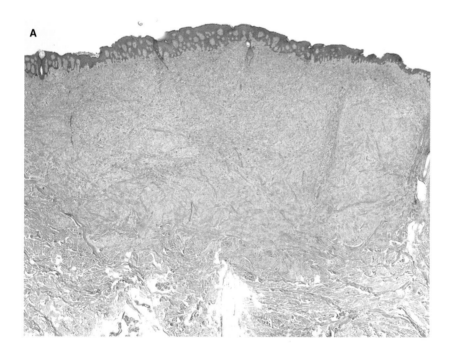

FIGURE 4-8   (A) Leiomyosarcoma. Irregular spindle-cell tumor in the dermis with focal infiltrative borders. (B) Higher magnification showing the atypical and pleomorphic spindle cells (cigar shaped). (C) Strong expression with Desmin.

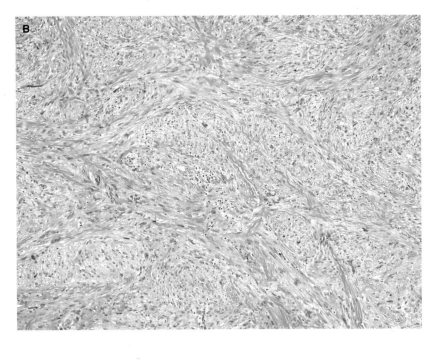

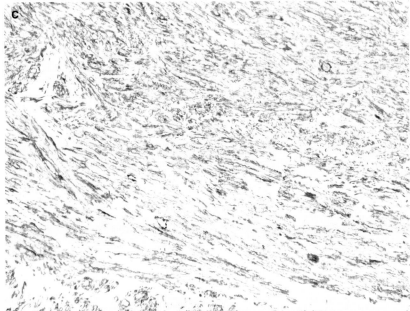

FIGURE 4-8

FIBROUS AND MYOFIBROBLASTIC TUMORS

Keloid

Keloid is a reactive lesion that represents exuberant scar formation. Keloids rarely appear spontaneously, and the great majority develops as a result of local trauma. Clinically, they present as raised, well-circumscribed nodules. They may arise at any age; however, they are most common in African American adolescents and young adults. Common sites include the upper back, deltoid area, chest, and ear lobes (187, 188).

PATHOLOGY (FIGURE 4-9A, B)
- Keloids show broad, homogeneous, brightly eosinophilic collagen bundles in haphazard array.
- Fibroblasts are numerous along the collagen bundles.
- Keloids have reduced vascularity when compared with hypertrophic scars and normal healing wounds.
- The overlying epidermis may be atrophic.
- Early lesions may show a slight vascularity and foci of myxoid ground substance.

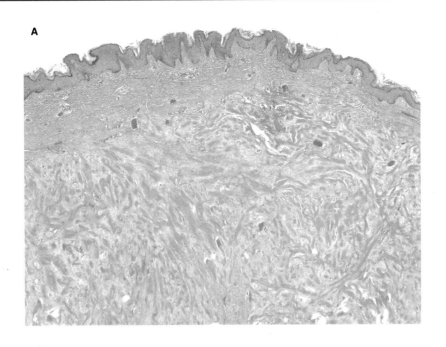

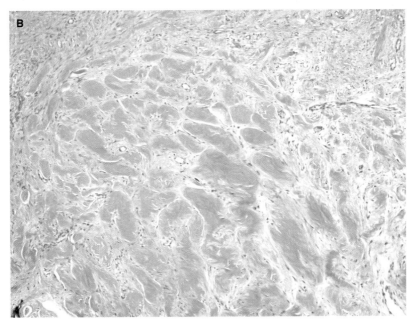

FIGURE 4-9

FIGURE 4-9   (A) Keloid. Thick and broad eosinophilic collagen bundles in the dermis. (B) Higher
magnification showing the homogeneous broad collagen bundles in the dermis. Note
the rare fibroblasts around the collagen bundles.

Nodular Fasciitis

Nodular fasciitis (NF) is a benign reactive proliferation of fibroblasts of unknown etiology. This lesion is most commonly seen in young or middle-aged adults. Common locations include the forearms, upper arm, and trunk. Clinically, it presents as a rapidly growing, subcutaneous tender nodule with a median diameter of 1.5 cm. Recurrences are quite rare, even after incomplete surgical excision, and thus, such recurrence should raise the possibility of misdiagnosis (189–191).

PATHOLOGY (FIGURE 4-10A, B)
- The tumor shows an unencapsulated, fairly circumscribed mass.
- Proliferation of plump spindle-shaped fibroblasts, which are usually arranged in haphazard array ("tissue culture" appearance)
- The spindle cells are set in a loose myxoid and collagenous stroma with feathery appearance.
- Many thin-walled blood vessels, with plump endothelial cells, ramify through the lesion, usually in a radial pattern.
- Commonly there are extravasated red blood cells and a sparse chronic lymphocytic infiltrate.
- Rare foamy histiocytes and multinucleate osteoclast-type giant cells
- The plump spindled cells are mitotically active, but such mitotic figures show normal morphology.
- Immunohistochemical studies show expression of smooth muscle actin (SMA), muscle-specific actin, and calponin, but desmin and h-caldesmon are usually negative, supporting the myofibroblastic (but not smooth muscle) differentiation of this neoplasm (191).

VARIANTS
- Intradermal fasciitis: Is a rare variant of NF that primarily arises in the dermis with only focal extension into the subcutaneous tissue. The histological changes are identical to NF.
- Intravascular fasciitis: It is a very rare variant that appears to originate from myofibroblasts within vessel walls. Histologically, it is very similar to NF, but it involves the full thickness and lumen of a peripheral blood vessel, mimicking vascular invasion (sometimes it shows a plexiform architecture).
- Proliferative fasciitis: This variant is more common in older patients, mostly on the lower extremities. The histomorphology of this variant is very similar to classic NF; however, there are many basophilic, ganglion-like giant cells.

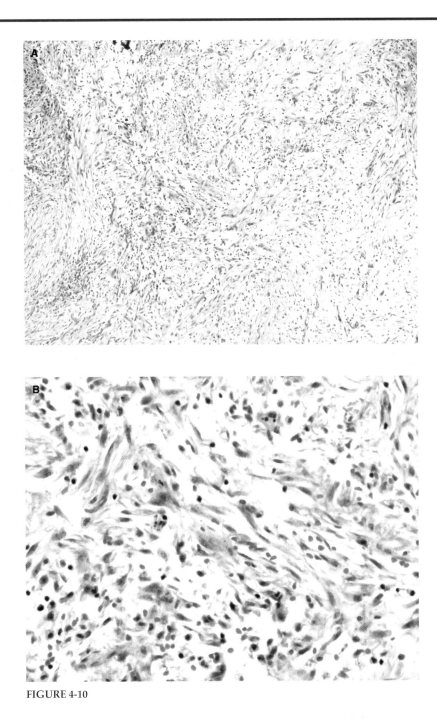

FIGURE 4-10

FIGURE 4-10 (A) Nodular fasciitis. Note the proliferation of spindle cells arranged in a tissue culture appearance. The stroma is myxoid and vascular. (B) Higher magnification showing the plump spindled cells. Note scattered mitotic figures.

Elastofibroma

Elastofibroma is a rare, deep, slow-growing tumor that is thought to represent a proliferation of collagen and abnormal elastic fibers with a predilection for the infrascapular fascia of older individuals, especially females. Most elastofibromas are unilateral and asymptomatic (192).

PATHOLOGY (FIGURE 4-11A–C)

- Elastofibromas are nonencapsulated, ill-defined lesions that blend with the surrounding connective and adipose tissue.
- Mostly acellular and composed of thickened collagen bundles admixed with many irregular, lightly eosinophilic fibers and some mature adipose tissue.
- Verhoeff elastic stain shows coarse and thick elastic fibers; sometimes distributed as irregular masses. Some fibers are branched while others show a characteristic, serrated edge.
- IHC: The cells are positive for CD34.

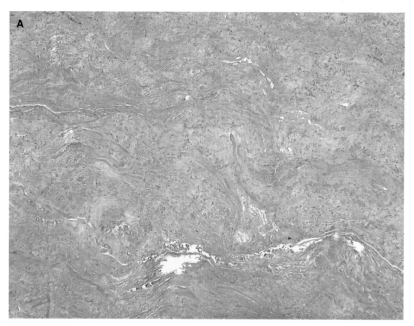

FIGURE 4-11

FIGURE 4-11 (A) Elastofibroma. Acellular, ill-defined lesion with thick collagen bundles. (B) Higher magnification of elastic fibers. Note the fragmentation and the beaded appearance. (C) Elastic stain (Verhoeff) showing the coarse and irregular elastic fibers.

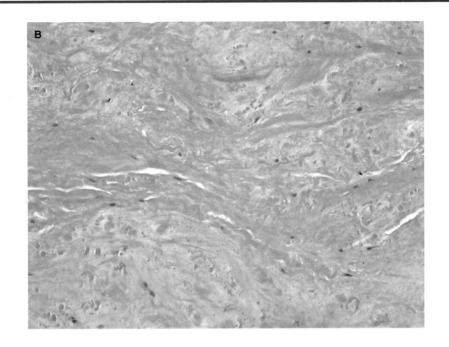

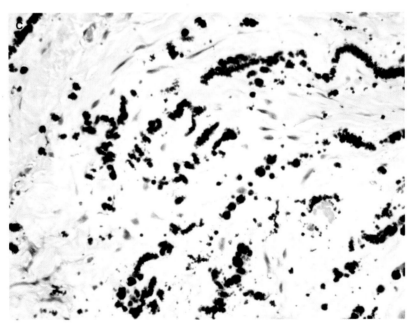

FIGURE 4-11

Nuchal Fibroma

Nuchal fibroma is a benign soft tissue tumor that arises mainly in the posterior neck of men between the third and fifth decades of life. Up to a third of lesions can occur in other locations including mostly the shoulder and back (nuchal-type fibroma). There is association with diabetes, scleredema, and multiple lipomas. In Gardner syndrome the lesions may occur in multiple sites. These tumors are asymptomatic and usually measure less than 3 cm in diameter. Nondestructive recurrences occasionally develop after excision (193, 194).

PATHOLOGY (FIGURE 4-12A, B)
■ Thick collagen bundles that focally replace the subcutaneous fat
■ The areas of collagen merge with the lower dermis.
■ Only scattered fibroblasts
■ Increased numbers of small nerve bundles
■ Common fat and nerve entrapment
■ Rarely, there is focal infiltration into the skeletal muscle.
■ IHC: Many of the cells are positive for CD34.

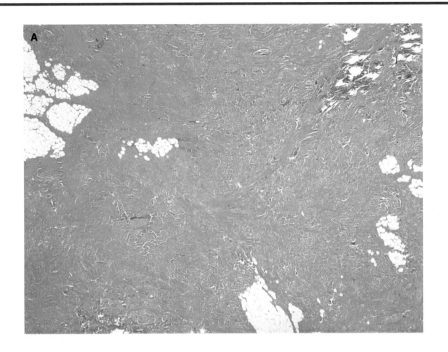

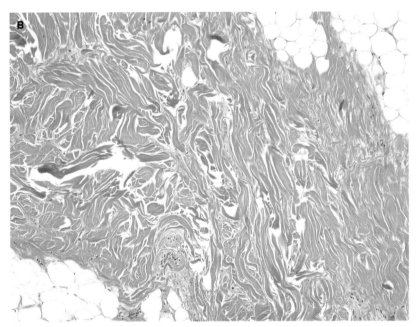

FIGURE 4-12

FIGURE 4-12   (A) Nuchal fibroma. Thick and hypocellular collagen bundles replacing the
subcutaneous fat. (B) Higher magnification showing the thickened collagen
entrapping the adipose tissue.

Gardner Fibroma

Gardner fibroma is a benign tumor of the superficial and deep soft tissue morphologically very similar to nuchal fibroma, presenting sporadically and/or in patients with Gardner syndrome. There is a predilection for childhood and adolescence. Most cases involve the back and paraspinal region. The tumor may be the first manifestation of Gardner syndrome. There are some overlapping features with nuchal fibroma; however, nuchal fibroma is more common in middle-aged males, on the posterior neck, and sometimes it is associated with diabetes mellitus (194, 195).

PATHOLOGY (FIGURE 4-13)
- Very similar to nuchal fibroma
- Hypocellular proliferation of haphazardly arranged collagen fibers with inconspicuous spindle cells
- There are small blood vessels and a sparse, mast-cell infiltrate.
- The collagen replaces the adipose tissue lobules.
- There is no increase in small nerve bundles, in contrast with nuchal fibroma.
- IHC: Expression of beta-catenin in up to 64% of the cases. The cells show nuclear reactivity for cyclin-D1 and c-myc.

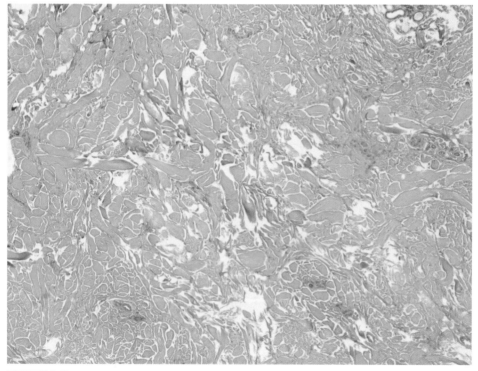

FIGURE 4-13

FIGURE 4-13   Gardner fibroma. Note the hypocellular proliferation of irregular collagen fibers.

Fibroepithelial Polyp (Acrochordon)

Fibroepithelial polyps (acrochordon, skin tag) are common connective tissue lesions. Usually, they present in adults, especially obese females, with a predilection for the neck, eyelids, underneath the breast, axillae, and groin. Perianal lesions are also common. These lesions are often multiple and can be associated with Birt–Hogg–Dubé syndrome, pregnancy and diabetes mellitus, the latter more likely to be if the lesions contain adipocytes (dermatolipomas, see above) (196, 197).

PATHOLOGY (FIGURE 4-14)

■ The polyp shows overlying epidermal hyperplasia.

■ Lesion may show horn cyst formation mimicking seborrheic keratosis (these lesion are most common on the neck and eyelids).

■ The connective tissue stalk is usually composed of well-vascularized, loosely arranged collagen.

■ If adipose cells are present in the stroma the lesion may be classified as dermatolipoma (see above).

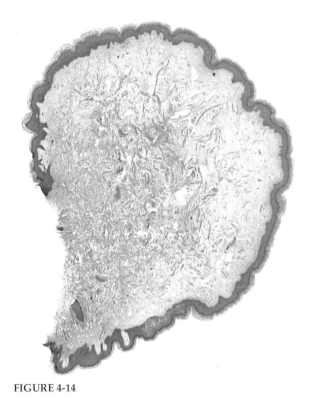

FIGURE 4-14

FIGURE 4-14   Acrochordon. Polypoid lesion with well-vascularized and loose stroma.

Pleomorphic Fibroma

Pleomorphic fibroma of the skin is clinically indistinguishable from a polypoid skin tag; however, histologically, it shows cells with bizarre hyperchromatic and pleomorphic nuclei. These atypical changes are likely to be the result of degeneration, as seen in other neoplasms (e.g., ancient schwannoma) (198).

PATHOLOGY (FIGURE 4-15A–C)
- ▪ Dome-shaped nodule with variable cellularity
- ▪ The spindle-shaped cells show striking nuclear pleomorphism.
- ▪ Multinucleation is a feature, but mitotic figures are very few and never atypical.
- ▪ IHC: The cells express actin, vimentin, and CD34, but not desmin or S100 protein.

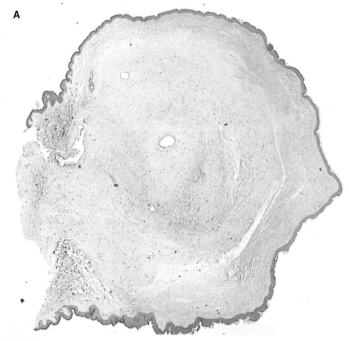

A

FIGURE 4-15

FIGURE 4-15 (A) Pleomorphic fibroma. Polypoid lesion with many spindle cells in the stroma. (B) Note the subtle spindle cells with pleomorphism. (C) Higher magnification showing the spindle cells with marked pleomorphism. Mitotic figures are not evident.

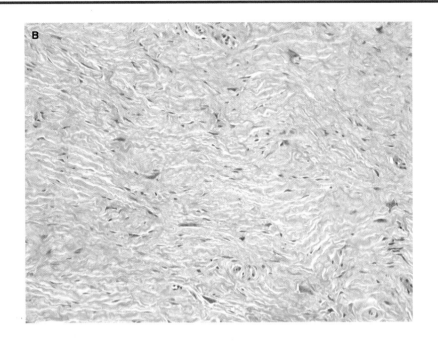

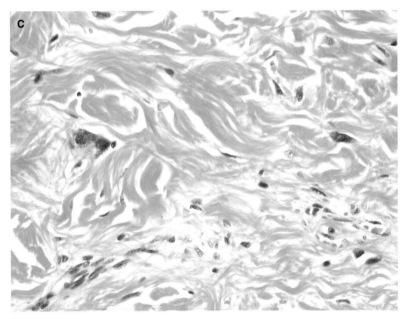

FIGURE 4-15

Sclerotic Fibroma (Storiform Collagenoma)

Sclerotic fibroma (storiform collagenoma, plywood fibroma) is a rare neoplasm that can present as a sporadic lesion or in a multifocal form in patients with Cowden syndrome. It has been suggested that sclerotic fibromas may represent a marker of this syndrome. Clinically, the lesions present as flesh-colored papules measuring 0.5 cm to 3 cm in diameter (199, 200).

PATHOLOGY (FIGURE 4-16)

- Well-circumscribed and unencapsulated hypocellular dermal nodule
- The overlying epidermis is attenuated.
- The tumor is composed of thickened and hyalinized collagen bundles arranged in a laminated fashion with intervening clefts (occasional focal storiform pattern).
- Rare spindle-shaped cells
- Some tumors may show more cellularity and scattered pleomorphic cells.
- Absence of elastic fibers
- Occasional stromal mucin deposition
- IHC: The tumor cells are positive for CD34, CD99, vimentin, and factor XIIIA.

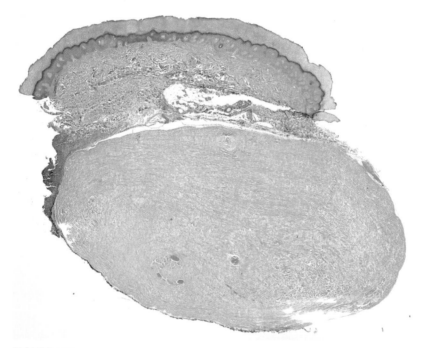

FIGURE 4-16

FIGURE 4-16   Sclerotic fibroma. Well-defined nodule in the dermis composed of hyalinized collagen bundles arranged in a laminated fashion.

Superficial Acral Fibromyxoma

Superficial acral fibromyxoma is rare benign tumor with a striking predilection for the fingers and toes; also on the heel and nails. Clinically, it presents as a small slow-growing solitary mass that had been present for months. Patients are usually young to middle-aged adults, and there is predilection for males (201, 202).

PATHOLOGY (FIGURE 4-17A, B)
- The tumor is a circumscribed dermal tumor (sometimes can involve the subcutaneous fat).
- It is composed of spindled or stellate cells arranged in a loose storiform or fascicular pattern set in a myxoid or collagenous stroma.
- The tumors have scattered small vascular channels.
- Frequent mast cells
- Mitotic figures are rare, and cytological atypia is mild or absent.
- IHC: The tumor cells express CD34, EMA, CD10, and CD99. The tumor cells are negative for SMA, desmin, keratins, or HMB-45.

(continued)

Superficial Acral Fibromyxoma (continued)

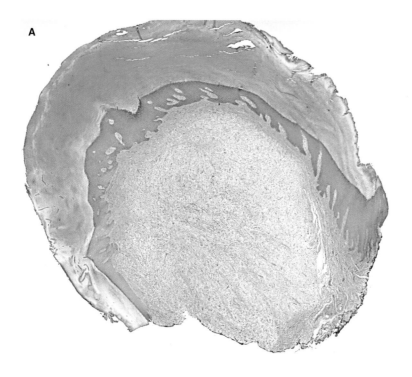

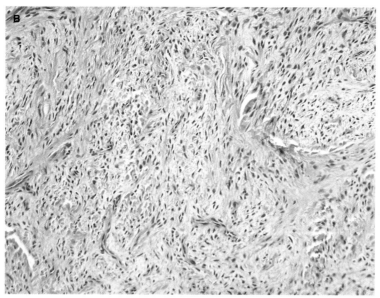

FIGURE 4-17

FIGURE 4-17   (A) Superficial acral fibromyxoma. Spindle cells in the dermis arranged in a loose fascicular myxoid stroma. (B) Higher magnification showing the bland spindled cells set in a myxoid and vascular stroma.

Superficial Angiomyxoma

Superficial angiomyxoma is a rare variant of myxoma. Clinically, it presents as a slowly growing nodule. The tumor presents more commonly on the head, neck, or trunk of adults. Frequently there is local recurrence after surgical excision. Carney complex is an autosomal dominant disorder associated with inactivating mutations in *PRKAR1A*. This complex consists of myxomas, lentigines on the lips, and endocrine changes. The myxomas described in the Carney complex are very similar if not identical to sporadic superficial angiomyxomas; however, angiomyxomas in Carney complex are usually seen in young adults, are multiple, and are more commonly located on the external ear, eyelid, and nipple. Carney complex should be considered if there are multiple superficial angiomyxoma or if it involves the external ear (203, 204).

PATHOLOGY (FIGURE 4-18A, B)

- Angiomyxomas are usually located in the dermis and subcutaneous tissue.
- It is composed of multiple ill-defined myxoid lobules with spindle-shaped and stellate cells set in a basophilic matrix.
- Commonly with many small blood vessels
- Commonly there is a sparse inflammatory infiltrate composed of lymphocytes and neutrophils.
- In almost half of the cases an epithelial component is noted and consists of epithelial strands, basaloid cells, or a keratin cysts.

(continued)

Superficial Angiomyxoma (*continued*)

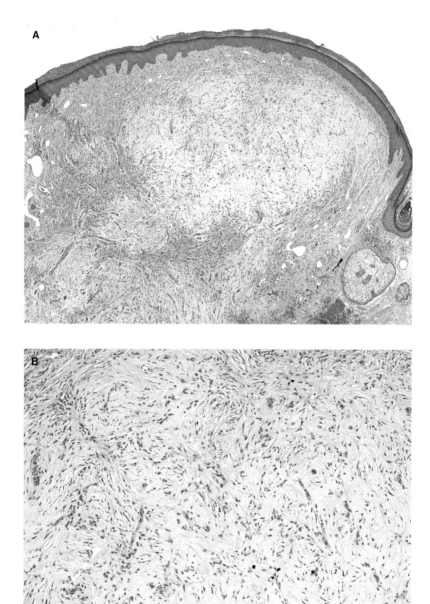

FIGURE 4-18

FIGURE 4-18   (A) Superficial angiomyxoma. Myxoid nodular lesion in the dermis composed of spindle cells and small vascular spaces. (B) Higher magnification showing the spindle and stellate cells. Note the marked myxoid deposits.

Acquired Digital Fibrokeratoma

Acquired digital fibrokeratoma is a rare benign neoplasm that most commonly develops on the distal extremities, especially fingers and toes, affecting males more often than females. Most of them are found in adults and present as slowly growing asymptomatic firm nodules. It may clinically resemble a supernumerary digit, which is usually congenital, located on the proximal portion of the fifth digit, and histologically contains abundant nerve bundles. Minor trauma or repetitive irritation has been suggested as a predisposing factor (205, 206).

PATHOLOGY (FIGURE 4-19A, B)
- Epidermis is orthokeratotic, hyperkeratotic, papillomatous, and acanthotic.
- Dermal core of thick collagen bundles oriented parallel in the vertical axis
- Variable numbers of stellate fibroblasts
- There is sometimes prominent cellularity, small vascular spaces, and elastic fibers.
- Only few inflammatory cells and no hair follicles
- Peripheral neural tissue is usually not present, in contrast to supernumerary digits.

DIFFERENTIAL DIAGNOSIS
Supernumerary digit may clinically resemble acquired digital fibrokeratoma; however, the latter is usually located on base of the fifth finger of neonates (congenital) or children, and histologically it shows numerous nerve bundles and paccinian corpuscles embedded in connective tissue.

(continued)

Acquired Digital Fibrokeratoma *(continued)*

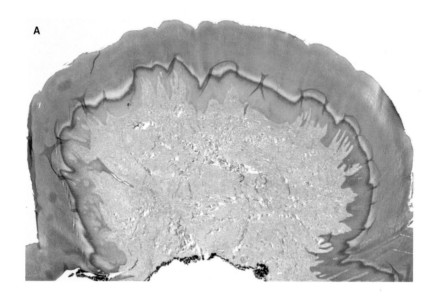

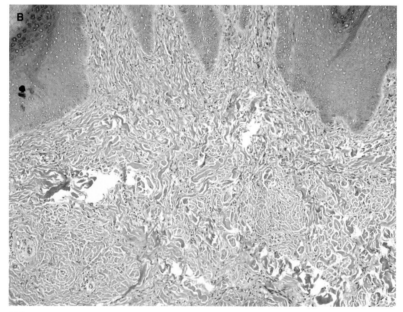

FIGURE 4-19

FIGURE 4-19   (A) Acquired digital fibrokeratoma. Polypoid lesion with hyperplastic and hyperkeratotic epidermis. (B) Note the characteristic mature collagen bundles, fibroblasts, and small blood vessels in the dermis.

Fibrous Hamartoma of Infancy

Fibrous hamartoma of infancy (FHI) is a rare, low-aggressive soft tissue tumor that usually occurs within the first 2 years of life; it may be discovered at birth. Clinically, it presents as a firm solitary mass located in the subcutaneous tissue or reticular dermis, usually measuring from 1 cm to 8 cm in diameter. Males are affected more often than females. FHI is most commonly found in the axilla, shoulder, upper arm, and back. Local recurrence is uncommon and the clinical course is typically excellent (207, 208).

PATHOLOGY (FIGURE 4-20A, B)
■ The tumor is ill defined and involves predominantly the deep dermis and subcutaneous fat.
■ There are three tissue components:
   A. Interlacing coarse bundles of fibrocollagenous tissue with vessels
   B. Fascicles of loosely arranged mesenchymal cells (myofibroblasts). These cells are positive for actin and calponin
   C. Interspersed mature adipose tissue
■ Myxoid areas with oval or stellate cells, sometimes arranged in a whorled pattern
■ Sparse stromal lymphocytic infiltrate
■ Rare mitotic figures
■ The overlying eccrine glands may show some changes including squamous syringometaplasia, duct dilatation, and intraluminal papillary formations.

(continued)

Fibrous Hamartoma of Infancy (*continued*)

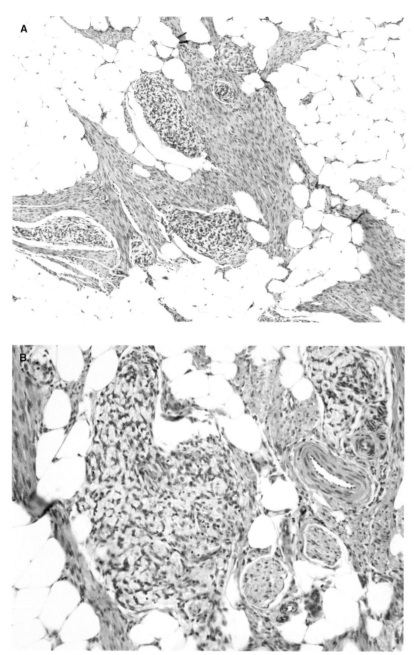

FIGURE 4-20

FIGURE 4-20   (A) Fibrous hamartoma of infancy. Note the fibrocollagenous tissue, the mesenchymal component and the interspersed mature fat. (B) Higher magnification showing the fascicles of loosely arranged mesenchymal cells. Note the vasculature in the background.

Infantile Digital Fibromatosis

Infantile digital fibromatosis (inclusion body fibromatosis) is an asymptomatic, nodular proliferation of fibrous tissue occurring almost exclusively on the dorsal and lateral aspects of the fingers or the toes. The tumors may be detected at birth or appear in the first year of life. The tumors often recur after excision but do not metastasize. Some lesions spontaneously regress over 1 to 10 years (209, 210).

PATHOLOGY (FIGURE 4-21A, B)
- The tumor extends from underneath the epidermis through the dermis and into the subcutis.
- Irregular interlacing fascicles of spindle-shaped myofibroblastic cells and collagen bundles
- The nuclei of the spindle cells are oval or spindle shaped, some with stellate forms.
- Characteristic "small perinuclear eosinophilic cytoplasmic inclusion bodies." These inclusions are actin positive.
- Rare mitotic figures but no cytologic atypia
- IHC: The tumor cells are positive for actin, calponin, and desmin. Sometimes, they may be positive for h-caldesmon and beta-catenin.

(continued)

Infantile Digital Fibromatosis *(continued)*

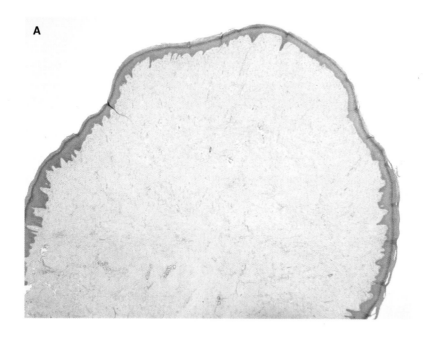

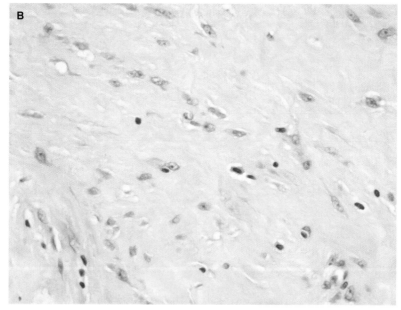

FIGURE 4-21

FIGURE 4-21　(A) Infantile digital fibromatosis. Polypoid lesion composed of bland spindled cells. (B) Note the rare, brightly eosinophilic intracytoplasmic inclusions.

Fibromatosis

Fibromatosis represents a wide spectrum of locally infiltrative neoplastic processes characterized by the proliferation of mature fibroblasts associated with mature collagen. Some of these entities are present at birth or develop in early childhood (e.g., juvenile fibromatosis), and others may appear in adulthood.

Palmar fibromatosis (Dupuytren contracture): Is most commonly seen in male adults. There is an association with diabetes and increased familial incidence. Clinically, it begins as a firm nodule in the distal palmar aponeurosis and eventually it affects the flexion at the metacarpophalangeal joints, especially in the ring finger, thus resulting in a claw-like deformity. Local recurrence is very common unless surgical intervention of the palmar fascia is performed (211).

Plantar fibromatosis (Ledderhose disease): Is the equivalent of palmar fibromatosis (see above). The age and sex distribution is roughly similar to palmar fibromatosis; however, a significant number of cases occur in children or adolescents. Clinically, it presents as single or multiple nodules on the medial aspect of the sole. Most cases are asymptomatic, but some patients may complain of burning sensation. Cytogenetically these lesions may show trisomy 8 and trisomy 14. Superficial fibromatosis are genetically distinct from deep fibromatoses as they lack mutations in the *CTNNB1* gene (beta-catenin). Local recurrence is quite common (211).

Desmoid fibromatosis: Represents a group of deep-seated fibrous neoplasms that can be seen in different clinical settings. The majority of cases are sporadic and solitary; however, some can be familial or associated with familial adenomatous polyposis (FAP). Per their anatomic location, desmoid tumors are classified into extra-abdominal (more common) cases), occurring in the abdominal wall, and intra-abdominal. All of these anatomical subsets more commonly occur between the second and fourth decades of life with a predilection for females. Mutations in *CTNNB1*, the gene encoding beta-catenin, are seen in approximately 85% of sporadic desmoid tumors. Local recurrence is common (212, 213).

PATHOLOGY (FIGURE 4-22A, B)

- Palmar fibromatosis: It is composed of cellular nodules of uniformly plump, proliferating myofibroblasts. It may show sparse mitotic activity. In its early phase, the tumor has very little collagenous stroma. In its chronic phase, the lesion is characterized by large amounts of hypocellular, hyalinized collagen. Scattered lymphocytes and macrophages may be present at the periphery of the tumor.

- Plantar fibromatosis: It is very similar to palmar fibromatosis; however, there are frequent lymphohistiocytic infiltrate and hemorrhage. Lesions tend to be more cellular, and there may be scattered multinucleated giant cells.

- Desmoid fibromatosis: It is composed by an admixture of plump spindled cells with tapering nuclei embedded in a variably hyalinized/myxoid collagenous stroma. There are conspicuous mitotic figures and peripheral collections of lymphocytes. Immunohistochemical studies show variable expression for actin and only rarely positive for desmin. There usually is nuclear expression of beta-catenin, albeit such observation is not entirely specific and can be seen in other lesions (e.g., solitary fibrous tumor, endometrial stromal sarcoma, and synovial sarcoma).

(continued)

Fibromatosis *(continued)*

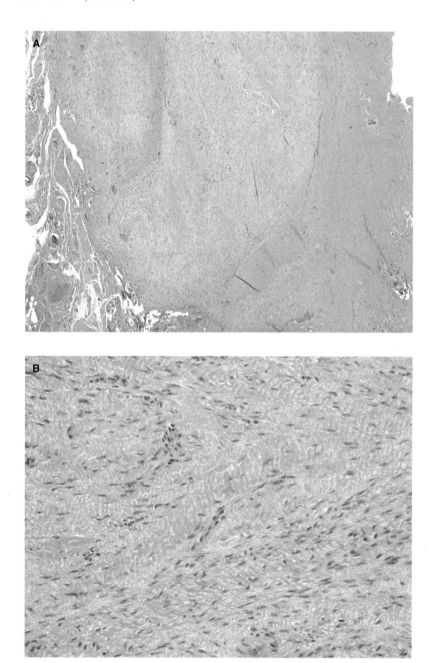

FIGURE 4-22

FIGURE 4-22   (A) Fibromatosis. Hypercellular nodules composed of uniformly plump, proliferating myofibroblasts. Note the hyalinized stroma. (B) Higher magnification showing spindle cells with elongated vesicular nuclei containing small central nucleoli.

Angiofibromas (Adenoma Sebaceum)

Adenoma sebaceum is a misnomer that is used for angiofibromatoid lesions found in most patients with tuberous sclerosis (TS). TS is an autosomal dominant syndrome affecting cellular differentiation and proliferation, which results in hamartoma formation in many organs. Facial angiofibromas (adenoma sebaceum) are characteristic in TS, and while occasionally present at birth, more often they appear during early childhood. They are dome-shaped, telangiectatic papules bilaterally and symmetrically distributed on the nose and cheeks. Other lesions include periungual fibromas (Koenen tumors), Shagreen patches (connective tissue nevi), and white hypopigmented and ash leaf–shaped macules on the trunk or limbs. Also common are oral fibromas, mostly gingival in location, and dental pits. TS can result from mutations of two separate genes: The first gene maps to chromosome 9, specifically 9q34 (*TSC1*; hamartin); the second gene maps to chromosome 16, specifically 16p13 (*TSC2*; tuberin) (214, 215).

PATHOLOGY (FIGURE 4-23)

- The epidermis shows some flattening of rete ridges.
- Common patchy basal melanocytic hyperplasia
- In the dermis, there is a network of collagen fibers with an onion-skin arrangement around follicles and blood vessels.
- Increased number of fibroblasts (plump, spindle shaped, stellate, and in some cases even multinucleate)
- There is often a sparse lymphohistiocytic infiltrate (including mast cells).
- The blood vessels are increased in number and are focally dilated.
- There is an atrophy and compression of adnexal structures.

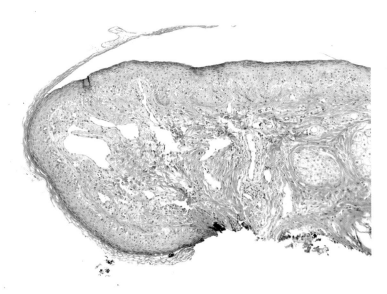

FIGURE 4-23

FIGURE 4-23   Angiofibromas ("adenoma sebaceum"). Irregular proliferation of fibrous tissue and ectatic blood vessels.

Fibrous Papule of the Nose

Fibrous papules are common, small, solitary, skin-colored papules, usually seen on the nose of middle-aged adults (216, 217).

PATHOLOGY (FIGURE 4-24)

- The overlying epidermis appears normal or slightly atrophic.
- The lesion is composed of a collagenous stroma with increased vascular channels.
- Scattered cells varying from spindle shaped to multinucleated are characteristic.
- There may be focal pigmentation of the overlying epidermis with prominent melanocytes resembling a melanocytic lesion.
- Occasional scattered pleomorphic cells that overlap with pleomorphic fibroma
- A few multinucleate "floret"-like cells may be present.
- By immunohistochemistry, the cells are positive for factor XIIIa and may also be positive for CD34.

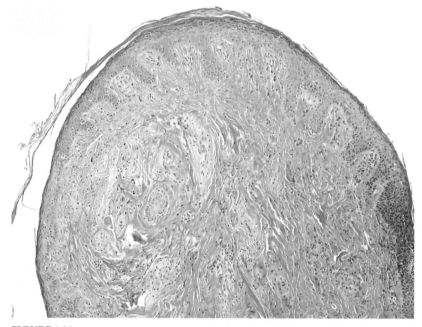

FIGURE 4-24

FIGURE 4-24   Fibrous papule of the nose. Polypoid lesion with dense collagenous stroma, vascular channels, and spindle cells.

Pearly Penile Papules

Pearly penile papules are common lesions that present as small rounded papules that are characteristically seen on the sulcus or corona of the glans penis. Often they present as rows or rings of papules. They are more commonly seen in uncircumcised young adult African Americans. The lesion histologically is analogous to other angiofibromas including angiofibromas, fibrous papule, subungual, and periungual fibroma (218).

PATHOLOGY (FIGURE 4-25)
■ Numerous vessels surrounded by dense connective tissue containing an increased number of plump and stellate "fibroblasts"

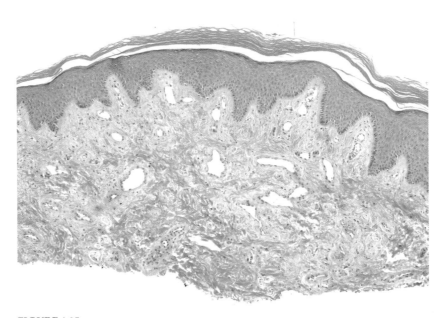

FIGURE 4-25

FIGURE 4-25 Pearly penile papules. Collagenous stroma with ectatic blood vessels. Identical histology to angiofibromas.

FIBROHISTIOCYTIC TUMORS

Multinucleated Cell Angiohistiocytoma

Multinucleate cell angiohistiocytoma is a benign fibrohistiocytic lesion that presents as multiple, localized, red-to-brown papules with predilection for the upper and lower limbs of middle-aged women (the dorsal aspects of the hands, fingers, wrists, and thighs) (219, 220).

PATHOLOGY (FIGURE 4-26A, B)
- Unremarkable epidermis
- In the superficial and mid dermis there is a proliferation of small ectatic narrow vessels.
- Fibrohistiocytic (epithelioid and spindle) cells scattered between collagen bundles
- Scattered multinucleate cells with angulated cytoplasm (they may have 3–10 nuclei)
- These multinucleated large cells are positive for vimentin and negative for CD68, CD31, CD34, and factor XIIIa. The interstitial fibrohistiocytic cells are positive for CD68 and factor XIIIA.

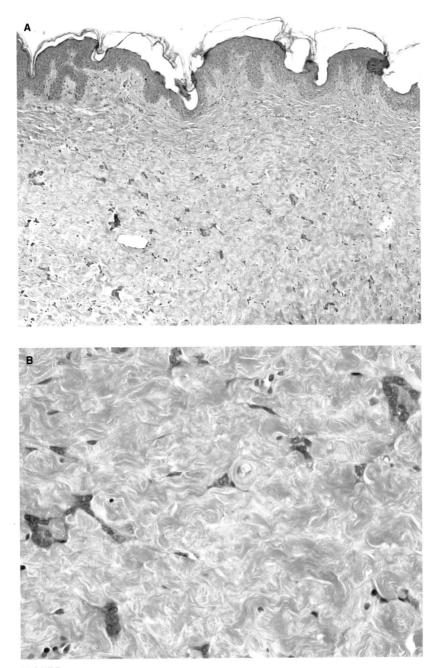

FIGURE 4-26

FIGURE 4-26   (A) Multinucleated cell angiohistiocytoma. Marked vascular and collagenous
proliferation with scattered, multinucleated giant cells. (B) High power of the
multinucleated giant cells.

Dermatofibroma

Dermatofibroma (fibrous histiocytoma) is a common benign fibrohistiocytic tumor of unknown etiology. Dermatofibromas frequently develop on the extremities, mostly the lower legs, but can be seen in any anatomic site. They occur most often in the middle aged and show a slight female predominance. Clinically, they most often present as a pigmented solitary nodules. There may be multiple tumors most frequently associated with autoimmune diseases such as systemic lupus erythematosus, Graves disease, and HIV infection (221, 222).

PATHOLOGY (FIGURE 4-27A–G)
- Ill-defined dermal lesion, sometimes extending into superficial subcutaneous fat (deep dermatofibroma)
- Interlacing fascicles of spindled cells set within a loose collagenous stroma. Other areas show dense, pink collagen fibers (i.e., keloidal collagen).
- In addition to the spindled cells there are foamy histiocytes, multinucleated giant cells, and small blood vessels.
- Most dermatofibromas display conspicuous mitotic figures, but they usually show a normal configuration.
- Frequent foci of chronic lymphocytes, macrophages, and hemosiderin
- A classic histopathologic feature is the presence of collagen bundles surrounded by tumor cells in the periphery of the lesions (collagen "entrapment").
- The overlying epidermis usually shows acanthosis and basal hyperpigmentation, seborrheic keratosis-like pattern, epidermal atrophy, or, rarely, pseudoepitheliomatous hyperplasia and focal acantholytic dyskeratosis (FAD). In some cases, there is basaloid hyperplasia resembling basal cell carcinoma or induction of skin adnexa resembling sebaceous hyperplasia.
- IHC: The cells express combination of "fibrohistiocytic" and myofibroblastic markers. Most lesions express CD68, factor XIIIA, and CD163. They may also express SMA, MSA, stromelysin, and D2–40. Some cases may display smooth muscle differentiation and such areas express desmin.

(*text continued on page 204*)

FIGURE 4-27   (A) Dermatofibroma. Ill-defined lesion with interdigitation of lateral borders with the adjacent dermis. (B) High power of the uniform, interlacing spindle cells embedded in a hyaline collagenous stroma. (C) Cellular dermatofibroma. Hypercellular lesion with fascicular growth pattern.

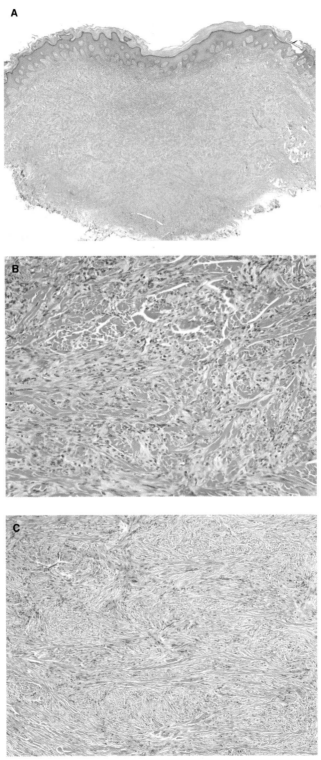

FIGURE 4-27

Dermatofibroma (continued)

VARIANTS

- Dermatofibroma with monster cells (atypical dermatofibroma): This variant is more commonly seen on the extremities. Histologically, the tumor shows the features of a more classic dermatofibroma; however, a number of cells have large pleomorphic nuclei with prominent nucleoli (monster cells). There may be atypical mitotic figures (up to one-third of cases).
- Cellular dermatofibroma (cellular fibrous histiocytoma): This variant has been most commonly reported in young adult males, and has a predilection for the limbs and head and neck. These lesions tend to be larger in size and have a high recurrence rate. Also, metastases to regional lymph nodes and lungs have been reported in some cases. Histologically, the tumor is hypercellular with a marked fascicular growth pattern and it frequently infiltrates the superficial subcutaneous tissue. Tumor cells have more ample eosinophilic cytoplasm, with "typical" mitotic figures. There may be central tumor necrosis. Immunohistochemistry may show variable expression for SMA and calponin.
- Aneurysmal fibrous histiocytoma: This is a rare variant of dermatofibroma. Clinically, it presents as a bluish nodule on the extremities of middle-aged adults, more commonly females. Since there may be extensive hemorrhage, some lesions may be clinically confused with a melanoma or vascular tumors. The rate of local recurrence is around 20%. Histologically, it is characterized by hemorrhagic irregular cleft-like and cystic spaces mimicking cavernous vascular channels with interstitial hemorrhage and hemosiderin deposition. The adjacent solid areas show the classic features of dermatofibroma.
- Epithelioid fibrous histiocytoma: This rare form is more commonly located on the proximal lower limb. It presents as a polypoid nodule that can be clinically mistaken for a pyogenic granuloma. Histologically, the tumors are polypoid and usually superficial. Frequently there is an epidermal collarette. The tumor is composed of round/angulated epithelioid cells with abundant eosinophilic cytoplasm and vesicular nuclei with small eosinophilic nucleoli. There are many small blood vessels. There may be focal xanthomatous and/or multinucleated giant cells. By immunohistochemistry the tumor cells commonly express factor XIIIa and CD163.
- Lipidized (ankle-type) fibrous histiocytoma: This variant presents as a polypoid yellow lesion, mostly on the lower leg. Histologically, the tumor is characterized by the presence of many foamy histiocytes and siderophages embedded in a hyalinized stroma (keloid-like).

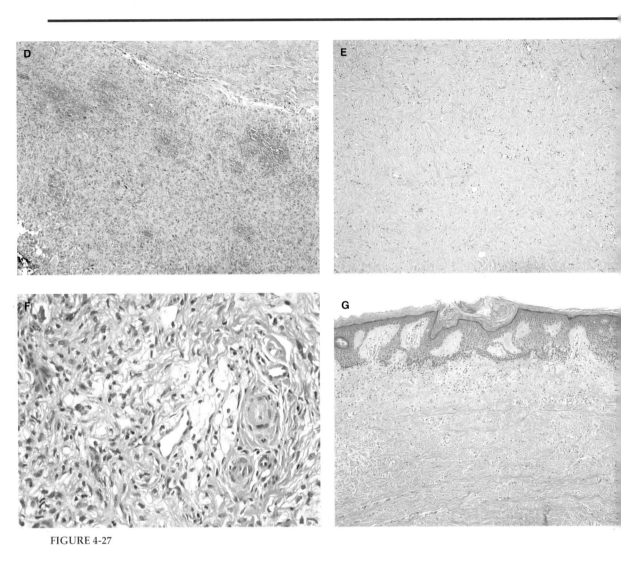

FIGURE 4-27

FIGURE 4-27   (D) Aneurysmal dermatofibroma. A dense cellular infiltrate with scattered hemorrhagic areas. (E) Sclerotic dermatofibroma. Note the marked sclerosing areas in the stroma of this lesion. (F) "Lipidized" dermatofibroma. Note the characteristic xanthoma cells admixed with the fibrohistiocyic cells. (G) Dermatofibroma with epidermal induction. Note the marked basal cell hyperplasia in this example of dermatofibroma.

Dermatofibrosarcoma Protuberans

Dermatofibrosarcoma protuberans (DFSP) is a locally aggressive cutaneous tumor with low to intermediate grade malignant potential. It has predilection for the trunk and proximal extremities of young and middle-aged adults, with slight male predominance. DFSP presents as a slow-growing, solitary or multiple, polypoid nodular lesion that ranges in size from 0.5 cm to 10 cm. Local recurrence is common (depending on the type of surgery used) and the risk of metastases is rare (<0.5% of cases, usually to the lungs). Usually, metastatic disease is preceded by multiple local recurrences and appears to be associated with fibrosarcomatous transformation. The fibrosarcomatous variant can be seen in 10% to 15% of cases. It is more aggressive, locally recurs in up to 75% of cases, particularly in acral lesions, and the rate of metastasis can be seen in up to 20% of cases. DFSP is characterized by a reciprocal translocation, t(17;22)(q22;q13) (*COL1A1* and *PDGFB* genes) (223–227).

PATHOLOGY (FIGURE 4-28A–E)
- DFSP is a dermal neoplasm that almost always extends into the subcutis (the subcutis is infiltrated in a lace-like pattern).
- The tumor is composed of fairly uniform spindled cells with elongated nuclei showing little or no pleomorphism and minimal pale cytoplasm.
- The cells spindle cells are arranged in a storiform or cartwheel pattern (sometimes centered on blood vessels).
- In contrast with dermatofibroma, there are usually only small amounts of intermingled collagen.
- Thin-walled capillaries

(*text continued on page 208*)

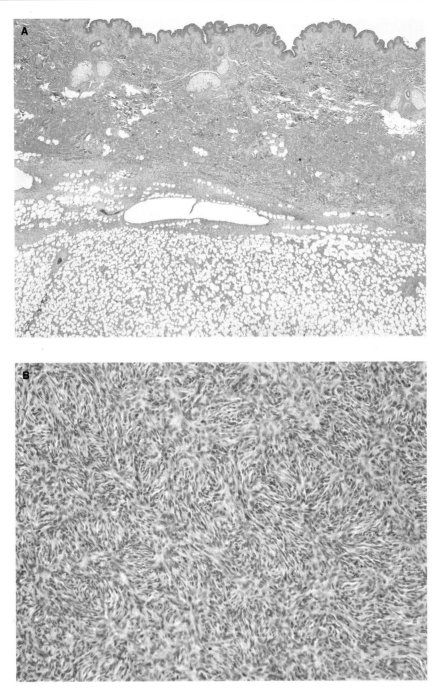

FIGURE 4-28

FIGURE 4-28   (A) Dermatofibrosarcoma protuberans. The deeper dermis shows a dense cellular infiltrate of uniform spindled cells extensively infiltrating the subcutaneous tissue (honeycomb). (B) Characteristic storiform pattern of the spindle cells.

Dermatofibrosarcoma Protuberans (continued)

- Only occasional, scattered mitotic figures, but they are more prominent in the fibrosarcomatous variant.
- Only rare histiocytes and multinucleate giant cells.
- Some cases may display prominent myxoid stroma.
- IHC: The tumor cells are strongly positive for CD34 and negative for factor XIIIa, S-100 protein, and CD117. CD99 is also positive in some cases. Anti-stromelysin and D2–40 are negative while they tend to be positive in dermatofibromas.
- Fibrosarcomatous change in DFSP: Fibrosarcomatous transformation can be seen either de novo or, more commonly, in recurrent classic DFSP. Histologically, the tumor is hypercellular with higher degree of nuclear atypia and higher mitotic count (>8 per 10 HPF) than typical DFSP. Focal loss of expression of CD34 is seen in the fibrosarcomatous areas. The *COL1A1-PDGFB* fusion transcripts can also be identified in these sarcomatous areas supporting a common histogenesis between the two components.
- Myxoid DFSP: This variant shows extensive myxoid stroma. There are large myxoid paucicellular areas, surrounded by more typical areas with storiform pattern. This variant also has numerous thin-walled blood vessels.
- Pigmented DFSP (Bednar tumor): This variant has melanin-containing melanocytes scattered within an otherwise typical DFSP. The amount of melanin pigment is quite variable.
- Giant cell fibroblastoma: This lesion is considered to be a variant of DFSP that most commonly involves young children. They occur in the same anatomic location as classic DFSP (trunk) and are characterized by a relatively hypocellular proliferation of spindle cells arranged in large areas with cystic degeneration forming pseudo-vascular spaces. These spaces are lined by cells with the same type of nuclei as the stromal cells. In the stroma, lending to the name of this entity, there are large, multinucleated, giant cells.

FIGURE 4-28   (C) Dermatofibrosarcoma protuberans. Subcutaneous fat involved by the spindle cells (honeycomb, lace-like appearance). (D) Note the fairly uniform spindled cells with elongated nuclei showing little or no pleomorphism. (E) Tumor cells are strongly positive for CD34.

Chapter 4: Connective Tissue Tumors

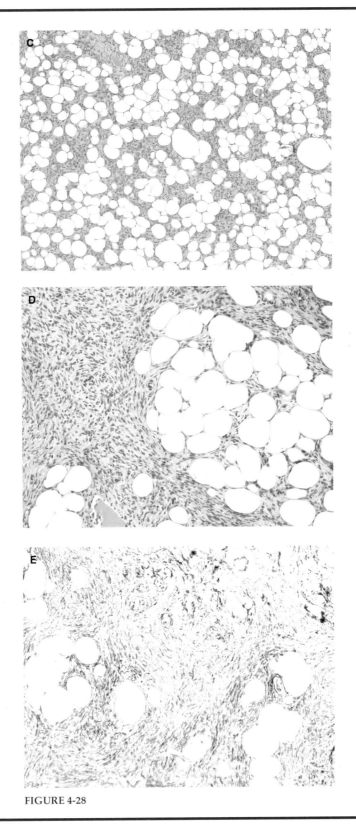

FIGURE 4-28

Fibrohistiocytic Lesion With Atypical Features

This uncommon lesion shares some features with DFSP. It occurs mostly in middle-aged individuals, more commonly on the trunk. It may reach several centimeters in size. Due to the possibility of recurrence, it has been recommended a complete excision. Based upon the absence of abnormalities of the *COL1a* gene, it is likely that this lesion corresponds to a variant of dermatofibroma rather than a DFSP (228, 229).

PATHOLOGY (FIGURE 4-29A–D)

- ■ The overlying epidermis typically shows acanthosis and hyperpigmentation of basal keratinocytes, and there is keloidal collagen, thus characteristic of dermatofibroma.
- ■ There is storiform pattern and frequent infiltration of the superficial adipose tissue, sometimes with a "honey-comb" pattern, thus more consistent with DFSP.
- ■ IHC: There appear to be two cellular populations, one expressing factor XIIIa/CD163 and another expressing CD34.

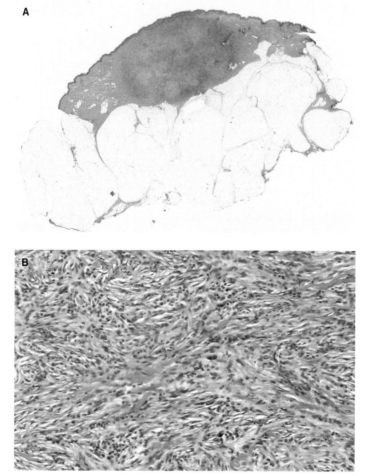

FIGURE 4-29

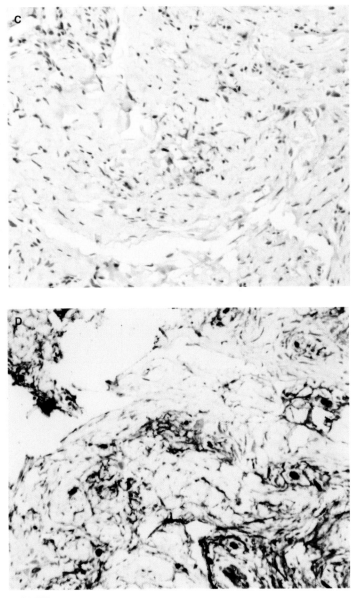

FIGURE 4-29

FIGURE 4-29   (A) Fibrohistiocytic lesion with atypical features. Spindle cell tumor in the dermis with storiform pattern and only superficial infiltration of the adipose tissue.
(B) Higher magnification showing spindle cells with similar appearance to a DSFP.
(C) Focal expression of factor XIIIA. (D) Focal expression of CD34 (same field as C).

Giant Cell Tumor of Tendon Sheath

Giant cell tumor of tendon sheath is a common benign tumor with a predilection for the volar surface of the fingers. It occurs particularly in young and middle-aged adults with a slight female predilection. Clinically, it presents as a lobulated, slow-growing mass that is firmly attached to the underlying structures. Local recurrence can be seen in up 30% of the cases. The most common cytogenetic abnormality in these tumors is t(1;2)(p13;q37) under the *COL6A3* promoter (230, 231).

PATHOLOGY (FIGURE 4-30A, B)
- The tumors are usually multilobulated and well circumscribed.
- Variable cellularity as sheets of rounded/polygonal cells with eosinophilic cytoplasm and vesicular nuclei
- Xanthomatous cells, siderophages, osteoclast-like multinucleated giant cells and lymphocytes
- The cells are set in a variably prominent collagenous stroma with cholesterol clefts and hemosiderin deposition.
- Mitotic figures may be numerous.
- IHC: The mononuclear cells are positive for CD68 and HAM56. Actin may be focally positive in the mononuclear cells. The giant cells are positive for CD68 and CD45.

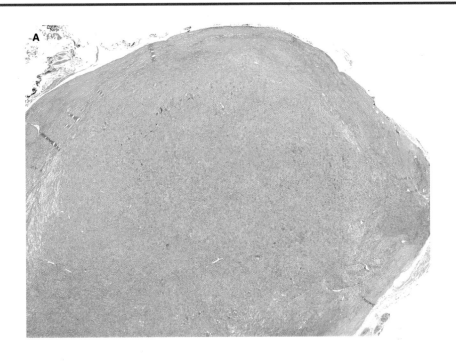

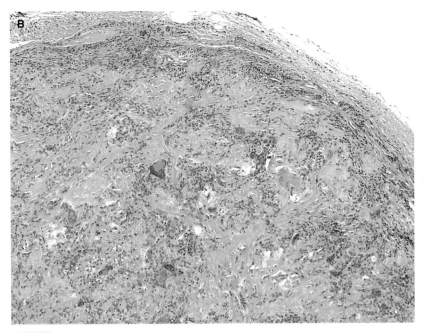

FIGURE 4-30

FIGURE 4-30   (A) Giant cell tumor of tendon sheath. Low magnification shows a well-defined pseudo-encapsulated tumor. (B) Note the presence of multinucleated giant and xanthomatous cells.

Angiomatoid Fibrous Histiocytoma

Angiomatoid fibrous histiocytoma (AFH) is a rare soft tissue tumor. It is more commonly seen in the subcutaneous tissues and rarely in the dermis of the extremities or trunk in children and young adults. Most cases behave in a relatively indolent manner. There is local recurrence in 2% to 12% of cases, more commonly associated with deep-seated lesions. Also, there are rare cases with distant metastases. Two specific translocations have been documented in AFH, t(12:16)(q13:p11) and t(12:22)(q13:q12), involving fusion of the *FUS* and *ATF-1* genes and fusion of the *EWSR1* gene with *ATF-1*, respectively. It is interesting that this translocation is also seen in clear cell sarcomas although these two lesions have clearly different clinical behavior (232–234).

PATHOLOGY (FIGURE 4-31A, B)
- This tumor is usually well circumscribed with a thick fibrous capsule.
- The capsule has a dense lymphoplasmacytic mantle that simulates a lymph node.
- The central portion of the tumor is composed of uniform, round, or short spindle-shaped eosinophilic cells with ovoid vesicular nuclei.
- Blood-filled cystic spaces and areas of hemorrhage
- Xanthoma cells, siderophages, and giant cells
- Cytological atypia and mitotic activity may sometimes be present and conspicuous but this does not correlate with behavior.
- IHC: The tumor cells are positive in about 50% of cases for desmin. Positivity for EMA, CD68, and CD99 is seen in up to 50% of cases. There may be HHF-35 and calponin expression.

FIGURE 4-31

FIGURE 4-31 (A) Angiomatoid fibrous histiocytoma. Well-circumscribed nodule composed of relatively uniform spindle cells. Note the marked lymphoid proliferation around the nodule. (B) Higher magnification of the tumor cells showing short spindle cells.

Atypical Fibroxanthoma

Atypical fibroxanthoma (AFX) is an uncommon tumor commonly seen in sun-damaged skin of the head and neck in elderly patients. Clinically, the tumors usually occur as a solitary nodule. Most common locations include the cheek, nose, and ear. In addition, AFX may arise in the setting of xeroderma pigmentosum and solid organ transplantation. AFX tends to follow an indolent clinical course. Although these tumors may be locally aggressive, metastases are only reported in less than 1% of cases. Genetic analysis of AFX has shown mutations of the *p53* tumor-suppressor gene, an alteration known to be induced by ultraviolet radiation (235–237).

PATHOLOGY (FIGURE 4-32A–F)
- Nonencapsulated dermal tumors that usually abuts the epidermis
- The majority of lesions are polypoid and often have an epidermal collarette.
- Occasionally ulcerated epidermis
- The deep margin is generally pushing rather than infiltrative.
- Superficial subcutaneous extension is exceedingly rare and more commonly seen in recurrent/aggressive tumors.
- Large, spindle-shaped, and anaplastic cells arranged in a haphazard fashion, and usually with a number of atypical mitotic figures
- Large histiocytic cells may form bizarre multinucleated giant cells that frequently contain lipid.
- Hemosiderin pigmentation is common, and this may cause clinical confusion with melanoma.
- Tumor necrosis, vascular, and/or perineural invasion are exceedingly rare in AFX, and if encountered an alternative diagnosis should be considered.
- The spindle cell variant of AFX is predominantly composed of spindle cells with only mild to moderate cytologic atypia.
- IHC: AFX is a diagnosis of exclusion. The histiocytic cells and the multinucleated cells are positive for CD68 and other histiocytic markers (CD163). CD10 is usually positive in AFX; however, many spindle cell neoplasms may show focal positivity for CD10, including melanoma and spindle cell carcinomas. The spindle cells can be focally positive for SMA and calponin. Other markers that are positive in AFX include CD99 and procollagen I (PC1). Tumor cells are negative for S-100 protein; as a possible pitfall, dendritic cells in the background are positive. Other melanocytic markers, as well as keratins, desmin, and h-caldesmon should be negative in AFX. Some authors accept focal, weak cytokeratin expression, but in our opinion such lesions should be considered as spindle cell carcinomas. In lesions lacking S100 or keratin expression, the combination of CD10 and PC1 expression supports a diagnosis of AFX.

DIFFERENTIAL DIAGNOSIS
As stated, AFX is a diagnosis of exclusion. Spindle cell squamous carcinoma (sarcomatoid carcinoma) or spindle cell melanoma should be ruled out. Thus, the immunohistochemical pattern should include markers for carcinoma (P63, high molecular weight cytokeratin, etc.) and melanoma (S100p, HMB45, MART-1). Anti-p63 is a useful marker as it is diffusely positive in sarcomatoid squamous cell carcinoma and is usually negative in AFX. Leiomyosarcoma should also be ruled out by performing smooth muscle markers, such as desmin.

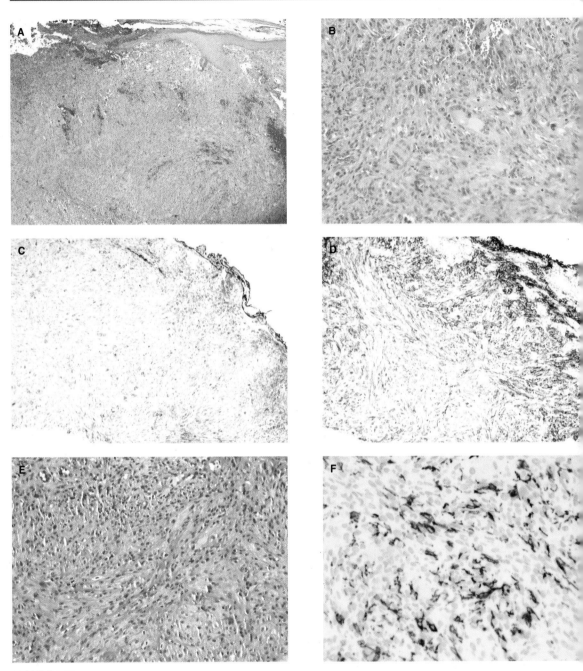

FIGURE 4-32

FIGURE 4-32   (A) Atypical fibroxanthoma. Ulcerated hypercellular epithelioid and spindle cell
neoplasm. (B) Higher magnification showing many atypical and pleomorphic cells
with histiocytic differentiation. Note the characteristic presence of multinucleated
giant cells. (C) Tumor cells are positive for CD68 (KP-1). (D) Tumor cells are positive
for CD10. (E) Spindle cell variant of AFX. Note the fascicles of spindle cells with
only mild cytologic atypia. (F) CD163 expression in the spindle cells, confirming the
histiocytic etiology.

Plexiform Fibrohistiocytic Tumor

Plexiform fibrohistiocytic tumor (PFT; or plexiform fibrous histiocytoma) is a rare lesion that mainly affects children and young adults. Female patients are affected more often. Clinically, the tumor commonly affects the upper extremities, particularly the forearm, fingers, hand, and wrist. It presents as a slow-growing, painless nodule that is situated in the dermis and subcutis. Preceding trauma has been reported in a few instances. There is a tendency for local recurrence. There are rare local lymph nodes and lung metastases (238–240).

PATHOLOGY (FIGURE 4-33A, B)

- The tumor is characterized by multiple infiltrative small nodules, or elongated fascicles that are characteristically arranged in a plexiform pattern.
- The tumor is mostly located at the junction between the dermis and subcutis (one-third of cases are purely dermal).
- Three distinct cell types: spindled fibroblast-like cells, mononuclear histiocyte-like cells, and osteoclast-like giant cells.
- Three main histologic patterns: (1) Clusters of mononuclear histiocyte-like cells and multinucleated giant cells in a plexiform arrangement, (2) clusters and fascicles of spindle fibroblast-like cells, and (3) mixed subtype composed of both patterns.
- Most cases show a focal lymphocytic infiltrate (more commonly in the fibroblastic subtype).
- Rarely cellular atypia and pleomorphism
- Low mitotic rate
- Occasional perineural and vascular invasion
- IHC: The histiocytic cells are positive for CD68. The fibroblastic cells are positive for vimentin, SMA, and calponin.

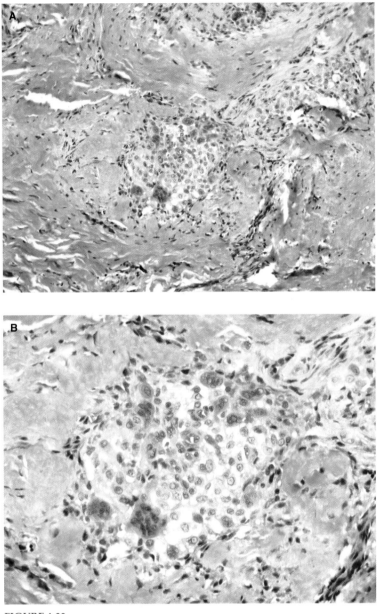

FIGURE 4-33

FIGURE 4-33   (A) Plexiform fibrohistiocytic tumor. Small infiltrative nodules composed of histiocytic, fibroblast-like and multinucleated giant cells. (B) Higher magnification showing the clusters of mononuclear histiocyte-like cells and multinucleated giant cells.

VASCULAR NEOPLASMS

Infantile Hemangioma

Infantile hemangioma is a common, benign, vascular tumor that has a clinical course characterized by marked early proliferation followed by spontaneous involution. Clinically, it presents as a flat red lesion, usually less than 5 cm in diameter, that gradually enlarges and develops a raised surface. The head and neck are by far the most commonly involved. Females are affected more often than males (241–243).

PATHOLOGY (FIGURE 4-34)

- In the early stage the lesions are characterized by nonencapsulated lobules and dense cords of plump endothelial cells.
- The early stage shows frequent mitotic figures.
- As the hemangioma proliferates, the vascular lumina increases in size.
- The involution phase shows an increase in apoptotic endothelial cells and a decrease in plump and mitotically active endothelial cells.
- As the involution phase progresses, the endothelial cells show a flattened appearance and the vascular lumina continue to enlarge until mature ectatic vessels remain. The lesion becomes more fibrotic with a decrease in vascular structures.
- IHC: Infantile hemangiomas express GLUT-1. This marker may aid in differentiating infantile hemangiomas from other vascular neoplasms or malformations such as congenital hemangiomas, kaposiform hemangioendothelioma (KHE), and tufted angioma.

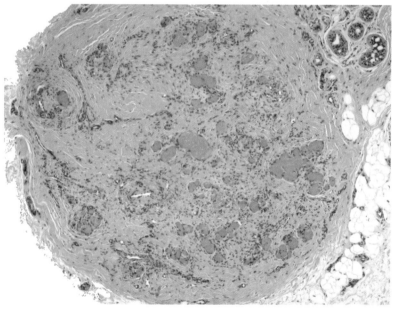

FIGURE 4-34

FIGURE 4-34   Infantile hemangioma. Nonencapsulated lobule of vessels of different sizes.

Verrucous Hemangioma

Verrucous hemangioma is an uncommon congenital vascular anomaly that presents at birth but sometimes may present in later adulthood. Verrucous hemangioma exhibits a gradual increase in size with age. Clinically, the lesions usually present as bluish-purple, partly confluent papules, and plaques typically unilateral and localized to the lower extremities. Satellite nodules may develop (244–246).

PATHOLOGY (FIGURE 4-35A, B)
- The epidermis shows marked papillomatosis and hyperkeratosis overlying an ill-defined proliferation of capillary-sized blood vessels mixed with ectatic lymphatics and veins.
- The vascular component can extend deeply into the reticular dermis and subcutaneous adipose tissue (distinguishing feature from angiokeratoma).

(continued)

Verrucous Hemangioma *(continued)*

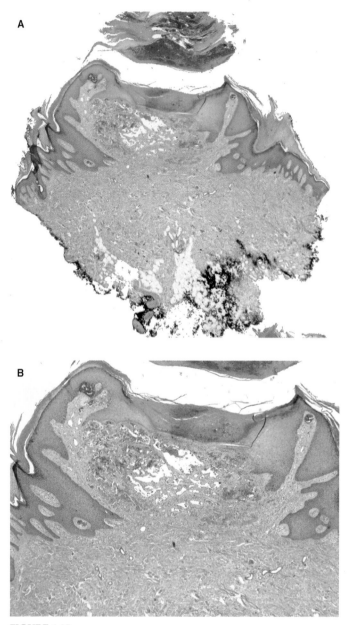

FIGURE 4-35

FIGURE 4-35   (A) Verrucous hemangioma. Note the marled verrucous hyperplasia of epidermis. In the deep dermis there are many capillaries with rare cavernous vascular spaces. (B) Higher magnification of the cavernous vascular spaces involving mainly the papillary dermis.

Cherry Angioma

Cherry angiomas are the most common cutaneous vascular proliferations. Typically they present in the third or fourth decades of life. Lesions may be found on any anatomic site, but they are predominantly seen on the trunk and proximal limbs. Most patients report an increase in number and size of individual lesions with advancing age. Clinically, lesions may have a variable appearance, ranging from a small red macule to a larger dome-topped or polypoid papule (247).

PATHOLOGY (FIGURE 4-36)

- The biopsy shows a small polypoid lesion with peripheral collarette.
- In the dermis, there is a network of dilated communicating channels with scant intervening connective tissue.
- These lesions show dilated and congested segments of capillaries in the dermis.

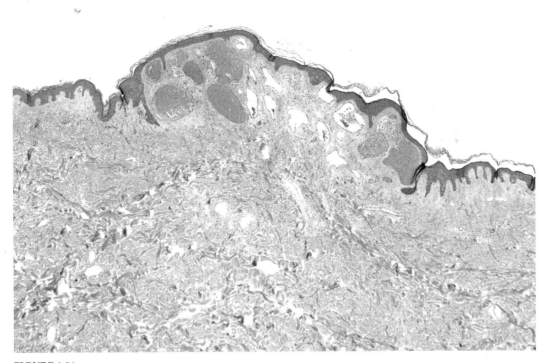

FIGURE 4-36

FIGURE 4-36   Cherry angioma. Note the dilated and congested vessels in superficial dermis.

Pyogenic Granuloma/Lobular Capillary Hemangioma

Pyogenic granuloma/lobular capillary hemangioma is a common benign vascular lesion of the skin and mucosa. The term pyogenic granuloma is a misnomer as it is neither an infectious nor granulomatous lesion. It may arise at any age and is more commonly seen in the oral mucosa (gingiva), lips, fingers, and face. Pyogenic granuloma often arises in pregnancy (also associated with oral contraceptives), particularly on the gingiva or elsewhere in the oral mucosa (granuloma gravidarum). Clinically, it presents as a glistening red papule or nodule that is prone to bleeding and ulceration. Local recurrence after excision is frequent, and in some cases it occurs as multiple satellite lesions that may be clinically diagnosed as a malignancy (248–250).

PATHOLOGY (FIGURE 4-37A, B)

- The lesion is usually polypoid and lobulated with an epidermal collarette.
- In the dermis there are many capillaries set in a loose edematous collagenous stroma.
- Endothelial cells have variably bland to plump nuclei and may be focally epithelioid.
- Mitoses may be numerous.
- Focal cytological atypia as a result of degeneration
- Common acute and chronic inflammatory superficial infiltrate (granulation tissue), particularly in ulcerated cases

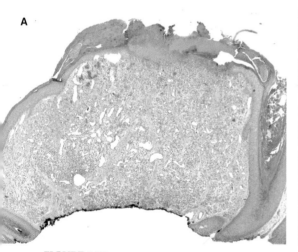 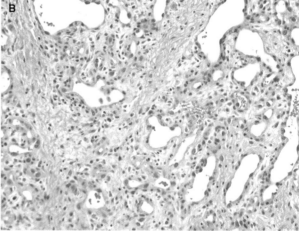

FIGURE 4-37

FIGURE 4-37 (A) Pyogenic granuloma. Polypoid lesion with ulcerated epidermis. There is marked granulation tissue with proliferation of capillary-sized blood vessels in the dermis. (B) Higher magnification of the capillary-sized blood vessels.

Arteriovenous Hemangioma

Arteriovenous hemangioma presents as a small, solitary, red papule with a predilection for the head and neck (lips, the perioral skin, the nose, and the eyelids) of middle-aged to elderly patients. Lesions measure less than 1.0 cm in diameter. It has an association with chronic liver disease (251, 252).

PATHOLOGY (FIGURE 4-38)
- The lesion is well circumscribed, nonencapsulated, and intradermal and is composed of thin- and thick-walled vessels (mostly veins).
- These vessels are lined by plump endothelial cells.
- The vessels have a fibromuscular wall, which contains variable elastic fibers.
- Most vessels have the features of veins. Arteries are difficult to identify.

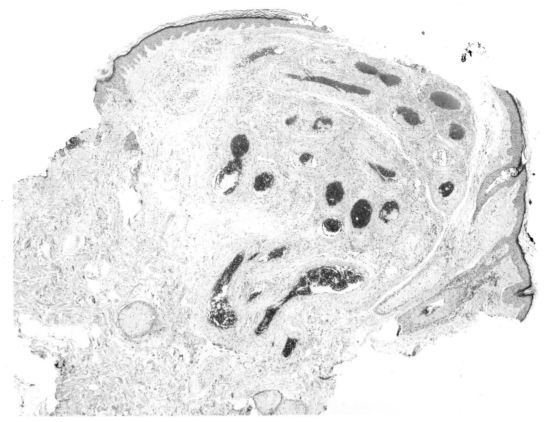

FIGURE 4-38

FIGURE 4-38   Arteriovenous hemangioma. There is a proliferation of thin- and thick-walled blood vessels (arteries and veins).

Microvenular Hemangioma

Microvenular hemangioma is an acquired vascular tumor. Clinically, it appears as a slowly enlarging, purple-to-red, dome-shaped papule or nodule that is usually located on the trunk or limbs of young to middle-aged adults. There may be multiple lesions (253–255).

PATHOLOGY (FIGURE 4-39)
- Proliferation of branching, thin-walled blood vessels lined by bland endothelial cells involving the papillary and reticular dermis
- Usually dissects the hyalinized collagen bundles and occasionally involves the subcutis.
- The arrector pili muscles can be infiltrated by vascular channels.
- By immunohistochemistry these lesions are positive for WT-1 and negative for D2–40 and GLUT-1.

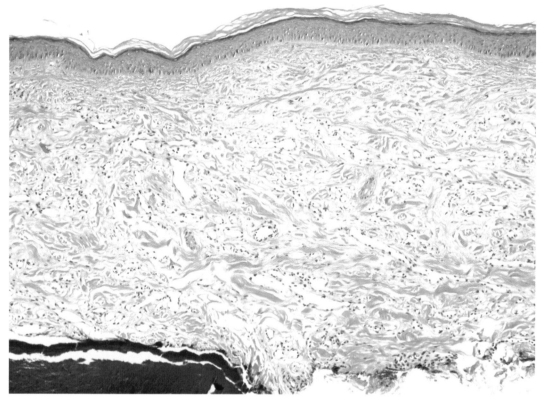

FIGURE 4-39

FIGURE 4-39   Microvenular hemangioma. Note the branching, irregular thin-walled vessels lined by bland endothelial cells containing plump nuclei.

Hobnail Hemangioma

Hobnail hemangioma (targetoid hemosiderotic hemangioma) is a benign vascular tumor that usually presents as a small solitary papule affecting the limbs or trunk of young or middle-aged people. The lesion shows male predilection. Clinically, the lesion is asymptomatic, usually less than 2 cm in diameter, and increases in size very slowly. It has a variable clinical appearance, and most examples present as annular lesions with a central violaceous papule surrounded by an eccentric ecchymotic ring that can exhibit a targetoid appearance. It has been reported in pregnancy (256–258).

PATHOLOGY (FIGURE 4-40A, B)
- Wedge-shaped vascular proliferation with the base toward the epidermis.
- The vascular channels are ectatic, irregular, thin-walled, and lined by plump endothelial cells with bland protruding nuclei and scanty cytoplasm (hobnail cells).
- Common papillary projections
- In the deep dermis and subcutis the vascular channels dissect collagen bundles surrounding the sweat glands.
- There is a variable mild inflammatory infiltrate around vessels and considerable extravasation of erythrocytes and hemosiderin (depending on the stage of the lesion).
- Superficial vessels may contain fibrin thrombi.

(continued)

Hobnail Hemangioma (*continued*)

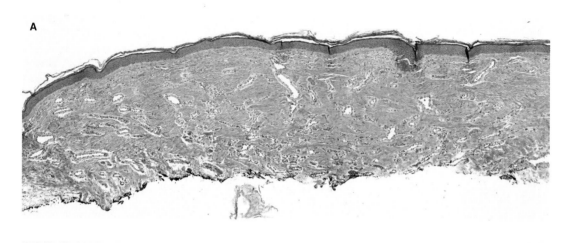

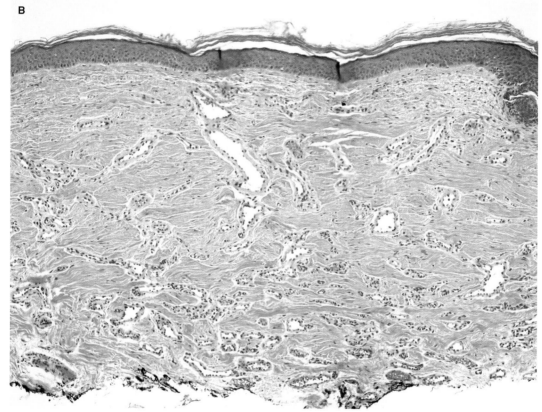

FIGURE 4-40

FIGURE 4-40 (A) Hobnail hemangioma. Subtle, wedge-shaped growth of thin-walled vascular channels. (B) Note the irregular vascular channels lined by endothelial cells with bland protruding nuclei (hobnail cells).

Acquired Elastotic Hemangioma

Acquired elastotic hemangioma is a rare benign vascular lesion. Clinically, it presents as a solitary, irregularly shaped, and slowly growing plaque with an angiomatous appearance. It usually arises on sun-exposed areas, such as the forearms, of middle-aged and elderly patients (259, 260).

PATHOLOGY
■ Band-like proliferation of capillary blood vessels in the upper dermis.
■ Blood vessels have thick walls with prominent endothelial cells (hobnail).
■ A narrow band of uninvolved papillary dermis is present.
■ Dermal solar elastosis

Angiokeratoma

Angiokeratomas are benign vascular lesions represented by dilated superficial blood vessels (capillaries) associated with secondary epidermal changes. There are several different variants:

- Angiokeratoma corporis diffusum: This type is characterized by multiple widespread clusters of red papules, especially in a bathing-trunk distribution. Originally thought to be synonymous with Anderson–Fabry disease (an X-linked genetic disorder that results from a deficiency of the lysosomal enzyme alpha-galactosidase A). However, this lesion can be associated with other enzymatic disorders and in people with normal enzyme activity (261, 262).
- Angiokeratoma of Fordyce: This type develops mainly on the scrotum of elderly men as single or multiple red papules. Other anatomic locations are penis, thighs, and the lower abdominal wall in men, and vulva in young adult females (263).
- Angiokeratoma of Mibelli: This type presents as warty lesions on bony prominences (especially fingers and toes) of children and adolescents. It is more common in females (264).
- Solitary or multiple angiokeratomas: This type has an ample age range and anatomical distribution, but the lower limbs are most commonly affected.
- Angiokeratoma circumscriptum: This type is the least common of the five. It presents as unilateral hyperkeratotic papules or nodules with predilection for the leg, trunk, or arm. Lesions commonly develop in infancy or childhood, and predominantly in females (265, 266).

PATHOLOGY (FIGURE 4-41)
- The lesion shows many dilated vascular spaces in papillary dermis.
- The overlying epidermis shows irregular acanthosis with elongation of the rete ridges and enclosing the vascular channels (appearing to be within the epidermis).
- A collarette may be formed at the margins of the lesions.
- Occasional thrombi
- In patients with Anderson–Fabry disease there is vacuolation of smooth muscle in arterioles and arteries, pericytes, and endothelial cells.

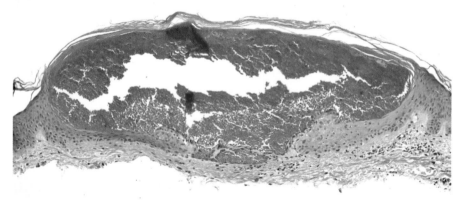

FIGURE 4-41

FIGURE 4-41   Angiokeratoma. Note the dilated capillaries in papillary dermis that appear to be within epidermis.

Spindle Cell Hemangioma (Hemangioendothelioma)

Spindle cell hemangioma (hemangioendothelioma) was initially considered to be a vascular tumor of low-grade malignancy (low-grade angiosarcoma); however, there are convincing data that this lesion may in fact represent a reactive vascular process or a malformation. The majority of cases arise before the age of 30. Clinically, the lesions may be single or multiple painful reddish papules. The hands and feet are the most common sites of involvement, but lesions may also occur on the trunk. Local recurrence of lesions is common after surgical removal (267–269).

PATHOLOGY (FIGURE 4-42)
- The lesion is poorly circumscribed and situated in the dermis and subcutis.
- The lesion is composed of thin-walled, congested cavernous vascular spaces that may have thrombi.
- Solid areas of spindle cells with slit-like vascular spaces (mimicking Kaposi sarcoma [KS])
- Many plump endothelial cells, either in groups or lining vascular channels
- Characteristic intracytoplasmic lumina
- The vascular spaces are lined by a single layer of bland endothelial cells.
- Rarely nuclear atypia or mitotic figures
- Common thrombosis and papillary projections resembling those seen with Masson tumor are commonly identified.
- Bundles of smooth muscle are quite often present around the blood vessels and in the spindled cell areas.
- At the periphery of many lesions, there are thick-walled, irregular blood vessels.

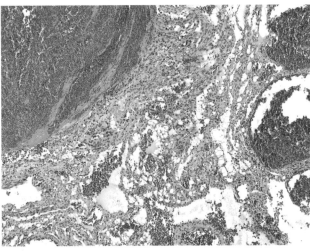

FIGURE 4-42

FIGURE 4-42   Spindle cell hemangioma. Note the large cavernous spaces admixed with bland spindle cells.

Cutaneous Epithelioid Angiomatous Nodule

Cutaneous epithelioid angiomatous nodule is a rare benign vascular tumor. It presents as a solitary (rarely multiple) violaceous papule usually on the trunk and extremities. There has been no lesion recurrence, progression, or metastasis reported to date (270, 271).

PATHOLOGY
- Circumscribed and located in the upper dermis (it may involve the deep dermis).
- It is composed of solid sheets of large endothelial cells with ample eosinophilic cytoplasm, enlarged nuclei, and prominent nucleoli.
- Tumoral cells containing prominent vacuoles within their cytoplasm are commonly seen.
- Occasional typical mitoses are present.
- In the background there may be mild fibrosis, hemosiderin deposition, and scattered inflammatory cells (occasionally with prominent eosinophils).

Epithelioid Hemangioma (Angiolymphoid Hyperplasia With Eosinophilia)

Epithelioid hemangioma (angiolymphoid hyperplasia with eosinophilia) is an uncommon idiopathic condition. It presents in adults as dome-shaped, smooth-surfaced isolated or grouped papules, plaques, or nodules. There is a slight predilection for males. Approximately 85% of lesions occur in the skin of the head and neck; most of them are on or near the ear, forehead, or scalp. While epithelioid hemangioma shares some histologic similarities with Kimura disease, they are generally regarded as separate entities. Epithelioid hemangioma lesions are superficial, whereas Kimura disease involves deeper tissues (nodes, salivary glands, and the subcutis). The pathogenesis of epithelioid hemangioma is not fully understood; it has been suggested to represent a benign vascular neoplasm or a reactive process to a preceding trauma. The latter is the favored interpretation (272–274).

PATHOLOGY (FIGURE 4-43A, B)
- The tumors are intradermal; however, they can rarely involve the subcutaneous fat.
- The lesion consists of a lobulated mass composed of numerous vascular spaces arranged in solid cords and nests.
- These vascular spaces are lined by large plump epithelioid endothelial cells with large nuclei, prominent nucleoli, and abundant eosinophilic cytoplasm.
- Some vessels may show cytoplasmic vacuoles.
- Intravascular proliferations of these cells may be seen in the lumina of larger vessels.
- The lesion is also characterized by a low mitotic index and absent nuclear atypia.
- Surrounding these small vessels is a variably prominent inflammatory cell infiltrate composed largely of lymphocytes, numerous eosinophils, and histiocytes. Sometimes the lymphocytes are arranged as germinal centers.
- Chronic lesions show stromal sclerosis.

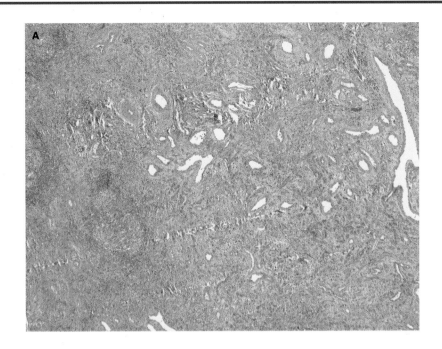

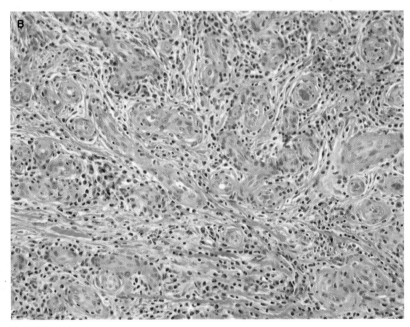

FIGURE 4-43

FIGURE 4-43 (A) Epithelioid hemangioma. Low magnification showing a vascular nodule with scattered lymphoid aggregates. (B) The vessels are lined by endothelial cells with histiocytoid appearance. Note the increased number of eosinophils in the background.

Glomeruloid Hemangioma

Glomeruloid hemangioma is a benign vascular tumor occasionally associated with POEMS syndrome (polyneuropathy, organomegaly, endocrinopathy, M-protein, and skin changes) and multicentric Castleman disease. Patients present with numerous vascular papules on the trunk and limbs and this may be the initial presentation of the disease (275–278).

PATHOLOGY (FIGURE 4-44)

■ The lesions shows dilated vascular spaces in the dermis, containing in their lumina clusters of capillaries resembling renal glomeruli (grape-like aggregates).

■ In between these capillaries there are plump endothelial cells that show a vacuolated cytoplasm (PAS-positive hyaline globules representing immunoglobulin).

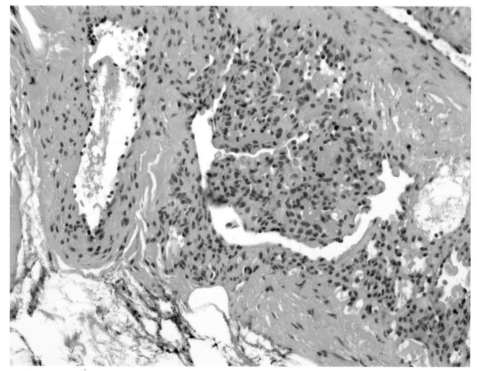

FIGURE 4-44

FIGURE 4-44   Glomeruloid hemangioma. High magnification showing grape-like aggregates of capillaries in the vascular lumina.

Venous Lake

Venous lakes are benign vascular lesions that manifest as dark blue-to-violaceous compressible papules caused by dilation of venules. They more commonly occur on sun-exposed skin, especially the lips, face, ears, and neck of elderly patients. Clinically, they sometimes can mimic malignant lesions, such as melanoma and pigmented basal cell carcinoma (279).

PATHOLOGY (FIGURE 4-45)
■ The lesion shows a single large dilated space or several interconnecting dilated spaces in superficial dermis.
■ The dilated channels have thin walls that are lined by a single layer of flattened endothelium.
■ Occasional thrombi.
■ Dermal solar elastosis.

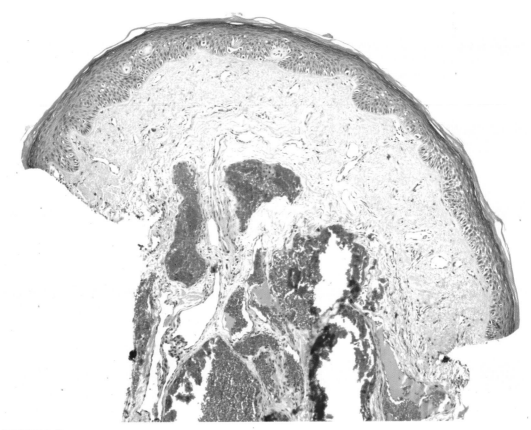

FIGURE 4-45

FIGURE 4-45   Venous lake. Note the dilated and congested veins in the dermis.

Intravascular Papillary Endothelial Hyperplasia (Masson Tumor)

Intravascular papillary endothelial hyperplasia is a benign lesion that represents a reactive proliferation of endothelial cells with papillary formations related to an organized thrombus. Clinically, it can present as a primary form in a thrombosed blood vessel (usually a vein). The secondary form presents as an incidental finding in association with other vascular lesions, such as cavernous hemangiomas, lymphangioma, etc. Clinically, they present as firm, sometimes painful nodules, most commonly seen on the fingers, head and neck, and trunk (280, 281).

PATHOLOGY (FIGURE 4-46A, B)

- In most cases the lesion arises within the lumen of a vein; however, it can also be seen associated with a vascular abnormality.
- Multiple small papillary processes covered by a single layer of flattened or plump endothelium
- The papillary endothelial cells show no atypia. Mitoses are infrequent.
- The core of the papillae consists of fibrin or hypocellular collagenous connective tissue with small capillaries (depending on the stage of organization).
- The papillae may be seen attached to the internal surface of the vessel wall or apparently lying free in the lumen.
- Adjacent associated thrombus

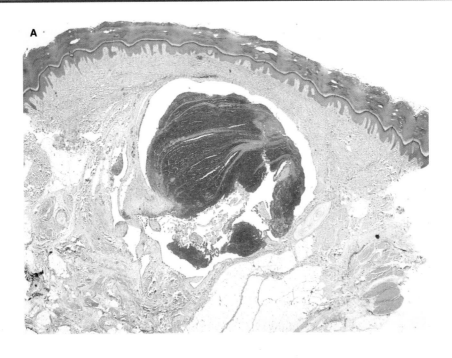

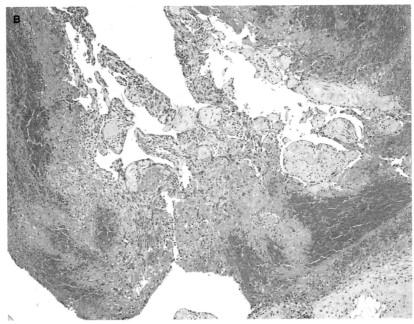

FIGURE 4-46

FIGURE 4-46   (A) Intravascular papillary endothelial hyperplasia (Masson tumor). Low
magnification of a thrombosed angioma. (B) Higher magnification showing small
papillae present within the lumen covered by flat endothelial cells.

Lymphangioma

Lymphangiomas are uncommon benign malformations of the lymphatic system. The classification of lymphangiomas lacks a standard definition but mostly includes: lymphangioma circumscriptum (superficial variant), cavernous lymphangioma (deep variant), cystic hygroma, and acquired progressive lymphangioma (282, 283).

Lymphangioma circumscriptum: It is the most common form characterized by a localized collection of numerous small vesicles, which can form larger confluent masses. They most often arise during infancy. The sites of predilection are the proximal extremities, trunk, axilla, and oral cavity (especially the tongue). Lymphangioma circumscriptum has a high recurrence rate after excision.

Cavernous lymphangioma: Cavernous lymphangiomas are rare and usually congenital or infantile. The most common sites are the head and neck region (especially the tongue) and extremities. It presents as a deep-seated lesion in the dermis, forming a painless swelling. This lesion tends to recur after simple excision.

Cystic hygroma: This lesion most likely represents a variant of cavernous lymphangioma. It presents as a large cystic mass, most often in the neck, axillae, or inguinal region. It is also prone to local recurrence unless widely excised.

Acquired progressive lymphangioma: This is a rare lesion. It is more commonly seen in adults. Particularly involves the extremities, especially the upper extremities. Clinically, it presents as a solitary erythematous patch that gradually increases in size.

PATHOLOGY (FIGURE 4-47)

- Lymphangioma circumscriptum shows large dilated lymph channels that cause expansion of the papillary dermis. These channels are numerous in the upper dermis and often extend into the deep dermis and subcutis. These deeper vessels have a thick wall that contains smooth muscle. The lumen is filled with lymphatic fluid.
- Cavernous lymphangioma shows in the dermis or subcutaneous fat as numerous dilated lymphatic channels lined by a single layer of endothelial cells. The vessel walls are lined by an incomplete layer of smooth muscle. The surrounding stroma consists of loose or fibrotic connective tissue with a lymphohistiocytic infiltrate. The vascular lumina may be filled with lymphatic fluid.
- Cystic hygroma: It is identical to cavernous lymphangioma.
- Acquired progressive lymphangioma: This variant shows marked involvement of the superficial dermis (occasionally also deep dermis and subcutis). The lesion is characterized by irregular, thin, vascular channels lined by a single layer of flat endothelial cells infiltrating collagen bundles. Vascular spaces may have a layer of smooth muscle and there may be focal papillary projections into the vessel lumina.

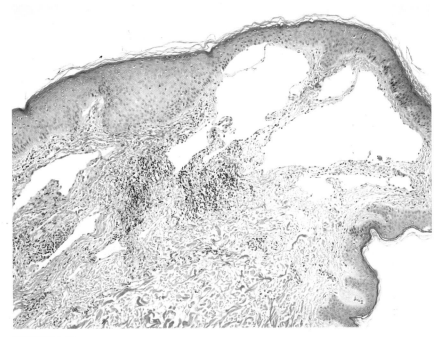

FIGURE 4-47

FIGURE 4-47   Lymphangioma. Note the dilated thin-walled lymphatic channels present in papillary dermis.

Eccrine Angiomatous Hamartoma

Eccrine angiomatous hamartoma (EAH) is a rare benign condition characterized histologically by increased numbers of eccrine structures and numerous capillary channels. Patients usually present with a solitary congenital nodule on the extremities that may be painful and that may show hyperhidrosis. The clinical presentation ranges from a simple angiomatous nodule to erythematous purpuric patches (284, 285).

PATHOLOGY
- Circumscribed, unencapsulated, dermal proliferation of well-differentiated eccrine secretory and ductal elements, in close association with well-differentiated, thin-walled angiomatous channels.
- The lesion is located in mid and deep dermis.
- EAH has been associated with a number of other histological elements including lipomatosus component, mucinous changes, apocrine glands, etc.
- The epidermis is normal; however, it may show verrucous hyperplasia.

Glomus Tumor

Glomus tumors are neoplasms that arise from the glomus apparatus, which is a thermoregulatory shunt mostly located on the fingers and toes. Clinically, it presents in young adults as small, blue-red painful papules of the distal extremities, more commonly in subungual sites. The majority of glomus tumors are benign but there are rare, frankly malignant cases (286, 287).

PATHOLOGY (FIGURE 4-48A–C)
- Well-defined (sometimes encapsulated) dermal neoplasm.
- Small vessels surrounded by aggregates of an organoid mantle of uniformly round glomus cells.
- These cells have a pale eosinophilic cytoplasm, clearly defined cell borders, and central dark-staining nuclei.
- The tumor cells and vessels are embedded in a fibrous stroma and some tumors may contain myxoid stroma.
- Rarely are there mitotic figures. Pleomorphism is not a feature of these tumors.
- Small nerve fibers and mast cells can be identified in the tumor stroma.
- IHC: The tumor cells are positive for SMA, MSA, and only rarely positive for desmin (in glomangiomyomas).

VARIANTS
- Glomangioma: It is a common variant of glomus tumor. The vascular component is prominent showing dilated lumina with a cavernous appearance. The glomus cells are distributed as a flattened monolayer to multiple rows of surrounding cuboidal glomus cells.
- Glomangiomyoma: Similar to glomangioma but it also contains fascicles of smooth muscle cells.
- Symplastic glomus tumor: This variant shows focal high nuclear grade in the absence of any other malignant features.

(continued)

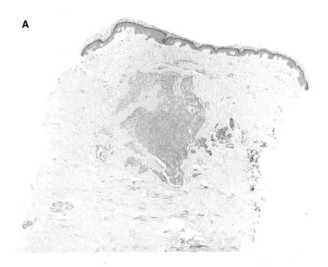

FIGURE 4-48 (A) Glomus tumor. Tumor in dermis composed of uniform small cells.

Glomus Tumor *(continued)*

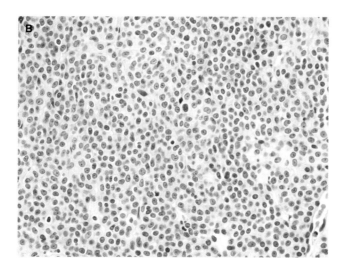

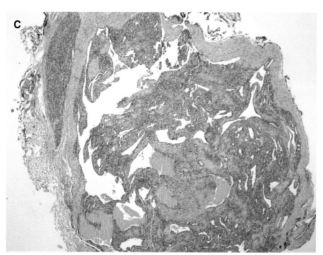

FIGURE 4-48

FIGURE 4-48   (B) Glomus cells have a characteristic uniform contour with round regular small nuclei. Note the rare blood vessel in the background. (C) Glomangioma. Note the vascularity of the lesion along with glomus cells.

Reactive Angioendotheliomatosis

Reactive angioendotheliomatosis (RAE) is an uncommon, reactive, cutaneous vascular proliferation that presents with distinctive clinical features consisting of infiltrated red-to-blue, patches and plaques. The lesions may appear on any anatomic site with a wide age range. RAE may be associated with a variety of conditions, including disseminated intravascular coagulation, cryoglobulinemia, infections, paraproteinemia, leukemia, rheumatoid arthritis, etc (288–291).

PATHOLOGY
- Lesions are mainly in dermis and only rarely involve the subcutis.
- The lesion is characterized by a benign intraluminal proliferation of endothelial cells.
- Some of these endothelial cells may obliterate the vasculature lumina.
- Glomeruloid appearance of the endothelial cells
- Cytological atypia can be apparent, but never prominent.
- IHC: The endothelial cells express CD34 and CD31.

Intravascular Histiocytosis

Intravascular histiocytosis is a rare disorder that is highly associated with rheumatoid arthritis. More commonly presents in middle-aged to elderly females with predilection for the upper and lower extremities. Clinically, it shows irregular patches of erythema, sometimes with livedo-like features, in close proximity to the involved joint. In most patients there is no underlying disease, but some lesions have been reported in the region of the metal implants of a knee joint replacement (292–294).

PATHOLOGY (FIGURE 4-49A, B)

- The biopsy shows dilated thin-walled vascular spaces in reticular dermis.
- These vascular spaces contain aggregates of histiocytic cells that show pale cytoplasm and vesicular nuclei.
- The histiocytes can be admixed with lymphocytes and neutrophils.
- There is a subtle perivascular inflammatory infiltrate composed of lymphocytes and plasma cells.
- Absence of cytological atypia
- IHC: The histiocytic cells are positive for CD68.

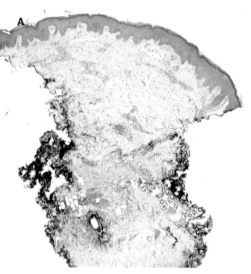
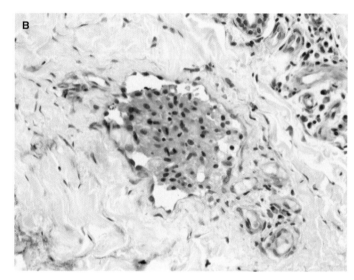

FIGURE 4-49

FIGURE 4-49   (A) Intravascular histiocytosis. Low power showing rare dilated, irregular thin-walled vascular channels in reticular dermis. (B) Higher magnification showing many histiocytic cells within the lumen of a dermal vessel.

Epithelioid Hemangioendothelioma

Epithelioid hemangioendothelioma is a rare vascular tumor of endothelial cell origin, which represents an intermediate-grade malignancy in terms of morphology and clinical behavior based on the potential for metastatic spread. Most cases occur in soft tissues of the limbs and bone; however, it can involve other organs, such as liver and lung. Cutaneous epithelioid hemangioendothelioma are exceedingly rare. Most cases present in adults. Cytogenetic analyses in some cases have shown a t(1;3)(p36.3;q25) (295–297).

PATHOLOGY
- There is a relatively well-circumscribed proliferation of nests and cords of plump, epithelioid to spindle-shaped endothelial cells in superficial and mid dermis.
- The cells have abundant pale-staining cytoplasm. Also, many of the cells contain cytoplasmic vacuoles with intraluminal erythrocytes.
- The intracytoplasmic lumina resembles signet-ring cell morphology.
- Cells may be arranged in thin cords in a fibromyxoid or hyalinized stroma resembling lobular carcinoma.
- Scattered dilated vascular channels are typically present at the periphery of the tumors.
- Cellular pleomorphism is typically minimal, and mitoses are often absent or at most present in very small numbers.
- IHC: The tumor cells are positive for factor VIII, CD31, and CD34. Some cases can be positive for SMA and rarely express cytokeratin.

Cutaneous Angiosarcoma

Cutaneous angiosarcoma is a rare, aggressive malignancy that can be seen in three different clinical settings: idiopathic cutaneous angiosarcoma of the head and neck, lymphedema-associated angiosarcoma, and postirradiation angiosarcoma. Also, cases have been reported in association with vinyl chloride exposure and xeroderma pigmentosum. Angiosarcoma arising in other organs may metastasize to the skin (298, 299).

- *Cutaneous angiosarcoma of the head and neck*: This lesion commonly involves the upper part of the face or the scalp of the elderly with an equal sex incidence. Clinically, they present as single or multifocal, blue to violaceous plaques or nodules. Thrombocytopenia may develop as a consequence of enlargement of the primary lesion (platelet consumption). Cases that are diagnosed earlier may have a better survival. It has been suggested that this variant may be partially induced by chronic sun exposure.
- *Lymphedema-associated angiosarcoma*: It is also named lymphangiosarcoma. This lesion commonly involves the arms of elderly females who have undergone radical mastectomy with axillary lymph node dissection and/or radiotherapy (Stewart–Treves syndrome). The tumors appear on average 12.5 years after surgery. Rare examples have been reported without association of lymph node dissection and without preceding edema.
- *Postirradiation angiosarcoma*: This variant is rare and can develop many years after radiotherapy for either benign (e.g., hemangiomas) or malignant conditions. It is most commonly associated with radiotherapy from breast or cervical cancer, usually after more than 5 years postradiation. Postirradiation angiosarcomas show high-level MYC amplification, reflecting gains in chromosome 8q24. These changes are not found in atypical vascular lesions (AVLs) associated with radiotherapy.

Note: All variants of cutaneous angiosarcoma have a poor prognosis, frequent local recurrences, rapid dissemination, and death in the majority of cases. Poor prognosis tends to be associated in tumors that have necrosis, epithelioid morphology, larger size, extensive depth of invasion, higher mitotic rate, and older age (>70 years).

PATHOLOGY (FIGURE 4-50A–D)
- The tumor shows a poorly circumscribed infiltrative intradermal lesion composed of anastomosing vascular channels of varying caliber.
- The vessels are lined by single or multiple layers of plump, pleomorphic and mitotically active endothelial cells. These endothelial cells may form papillae or solid nests within vascular lumina.
- The vascular proliferation characteristically dissects collagen bundles.
- In some instances lesions have a solid, undifferentiated, spindled cell appearance.
- Common lymphocytic aggregates
- Some cutaneous, non-HIV-associated angiosarcomas may simulate KS by showing irregular, branching vessels with promontory sign and plasma cells.
- IHC: In poorly differentiated examples, especially the epithelioid variant, can be difficult to diagnose without the aid of ancillary studies. These tumors are positive for factor VIII, CD31, CD34, and FLI-1.
- Epithelioid angiosarcomas are positive for cytokeratin (50%–60%) and EMA (25%).

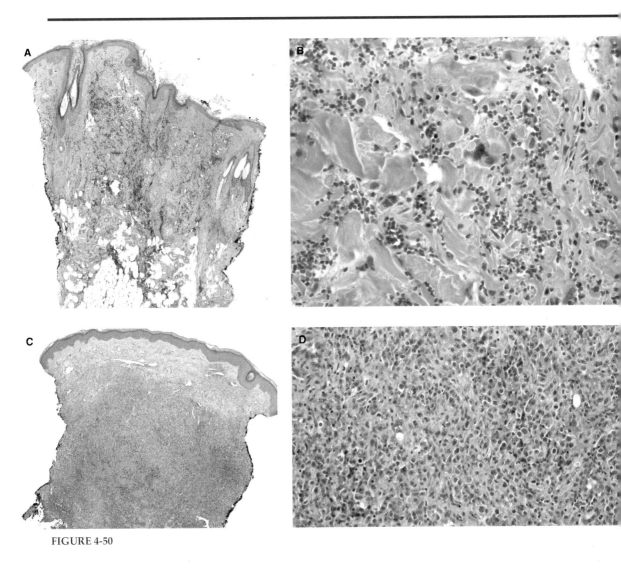

FIGURE 4-50

FIGURE 4-50   (A) Angiosarcoma. Low power shows an ill-defined infiltrative intradermal lesion with numerous anastomosing vascular spaces. (B) Note the pleomorphic and hyperchromatic endothelial cells. (C) Epithelioid angiosarcoma. Epithelioid malignant tumor in the dermis with scattered hemorrhagic areas. (D) Note the atypical epithelioid cells. This variant can be easily confused with other malignant neoplasms such as melanoma.

Atypical Vascular Lesion

Atypical vascular lesions (AVL) usually develops months or years after radiotherapy and/or postmastectomy for breast carcinoma. Clinically, it presents as one or more small, flesh-colored papules or erythematous patches that arise in radiated skin. The interval time between radiotherapy and the appearance of the lesions is usually shorter than that seen in angiosarcomas. Most AVLs pursue a benign course, but there are rare reports of progression to angiosarcoma, usually after multiple recurrences, suggesting that AVL may be a precursor to or incipient angiosarcoma (300–302).

PATHOLOGY (FIGURE 4-51A, B)
- The majority of lesions show irregular, anastomosing lymphatic-like vascular channels lined by a single layer of endothelial cells.
- The lesions are located in superficial and/or deep dermis. Rare examples have been described involving the subcutaneous fat.
- The lesions usually do not show an infiltrative growth pattern.
- The cells lining the channels can have a hobnail appearance with bland cytomorphology.
- Papillary projections may be seen.
- Mitotic figures are not characteristic.
- Note: Separating well-differentiated angiosarcoma from AVL can be extremely difficult, especially in small samples. Because areas within and adjacent to angiosarcoma can be indistinguishable from AVLs, it is thus essential to correlate the biopsy with the clinical presentation. Size is very important in separating these entities as most AVLs are small (average size 0.5 cm) and angiosarcomas are usually much larger (average size 7.5 cm). AVLs typically lack multilayering of endothelial cells, prominent nucleoli, mitoses, and hemorrhage. In AVLs, there is no destruction of adnexa or extension into the subcutaneous tissue. Recently, it has been suggested that only angiosarcomas, and not AVLs, show clusters of endothelial cells apparently "floating" within vascular lumina and unattached to the wall. Also, myc amplification is not detected in AVLs.

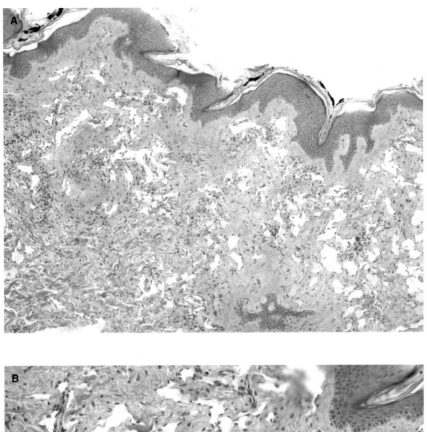

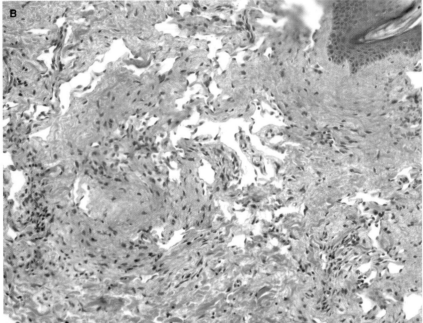

FIGURE 4-51

FIGURE 4-51 (A) Atypical vascular lesion of the breast. Note the dilated anastomosing vessels in superficial dermis with only minimal nuclear atypia. (B) High power of the dilated vascular channels.

Kaposi Sarcoma

Kaposi sarcoma (KS) is an endothelial cell neoplasm regarded as a low-grade malignant vascular tumor. However, some authors propose it is a reactive process. Human herpesvirus type 8 (HHV8) is the etiological agent. The exact mechanism regarding HHV8 transmission in non-HIV patients remains unclear; however, it is possibly sexual, horizontal, or parenteral. KS has a highly variable clinical course, ranging from isolated indolent and asymptomatic lesions to extensive organ involvement. KS characteristically develops in three stages: patch, plaque, and nodular. The initial patch stage lesions appear as flat, red dermal lesions. The lesions typically progress to the second phase, the plaque stage, and appear indurated, with an erythematous or violaceous color. Progression to the third stage, nodular, is characterized by multiple dermal nodules. There are four distinct subtypes: classic type, African type, immunosuppression-associated KS, and an AIDS-related (epidemic) KS (303–305).

- *Classic type*: This type is more commonly seen in Mediterranean and Jewish populations. Patients are typically elderly males and show a predilection for the distal extremities (lower leg and feet). This type of KS follows a prolonged indolent course, but patients have an increased risk of developing lymphoproliferative disorders.
- *African type*: This type of KS is more commonly seen in parts of tropical Africa (Zaire and Uganda). In this region, KS is endemic. Within this category there are lesions that arise on the limbs of middle-aged men and tend to show an indolent course. A subtype includes lesions that arise in young children that present with visceral or lymph node involvement and very poor prognosis.
- *Immunosuppression-associated KS*: This type is rare and usually presents in patients with organ transplant (kidney), long-term steroid use, and chemotherapy. The course of the disease is usually indolent.
- *AIDS-related (epidemic) KS*: This type classically presents in young adults and is most common in homosexual and bisexual men. The lesions disseminate widely and may result in an aggressive course; however, with the use of highly active antiretroviral therapy, the incidence and severity of KS in HIV individuals has dramatically decreased.

PATHOLOGY (FIGURE 4-52A–E)
- *Patch stage*: This phase is characterized by an increase of irregular, jagged vessels arranged mainly parallel to the epidermis. The vessels are thin walled and lined by inconspicuous or plump endothelial cells. These vessels dissect collagen bundles and surround adnexal structures and vessels (the promontory sign). The background shows an admixture of lymphocytes and plasma cells. Red cell extravasation and hemosiderin deposition is common.

(text continued on page 252)

FIGURE 4-52   (A) Kaposi sarcoma. Patch stage showing a subtle population of spindled cells and vessels. Note the extravasated red blood cells in the background. (B) Higher magnification showing vessels dissecting the collagen bundles. Vessels are lined by plump endothelial cells. (C) Nodular stage showing dermal nodules of endothelial cells.

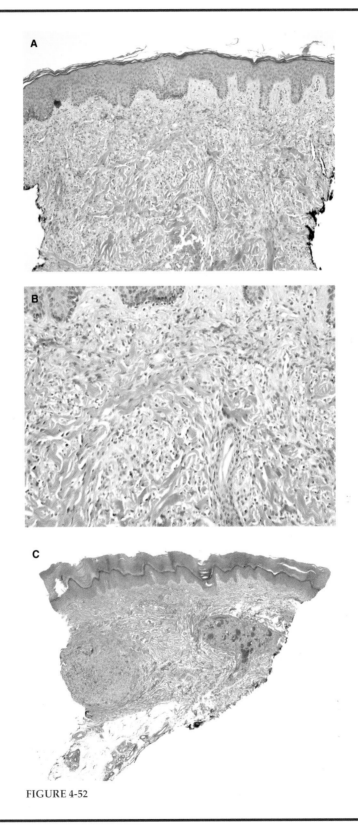

FIGURE 4-52

Kaposi Sarcoma (*continued*)

- *Plaque stage*: This phase shows more prominent dermal vascular proliferation, with variable lumina (slit-like appearance). Eosinophilic-spindled cells are characteristically seen in the dermis and around the vessels with variable nuclear pleomorphism. Mitotic figures are present, usually not prominent. Erythrocytes can be identified within vascular lumina and extravasated in the stroma. Dilated thin-walled vessels are found at the periphery of the tumor. Lymphoplasmacytic inflammatory response in seen in the background.
- *Nodular stage*: This phase shows a well-defined dermal nodules composed of eosinophilic spindle cells. Between the spindle cells there are numerous slit-like vascular spaces. Many ectatic vessels are still present at the periphery of the nodule. Conspicuous mitotic figures and lymphoplasmacytic infiltrate.
- NOTE: Characteristic amorphous eosinophilic, PAS-positive, diastase-resistant hyaline globules located in between the spindle cells or within the cells.
- IHC: The spindle cells are positive for CD34 and CD31. HHV8 is positive.

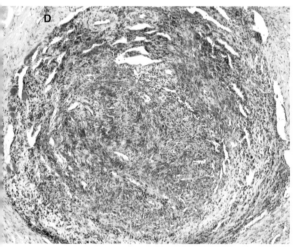 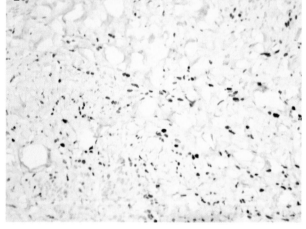

FIGURE 4-52

FIGURE 4-52   (D) Kaposi sarcoma. Higher magnification showing the spindled cells admixed with extravasated red blood cells. (E) Expression of HHV-8 by endothelial cells.

Kaposiform Hemangioendothelioma

Kaposiform hemangioendothelioma (KHE) is a rare, aggressive vascular proliferation in infants and young children; however, adults can be rarely affected. KHE was initially described in the retroperitoneum or deep soft tissues. Usually it presents in the skin as an isolated lesion more commonly located on the extremities and head and neck area. KHE is characterized by locally aggressive and destructive growth. An association of Kasabach-Merritt syndrome is seen in more than 50% of cases (306–309).

PATHOLOGY (FIGURE 4-53A, B)
- The tumor is composed of ill-defined lobules and/or sheets of packed spindle cells or rounded endothelial cells and pericytes.
- The cellular areas have an infiltrative pattern in the dermis, subcutaneous fat, and muscles.
- Microthrombi are commonly seen (at the periphery of tumor lobules).
- There is only focal cellular pleomorphism and mitotic figures are infrequent.
- There are areas with dilated, thin-walled vessels resembling lymphangioma.
- Other areas show irregularly shaped, branching, capillary-like vessels resembling KS or capillary hemangioma.
- IHC: The tumor cells are positive for CD31, CD34, FLI1, and Prox1.

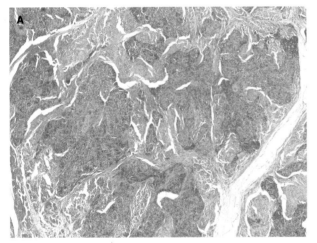
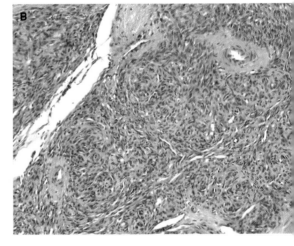

FIGURE 4-53

FIGURE 4-53   (A) Kaposiform hemangioendothelioma. Low power shows ill-defined lobules of packed spindle cells. (B) Higher magnification showing the vascular spindle cells reminiscent of a Kaposi sarcoma. Note the microthrombi formation.

NEURAL NEOPLASMS

Neurofibroma

Neurofibroma (NF) is common neural neoplasm. The majority of cases present as pedunculated solitary lesions. Patients with multiple lesions may have neurofibromatosis type I (NF-1, von Recklinghausen disease) (310). This is a genodermatosis inherited in an autosomal dominant fashion. The gene for NF1 has been cloned to chromosome 17q11.2 and the encoded protein is called neurofibromin (311).

PATHOLOGY (FIGURE 4-54A, B)
- Dermal lesion (sometimes the subcutis is involved)
- Hamartomatous proliferation composed of four types of cells: neurons, Schwann cells, perineural cells, and fibroblasts
- Delicate fascicles of spindled cells with scanty indefinite pale cytoplasm and elongated wavy nuclei
- Collagenous or myxoid stroma
- Occasional floret-like multinucleated giant cells
- Scattered inflammatory cells, especially mast cells
- IHC: S100p positive in the large majority of cases; also some cases are CD34 positive. The intervening axons are highlighted by antineurofilaments and antiperipherin.

VARIANTS
- Atypical NF: This is an unusual morphologic variant that shows nuclear pleomorphism and variably increased cellularity. Similar to standard NF, the cells should not display mitotic figures. This variant has been reported to be more commonly associated with NF-1. Despite the presence of cytologic atypia, there is no short-term risk of recurrence or malignant transformation.
- Plexiform NF: This is a distinct variant that is almost always associated with NF-1. It shows irregular cylindrical or fusiform enlargement of thick nerves, often with extensive myxoid change within a background of more typical NF.
- Diffuse NF: This variant is associated with NF-1 in up to 20% to 30% of cases. It shows a poorly defined lesion composed of Schwann cells that have short fusiform or rounded nuclei and characteristically are arranged resembling Meissnerian corpuscles. The stroma tends to be uniformly collagenous. The lesions diffusely infiltrate the deep reticular dermis and subcutaneous tissue.

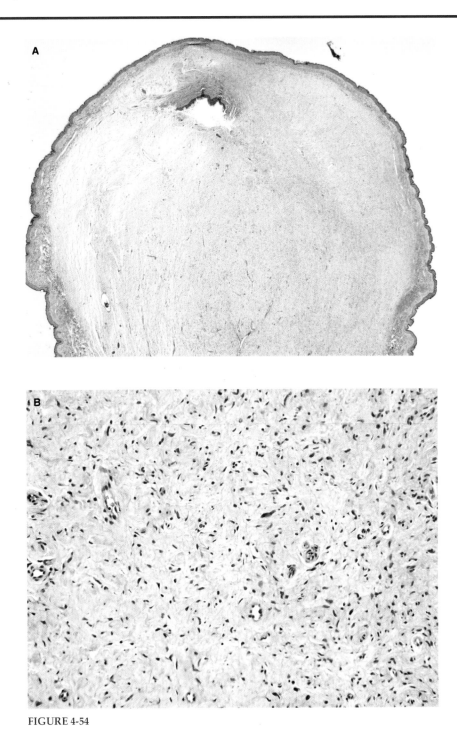

FIGURE 4-54

FIGURE 4-54   (A) Neurofibroma. Unencapsulated lesion in the dermis composed of spindle cells within a lightly stained stroma. (B) Higher magnification showing the ill-defined cells with eosinophilic cytoplasm and wavy-shaped nuclei.

Schwannomas

Schwannomas are uncommon cutaneous lesions. Clinically, they present as solitary tumors localized on the limbs of adults. Multiple tumors are uncommon and can occur in different clinical settings: (A) in association with NFs in von Recklinghausen disease (NF-1); (B) in neurofibromatosis type 2 (NF-2), due to mutations in the NF2 gene, located at 22q12.2 (acoustic schwannomas, meningiomas, etc.); and (C) in schwannomatosis (multiple cutaneous schwannomas) (312, 313).

PATHOLOGY (FIGURE 4-55A, B)

■ The tumors are well defined and encapsulated, usually confined to the subcutaneous or deeper tissues (primary intradermal origin is rare).

■ They are composed of two types of tissue: Antoni A and Antoni B areas.

   ■ Antoni A: Hypercellular component with fairly closely packed spindle cells (Schwann cells) with tapering, elongated, and wavy nuclei. Nuclear palisading is a characteristic feature, forming Verocay bodies.

   ■ Antoni B: Loose meshwork of myxoid tissue with widely separated Schwann cells. There are lipid-laden macrophages, dilated blood vessels with thick hyaline walls, hemorrhage, and sometimes calcification.

■ IHC: The tumor cells are positive for S100p. In contrast with NF, schwannomas have only rare axons and they are located at the periphery of the lesion.

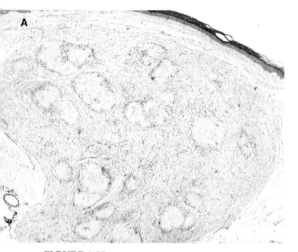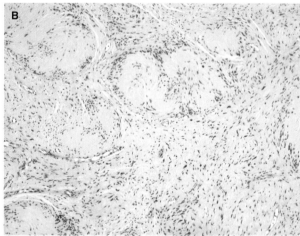

FIGURE 4-55

FIGURE 4-55   (A) Schwannoma. Well-defined tumor in the dermis. Note the Verocay bodies. (B) High power showing the Verocay bodies in the interlacing bundles of spindle-shaped cells.

Palisaded Encapsulated Neuroma

Palisaded encapsulated neuroma (PEN), also known as solitary circumscribed neuroma, is actually a misnomer since the lesions are not really encapsulated. It is an uncommon tumor that presents as a solitary skin-colored papule on the face of middle-aged individuals. The average size is 0.5 cm in diameter (314, 315).

PATHOLOGY (FIGURE 4-56A, B)

- Single, well-circumscribed, albeit not truly encapsulated, nodule confined to the dermis (some tumors can be multinodular)
- Spindle cells with wavy nuclei and pale cytoplasm
- Fascicles separated by a loose matrix. Characteristic artifactual clefting between the fascicles
- Some cases show degenerative changes including epithelioid appearance.
- Usually, a nerve can be noted at the base of the lesion.
- IHC: To distinguish among NF, schwannoma, and PEN, analysis of number and location of axons with anti-neurofilaments or anti-peripherin may be helpful. PEN has a 2:1 axon to other cell ratio, NF has a 4:1, and schwannoma only shows rare axons and they are located peripherally.

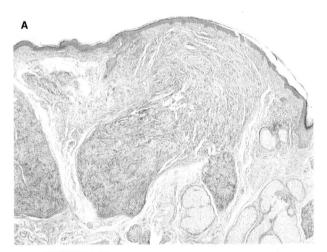 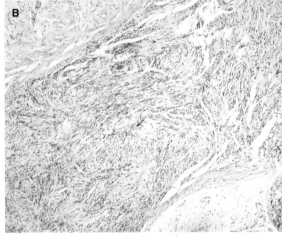

FIGURE 4-56

FIGURE 4-56   (A) Palisaded encapsulated neuroma. Multinodular tumor in the dermis composed of uniform spindle cells. (B) High power showing the pale-staining spindled cells with uniform elongated nuclei. Note the clefting in the background.

Perineurioma

Cutaneous perineurioma is a rare neoplasm. Clinically, it presents as a small skin-colored nodule mainly on the lower limbs of middle-aged adults, with predilection for females (316, 317).

PATHOLOGY (FIGURE 4-57A, B)
- Well-circumscribed, often dumbbell-shaped dermal tumor
- Bland, short, spindle-shaped cells arranged in fascicles, forming characteristic concentric collections in a whorling and a storiform pattern (onion-bulbs)
- Tumor cells may have epithelioid morphology.
- Variable hyalinization of the collagen is present and some cases show scattered, mononuclear inflammatory cells.
- IHC: The tumor cells are strongly positive for EMA and vimentin, but negative for S-100p. Some cases show focal and sometimes diffuse positivity for CD34.

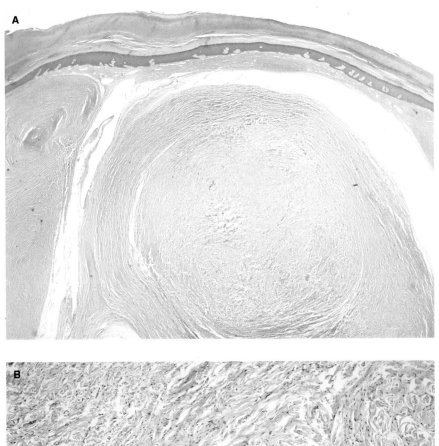

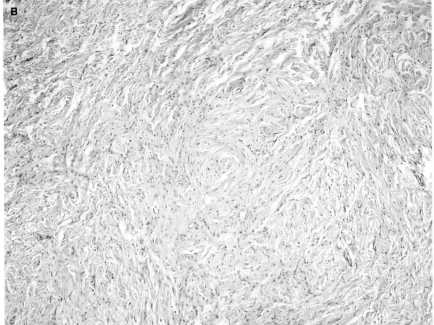

FIGURE 4-57

FIGURE 4-57   (A) Perineurioma. Low magnification shows a well-defined dermal tumor composed
of spindle cells arranged in whorling pattern. (B) Higher magnification shows
characteristic concentric collections in a subtle storiform pattern (onion-bulbs).

Granular Cell Tumor

Granular cell tumor is a benign neoplasm of disputed etiology. It more commonly presents in middle-aged to elderly patients, and shows predilection for females. It can be found in many anatomic sites, but most commonly occurs on the tongue, trunk, or extremities (318, 319).

PATHOLOGY (FIGURE 4-58A–C)

■ Nonencapsulated ill-defined lesion composed of sheets and nests of large round cells with prominent granular eosinophilic cytoplasm (PAS positive and diastase resistant)
■ Mostly dermal based but there is frequent extension into the upper subcutis
■ The tumor cells have characteristic large cytoplasmic granules, surrounded by a clear halo (pustulo-ovoid bodies of Milian).
■ There may be scattered mitotic figures.
■ The epidermis shows characteristic pseudoepitheliomatous hyperplasia; such cases may be interpreted to be invasive SCC in superficial biopsies.
■ IHC: Tumor cells are positive for S100p, CD68, and NSE. MART-1 can be positive in some cases.

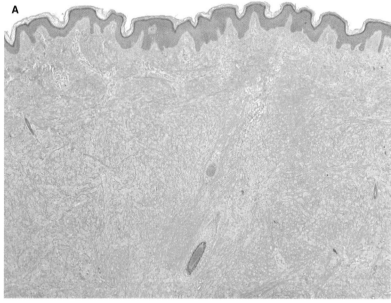

FIGURE 4-58

FIGURE 4-58   (A) Granular cell tumor. Ill-defined tumor in the dermis composed of large round cells with eosinophilic granular cytoplasm. (B) High power showing the large cytoplasm with a granular appearance. (C) Strong expression of S100 protein by the tumor cells.

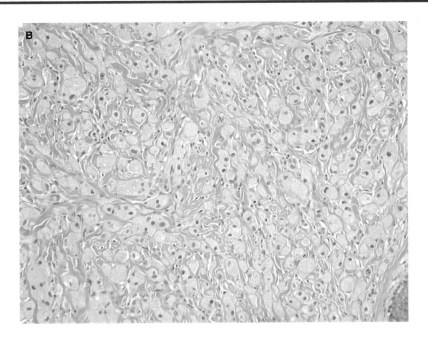

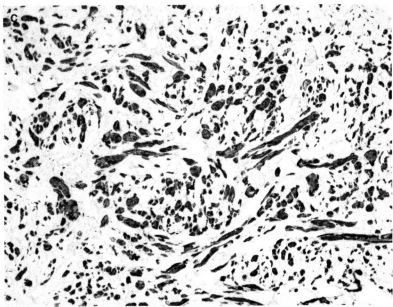

FIGURE 4-58

Nerve Sheath Myxoma

Nerve sheath myxoma, also known as myxoid neurothekeoma, is a peripheral nerve sheath tumor with a strong predilection for the extremities, fingers, and knees. It is more commonly seen in the fourth decade of life and shows a predilection for males. They may recur when incompletely excised (320–322).

PATHOLOGY (FIGURE 4-59)
- Well-defined multinodular lesions bordered by a band of dense fibrous connective tissue
- Mainly in the dermis and subcutaneous fat
- Characteristic dense myxoid matrix and scant intralesional collagen
- The lobular myxoid areas contain spindled, stellate-shaped, ring-shaped, and epithelioid Schwann cells.
- Scattered mitotic figures are common, without atypical forms.
- IHC: The tumor cells are usually positive for S-100 protein, GFAP, and CD57, thus supporting a nerve sheath differentiation.

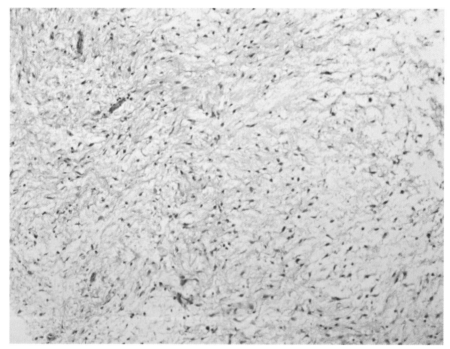

FIGURE 4-59

FIGURE 4-59   Nerve sheath myxoma: Dense myxoid matrix with spindle cells.

Cellular Neurothekeoma

Cellular neurothekeomas are rare cutaneous tumors of disputed etiology. These tumors usually present on the head, neck, and upper extremities. They are more commonly seen in children and young adults with predilection for females. Clinically, they present as long-standing asymptomatic nodule that measure up to 6 cm in diameter. There is no good evidence that cellular neurothekeomas show nerve sheath differentiation, so several authors have proposed that they have fibrohistiocytic differentiation. Despite sometimes showing atypical cytologic features, cellular neurothekeomas consistently behave in a benign fashion and only occasionally recur (generally in the setting of incompletely excised lesions located on the face) (323–325).

PATHOLOGY (FIGURE 4-60A, B)

- Poorly defined, micronodular or lobulated growth in the dermis with frequent extension into the superficial subcutis
- The lobules are composed of epithelioid and spindled cells with abundant, pale, eosinophilic cytoplasm with vesicular nuclei and mild or no cytologic atypia; however, up to 25% of cases show marked pleomorphism.
- Common, normal-shaped mitotic figures (occasionally >5/10 HPF)
- Collagen around the tumor cells sometimes appears sclerotic.
- Myxoid change can be prominent (so-called myxoid variant).
- IHC: The tumors are strongly positive for NKI-C3, NSE, S100A6, PGP9.5, and MITF, and nearly 60% show expression of SMA. Always negative for S100p or other melanocytic markers. None of these markers is specific for cellular neurothekeomas.
- Large tumor size (>2 cm) and atypical histologic features, such as high mitotic rate, pleomorphism, and infiltration of fat seem to have no clinical significance.

(continued)

Cellular Neurothekeoma (*continued*)

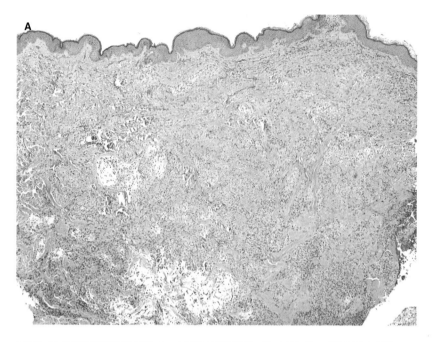

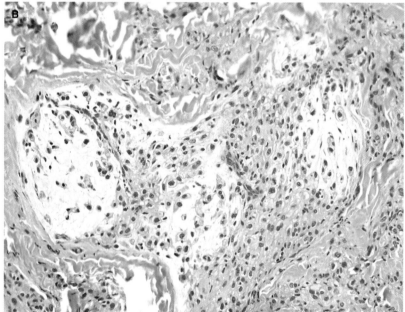

FIGURE 4-60

FIGURE 4-60   (A) Cellular neurothekeoma. Irregular dermal neoplasm composed of nests and fascicles of epithelioid and spindle cells. (B) Higher magnification showing the epithelioid cells with abundant pale and eosinophilic cytoplasm. Note the focal myxoid changes in the background.

Pigmented Lesions of the Skin

5

Lentigo Simplex

Lentigo simplex is a common pigmented lesion. It is small, brown, well defined, and may be found anywhere on the body. Lentigines are clinically important when they are associated with systemic conditions, such as Peutz–Jeghers, LEOPARD, and Carney syndromes (326).

PATHOLOGY (FIGURE 5-1)

■ Show a slight elongation of the rete ridges associated with a subtle increase in number of basal melanocytes.

■ There is mild cytologic atypia of melanocytes.

■ There may be melanophages in the papillary dermis.

■ Note: Some lesions may be in transition between lentigo and junctional nevus, sometimes designated "jentigos."

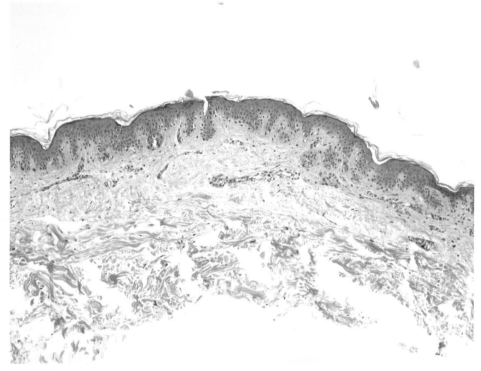

FIGURE 5-1

FIGURE 5-1   Lentigo simplex. Note the mild elongation of rete ridges with only rare basal melanocytes.

Solar Lentigo

Solar lentigos, also known as actinic lentigos, are benign, brown to black macules that commonly develop on sun-damaged skin of middle-aged to elderly individuals. These lesions are considered a clinical marker of past severe sunburn and aged skin. Ink-spot lentigo is a rare variant of lentigo, and it is particularly important because clinically it may be confused with melanoma given the irregular and reticulated appearance (327).

PATHOLOGY (FIGURE 5-2)
- The lesions are associated with solar elastosis.
- They are characterized by elongation of the rete ridges in a bud-like fashion.
- Elongated rete ridges as finger-like projections with basal hyperpigmentation and connection with adjacent rete ridges to form a reticulate pattern ("dirty finger" architecture).
- There may be slightly increased numbers of benign-appearing melanocytes at the base of the clubbed rete ridges.
- Occasional melanophages in the papillary dermis
- Cases with atypia of keratinocytes should probably be called pigmented actinic keratosis.
- Solar lentigos may undergo regression with a heavy lichenoid inflammatory infiltrate in the papillary dermis along with interface damage of the dermal epidermal junction. Such lichenoid infiltrate can be seen also in seborrheic keratosis and actinic keratosis (i.e., benign lichenoid keratosis).

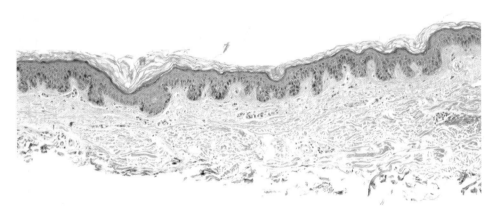

FIGURE 5-2

FIGURE 5-2   Solar lentigo. Hyperpigmented basal keratinocytes (dirty finger pattern).

Labial Melanotic Macule

Labial melanotic macule is most commonly found on the lips; however, similar lesions are also seen at other mucosal sites such as on the genitalia and hard palate. Clinically, they present as tan-brown macules, measuring less than 1.5 cm in diameter (328, 329).

PATHOLOGY (FIGURE 5-3)
- Prominent hyperpigmentation of the basal layer, usually at the tips of the rete ridges.
- Mild acanthosis
- Slightly increased, benign-appearing melanocytes
- Melanophages in the lamina propria
- Recently it has been described that some lesions with this morphology actually correspond to early stages of mucosal melanoma. For this reason it is important to correlate the histologic features with the clinical impression. If the biopsy is a sample of a large, pigmented lesion, be cautious when interpreting such a lesion.

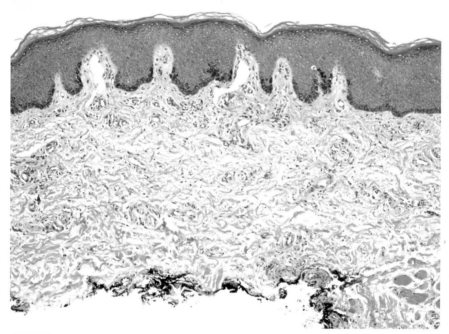

FIGURE 5-3

FIGURE 5-3   Labial melanotic macule. Acanthotic epidermis with hyperpigmentation at the tips of rete ridges.

Becker Nevus

Becker nevus is a benign, androgen-dependent lesion that is usually acquired; however, some cases are congenital. The lesions have an onset during or after puberty and are more commonly seen in males. Clinically, they present as unilateral, tan brown macules with hypertrichosis. They are more common in the chest, shoulder, or upper arm but can occur in any anatomic location (330, 331).

PATHOLOGY (FIGURE 5-4)

- The epidermis shows mild hyperkeratosis, acanthosis, papillomatosis, and elongation of the epidermal ridges with increased pigmentation in the basal layer.
- Some cases show flattening of the epidermis and fusion of elongated rete ridges.
- Melanocytes often appear mildly increased in number within epidermis, and in superficial dermis there are melanophages.
- In some cases the reticular dermis shows large numbers of enlarged, smooth muscle bundles.
- Increased number of hair follicles and sebaceous glands.

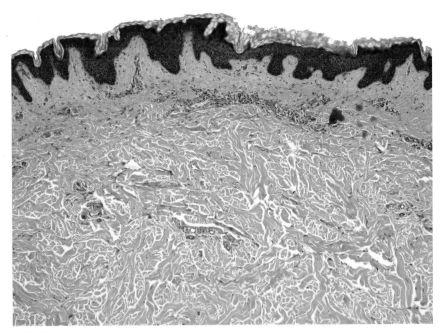

FIGURE 5-4

FIGURE 5-4   Becker nevus. Mild acanthosis and papillomatosis of epidermis. Note the subtle superficial perivascular chronic inflammatory cell infiltrate.

Melanocytic Nevi

Melanocytic nevus is a benign melanocytic proliferation that usually presents in childhood and adolescence but can also be congenital. Melanocytes are normally present in the basal layer of the epidermis and with certain forms of stimulation, such as sun exposure, the density of melanocytes in normal epithelium may increase. Melanocytic nevi represent proliferations of melanocytes that are in contact with each other, forming small collections, that is, nests. Malignant transformation can be seen in these lesions; however, this is a rare phenomenon. Large congenital melanocytic nevi have a greater risk of progression to malignancy. Melanocytic nevi are more common in individuals with pale skin and light-colored eyes. Acquired melanocytic nevi are generally less than 1 cm in diameter and evenly pigmented. Congenital melanocytic nevi vary considerably in size and are classified as small (<1 cm), intermediate (1–3 cm), or large/giant (>3 cm) (332–334).

There are two concepts regarding the etiology of melanocytic nevi. Most authors consider that melanocytes first proliferate in the epidermis (junctional nevi) and then colonize the dermis (compound and intradermal nevi). However, other authors have suggested that melanocytic nevi may come from perineural cells that develop melanocytic features, including melanin production (335).

PATHOLOGY

- Junctional nevus: Well-formed nests of melanocytes, mainly located at the dermal epidermal junction (usually within the tips on the rete ridges). The melanocytes are oval to cuboidal in shape, with clear cytoplasm containing a variable amount of melanin pigment (Figure 5-5).

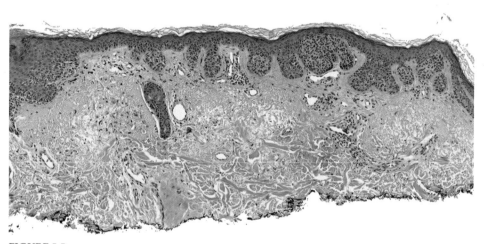

FIGURE 5-5

FIGURE 5-5   Junctional nevus. Uniform and regular melanocytic nests in epidermis.

■ Compound nevus: This type has both a junctional and an intradermal component. The melanocytes in the upper dermis are usually epithelioid in shape with melanin pigment in the cytoplasm, and deeper cells are often smaller and contain less melanin ("maturation" phenomenon). As a rule, the junctional component does not usually extend beyond the dermal component in the majority of acquired nevi (as seen in dysplastic nevus); however, "shoulder" can sometimes be present in a compound nevus, particularly in genital regions and in congenital lesions, and thus its presence alone does not establish a diagnosis of dysplastic nevus. The overlying epidermis sometimes may show marked acanthosis with hyperkeratosis, thus imparting a seborrheic keratosis-like appearance. These nevi have been termed keratotic melanocytic nevi (papillomatous melanocytic nevi) (336). Mitotic activity can rarely be identified in the dermal component of an acquired melanocytic nevus (but not forms), especially in nevi in pregnant women (Figure 5-6).

(text continued on page 272)

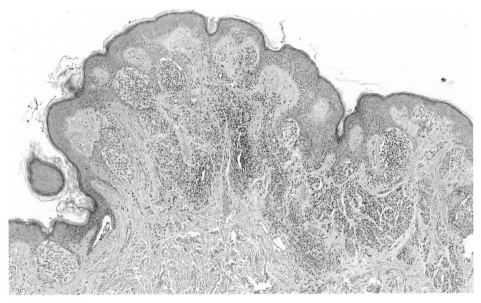

FIGURE 5-6

FIGURE 5-6   Compound nevus. Note both the junctional and intradermal component.

Chapter 5: Pigmented Lesions of the Skin

Melanocytic Nevi (*continued*)

■ Intradermal nevi: In this type the melanocytes are confined to the dermis. The cells usually show intranuclear pseudo-inclusions. Multinucleate melanocytes can be identified throughout the lesion. In the deeper parts of the lesion the nevus cells may adopt a spindle/neuroid appearance and may be arranged in structures resembling Meissner corpuscles. The presence of pseudo-vascular spaces may give an angiomatous-like appearance (Figure 5-7A–E).

(*text continued on page 274*)

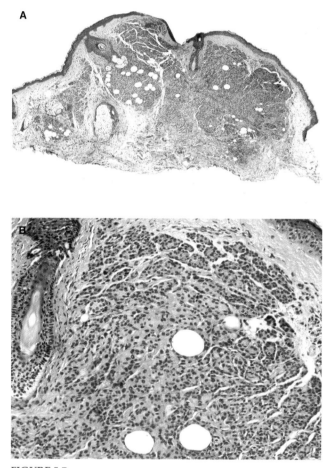

FIGURE 5-7

FIGURE 5-7   (A) Intradermal nevus. Low magnification showing intradermal melanocytes with normal maturation toward the base of the lesion. (B) Higher magnification showing epithelioid melanocytes with lack of cytologic atypia. (C) Note the characteristic stroma that is focally myxoid and edematous. (D) Some intradermal nevi will show characteristic multinucleated melanocytes. (E) Note the marked neurotization in this intradermal nevus.

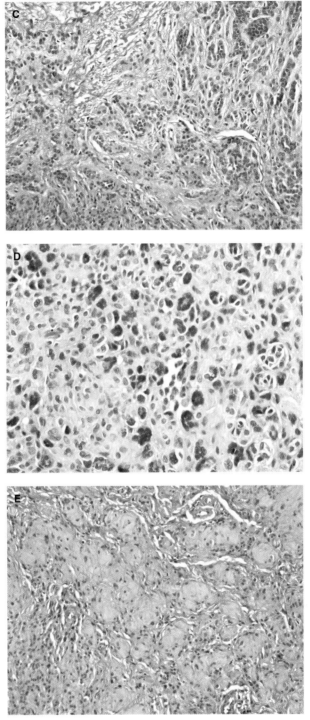

FIGURE 5-7

Melanocytic Nevi (*continued*)

VARIANTS

■ Congenital nevi: These nevi are present at birth and may be multiple. They are classified according to their size as small (up to 1.5 cm), medium (from 1.5 cm to 20 cm) and large (>20 cm). Histologically, they usually extend deeply into the dermis and sometimes into the subcutaneous tissue. They characteristically involve the arrector pili muscle and surround adnexal structures (Figure 5-8).

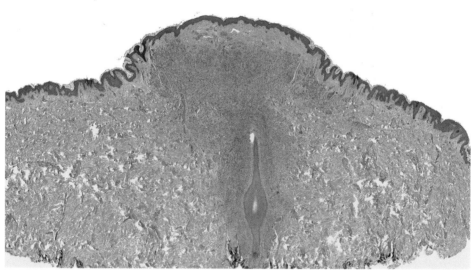

FIGURE 5-8

FIGURE 5-8   Congenital intradermal nevus. Note the marked accentuation of the melanocytes around the hair follicle.

■ Sutton (Halo) nevi: This variant can be junctional, compound, or intradermal but is more commonly compound. The term Meyerson is used when there is an eczematous halo surrounding the nevus. It occurs more often in young adults. Sutton is used when the lesion presents as a pigmented nevus surrounded by a hypopigmented border. It arises most frequently in the second decade and is more commonly seen on the back. Histologically, the nevus is usually compound and infiltrated by lymphocytes and histiocytes with occasional plasma cells. Epithelioid histiocytes can sometimes be found within the inflammatory cell infiltrate (Figure 5-9A–C).

(text continued on page 276)

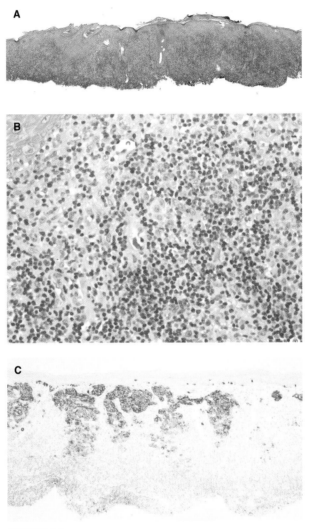

FIGURE 5-9

FIGURE 5-9   (A) Halo nevus. Note the compound nevus with a dense lichenoid inflammatory infiltrate. (B) Higher magnification showing melanocytes admixed with many lymphocytes. (C) MART-1 immunohistochemistry stain highlights the melanocytes.

Melanocytic Nevi (*continued*)

■ Balloon cell nevus: This type results from melanosome degeneration resulting in cytoplasmic vacuolation. The lesion shows no particular characteristic clinical features. Histologically, it is composed by large nevus cells, with clear foamy cytoplasm and a central nucleus. Multinucleate balloon cells are often present. The diagnosis should be made to lesions containing a predominance of balloon cells (>50%), as nevi may show few foci of balloon cell change (Figure 5-10A, B).

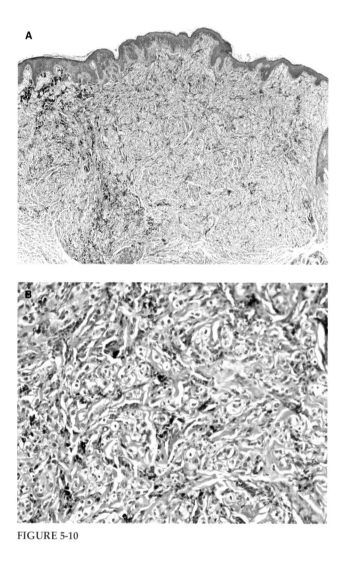

FIGURE 5-10

FIGURE 5-10 (A) Balloon cell nevus. Compound nevus with many cells that have a foamy cytoplasm. (B) Higher magnification showing the melanocytes with ample foamy cytoplasm.

- Recurrent nevus ("pseudomelanoma" of Ackerman): It refers to the appearance of a melanocytic lesion after incomplete excision of a previous benign or dysplastic nevus. Usually it is seen after a shave biopsy or after trauma (irritation) and laser treatment. Histologically, the lesion usually shows remnants of the previous nevus and a dermal scar. In the epidermis, the melanocytes show mild to moderate nuclear pleomorphism, and there may be focal pagetoid spread, but it should be circumscribed to the area immediately above the scar. The rete ridge pattern overlying the scar is usually effaced. These lesions may display an abnormal pattern of expression of HMB45 antigen, since the dermal component may become strongly positive (337) (Figure 5-11A, B).
- Melanocytic nevi at special sites: Nevi at special sites (scalp, ear, breast, genital, flexural areas) usually show histological features similar to acquired nevi seen elsewhere; however, a subset of such nevi may show histological features that can mimic melanoma. These changes include architectural as well as cytological abnormalities such as large nests of melanocytes with variation in shape, dyscohesive nests, and mild atypia of melanocytes. Mitotic figures are not characteristic in such lesions.

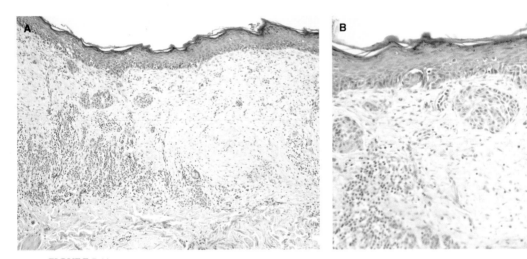

FIGURE 5-11

FIGURE 5-11   (A) Recurrent nevus. Note the scar in the dermis and the remnant nevus. (B) There are architectural changes in the epidermis including the cytologic atypia, discohesion, and single cell proliferation.

Acral Nevi

Acral nevi can show either similar or identical histologic changes to acquired nevi, or they can show unusual features (possibly related to the presence of skin markings and anatomic site), which can be interpreted as melanoma (338–340).

PATHOLOGY (FIGURE 5-12A, B)
- These nevi tend to be symmetric.
- Lentiginous and nested component along the dermal–epidermal junction
- The nests are variable in size and shape and are vertically orientated.
- Characteristic transepidermal elimination of nests
- Retraction artifact around the melanocytic nests
- The melanocytes have pale-staining cytoplasm and vesicular nuclei, showing only mild atypia.
- Tendency of melanocytes to be scattered throughout the entire thickness of the epidermis, giving the impression of pagetoid spreading, is not uncommon. Proliferation through higher levels of the epidermis may extend laterally beyond the limits of the intradermal component. This phenomenon is more commonly seen in young patients.
- Evenly distributed pigmentation in the stratum corneum
- The dermal component shows normal maturation with depth.
- Note: Pagetoid upward migration can be prominent in some cases ("MANIAC" nevi = melanocytic acral nevi with intraepidermal ascent of cells).

A

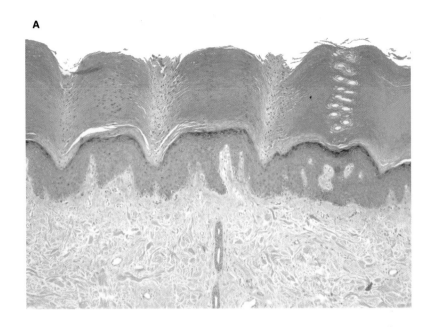

B

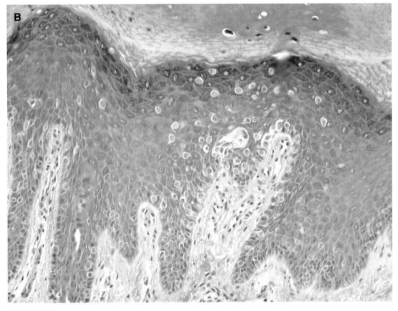

FIGURE 5-12

FIGURE 5-12   (A) Acral nevus (junctional): Small and symmetric junctional nevus with lentiginous growth and transepidermal elimination of melanocytes. Note the even distribution of pigmentation in the stratum corneum. (B) Melanocytic acral nevus with intraepidermal ascent of cells (MANIAC). This is an acral nevus in a young White patient that measured 4 mm. Note the characteristic intraepidermal growth of melanocytes with marked pagetoid upward migration.

Deep Penetrating Nevi

Deep penetrating nevus (DPN), also known as plexiform spindle cell nevus, is a distinct variant of melanocytic nevus. The most frequent sites of origin are the shoulder, face, and neck but it can also be located in other parts of the body. DPN generally presents between the second and third decades of life as a solitary dark, irregularly, papule of less than 1 cm in diameter and shows a slight female predominance (341–344).

PATHOLOGY (FIGURE 5-13A, B)

- A distinctive feature at scanning magnification is the sharply demarcated, circumscribed, often symmetrical wedge-shaped configuration of the lesion, with the base toward the epidermis and the tip toward the reticular dermis/subcutis.
- The lesion is usually compound with small intraepidermal nests.
- The lesion is composed of loose nests and vertically oriented fascicles of pigmented epithelioid and, less frequently, short spindle-shaped melanocytes.
- Frequent perineural extension and infiltration of the arrector pili muscle.
- Rare or no mitoses. The presence of more than occasional mitoses is suggestive of melanoma.
- Frequent nuclear vacuoles/pseudoinclusions

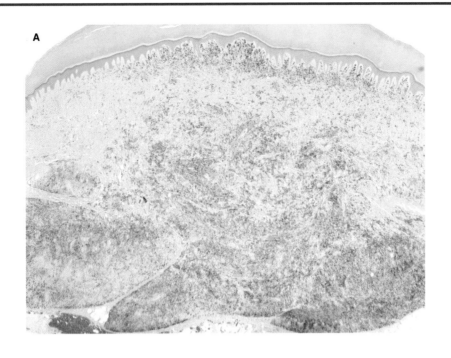

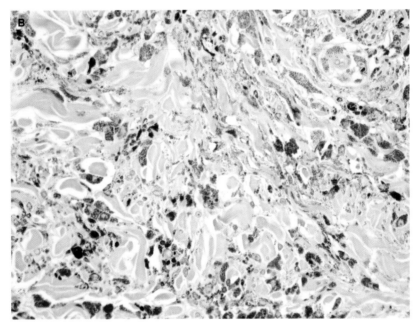

FIGURE 5-13

FIGURE 5-13 (A) Deep penetrating nevus. Loose nests and fascicles of pigmented epithelioid and spindle-shaped melanocytes in the dermis. (B) Epithelioid and spindle-shaped melanocytes with intermixed heavily pigmented melanophages.

Dysplastic Nevus (Clark Nevus)

Dysplastic nevi (Clark nevi) are acquired nevi with characteristic histologic and clinical features. Patients with multiple dysplastic nevi have an increased risk for melanoma, and dysplastic nevi themselves have at least some potential for malignant transformation. Dysplastic nevi are usually larger than ordinary nevi, irregular in shape, and often show uneven color with dark brown centers. The lifetime risk of a normal individual of developing a melanoma is approximately 0.6%; however, in patients with multiple dysplastic nevi, this risk increases close to 10%. Also, the risk of developing melanoma in patients with dysplastic nevus syndrome is more than 50% in melanoma-prone families (could be close to 100% in patients with at least two close relatives with melanoma) (345–348).

Dysplastic nevus syndrome: This syndrome refers to the familial or sporadic occurrence of multiple dysplastic nevi in an individual. These patients have a tendency to develop large numbers of dysplastic nevi (80 or more) and are associated with an increased incidence of melanoma. The familial variant is inherited as an autosomal dominant disease with incomplete penetrance and is associated with mutations of the *CDKN2A* gene on 9p21–22 (40% of families). Patients with dysplastic nevus syndrome have an increased risk of developing other neoplasms, especially pancreatic cancer (349, 350).

PATHOLOGY (FIGURE 5-14A–C)
- Dysplastic nevi can be junctional or compound.
- Dysplastic nevi are characterized by architectural disorder and cytological atypia.
- They show characteristic extension of the epidermal component beyond the lateral border of the dermal melanocytes ("shoulder" phenomenon).
- Fusion of the rete ridges (bridging).
- Intraepidermal lentiginous hyperplasia with marked elongation of the rete ridges.
- Melanocytes are located not only at the tips of the rete ridges forming nests but along the lateral sides of the rete as single cells (lentiginous hyperplasia).
- Nests are irregular in shape.
- Dusty pigmentation of melanocytes.
- Uncommon mitotic figures, restricted to the upper dermis.
- There may be focal pagetoid upward migration, and it is usually restricted to the center of the lesion (prominent pagetoid upward migration should raise the possibility of melanoma).
- Diverse degrees of cytologic atypia (mild, moderate, and severe)
- Characteristically lamellar and concentric fibroplasia of the papillary dermis
- Patchy superficial perivascular lymphohistiocytic infiltrate

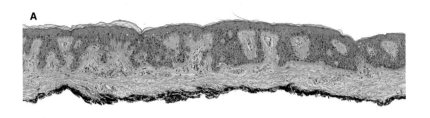

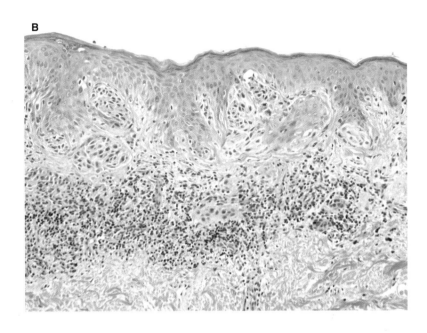

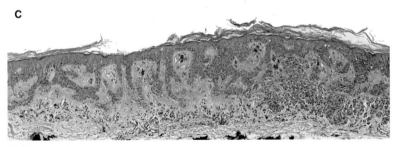

FIGURE 5-14

FIGURE 5-14   (A) Junctional dysplastic nevus. Note the bridging of rete ridges, single-cell
melanocytic proliferation, and the stromal changes (fibroplasia). (B) Junctional
dysplastic nevus. In this example note the host response (inflammatory infiltrate in
the dermis). (C) Compound dysplastic nevus. Shouldering phenomenon in addition to
bridging, single-cell proliferation, fibroplasia, and scattered melanophages.

Spitz Nevus

Spitz nevus is a biologically benign nevus that can be difficult to distinguish on histologic grounds from melanoma. Clinically, it presents as a solitary, rapidly growing, flesh-colored papule on the face, trunk, or extremities of children and adolescents (351–355).

PATHOLOGY (FIGURE 5-15A–C)

■ Most Spitz nevi are compound; however, they can be junctional or intradermal.

■ Lateral circumscription and symmetrical

■ The melanocytes are epithelioid or spindle cells, or a mixture of the two.

■ Some cases show prominent, pseudoepitheliomatous hyperplasia.

■ In lesions composed of spindle cells, the cells are arranged in fascicles and have a large ample eosinophilic cytoplasm with eosinophilic nucleoli.

■ The epithelioid cells can show bizarre shapes and are often arranged in vertically orientated nests ("hanging bananas"), often surrounded from the surrounding epidermis by a peripheral, retraction artifact.

■ Rare single melanocytes with pagetoid upward migration within the epidermis, especially at the center of the lesion.

■ There is maturation of nevus cells. The nevus cells in deeper dermis have a characteristic single-cell infiltrating ("Indian-file" distribution) among collagen bundles.

■ Kamino bodies (eosinophilic globules) are typically seen at the dermal epidermal junction (PAS positive). They are composed of laminin, type IV collagen, and fibronectin and, therefore, do not represent apoptotic keratinocytes.

■ Mitotic figures can be seen in the superficial dermal portion of the tumor (especially in younger patients). Mitotic figures seen in the deeper portion of the lesion should favor a diagnosis of melanoma.

■ Edema of the upper dermis and superficial telangiectatic vessels.

■ Superficial perivascular and a lichenoid inflammatory reaction.

■ Note: Irritated/traumatized Spitz nevi may display atypical features including intraepidermal spread at the lateral sides of the lesion. Thus the presence of previous trauma or irritation (parakeratosis, fibrin, and hemorrhage within the stratum corneum) should be taken into consideration before establishing a diagnosis of melanoma.

(*text continued on page 286*)

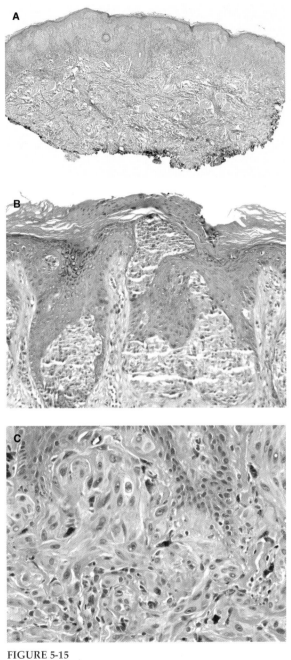

FIGURE 5-15

FIGURE 5-15   (A) Spitz nevus (compound). Low magnification shows striking symmetry.
Note the focal, subtle lichenoid inflammatory response at the base of the lesion.
(B) Large intraepidermal nests composed of spindle and epithelioid cells. Note there
is irritation and it is not uncommon to see pagetoid nesting in the center of the lesion.
(C) Epithelioid cells with bizarre shapes and prominent, central, single nucleolus
(ganglion-like).

Spitz Nevus *(continued)*

VARIANTS

■ *Desmoplastic Spitz nevus*: This is a rare variant of a Spitz nevus. It presents as a brown papule, most often on the extremities. Histologically, the lesion is centered in the dermis forming a wedge-shaped infiltrate of a subtle population of pleomorphic spindle and epithelioid cells with abundant, eosinophilic cytoplasm. Intranuclear cytoplasmic pseudoinclusions are often identified. The melanocytes characteristically mature with depth and disperse among collagen fibers. Mitoses are rarely seen. The stroma is extremely dense and sometimes hyalinized (Figure 5-16A, B).

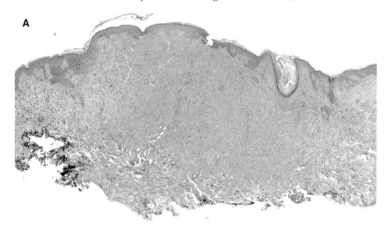

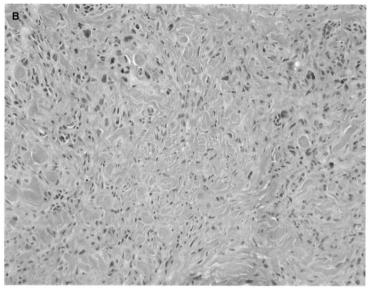

FIGURE 5-16

FIGURE 5-16   (A) Desmoplastic Spitz nevus. Subtle infiltrate of relatively small cells in the dermis in a wedge-shaped pattern. (B) High power shows spindle and epithelioid cells with eosinophilic cytoplasm. Note the rare intranuclear inclusions.

■ *Pigmented spindle cell nevus of Reed*: It is a benign melanocytic lesion and some authors classify this nevus as a variant of Spitz nevus. It is most commonly seen in younger patients and shows a female predominance. It is frequently located on the lower limbs (thigh), upper limbs, and trunk. Histologically, the lesion may be junctional or compound. It is symmetrical and sharply demarcated. The junctional nests have a characteristic pear-shaped configuration and are composed of clusters of plump, spindle cells with elongated vesicular nuclei. Some cases have dendritic melanocytes and Kamino bodies. The lesions are heavily pigmented (Figure 5-17A, B).

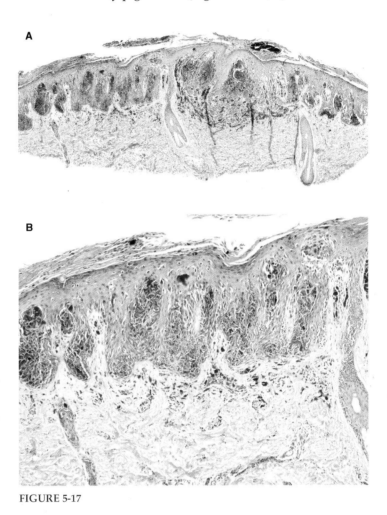

FIGURE 5-17

FIGURE 5-17   (A) Pigmented spindle cell nevus of Reed. Symmetrical and sharply demarcated compound lesion. Note the junctional nests have a pear-shaped configuration with marked pigmentation. (B) The nests have clusters of plump spindle cells.

Dermal Melanocytoses

"MONGOLIAN" SPOT

"Mongolian" spot is a slate-colored patch usually located on the sacral area of infants. It is usually present at birth or appears within the first weeks of life and typically disappears spontaneously within 4 years; however, it can persist for life. It is more common in certain races, particularly Chinese and Japanese. Larger lesions can be a marker of an underlying storage disease, such as Hurler syndrome, GM1 type I gangliosidosis, and mucolipidosis type II. These lesions are thought to represent arrested migration of melanocytes from the neural crest to the epidermis (356, 357).

PATHOLOGY
■ The lesion is composed of a subtle population of intradermal dendritic spindle cell pigmented melanocytes.

NEVUS OF OTA AND ITO

Nevus of Ota is a unilateral benign dendritic melanocytic lesion located in the distribution of the ophthalmic and maxillary divisions of the trigeminal nerve. It is more commonly seen in females. In most patients, the sclera and conjunctiva are also involved. Over half of these lesions are present at birth, but some cases may appear at puberty. Nevus of Ito is a rare lesion that is located in the supraclavicular and deltoid regions, and sometimes in the scapular area. This lesion can be seen in association with nevus of Ota (358, 359).

PATHOLOGY (FIGURE 5-18)
■ The epidermis can display hyperpigmentation and increased numbers of melanocytes (but no well-defined nests).
■ The lesion is located at dermis and composed of heavily pigmented, spindle-shaped, dendritic melanocytes.

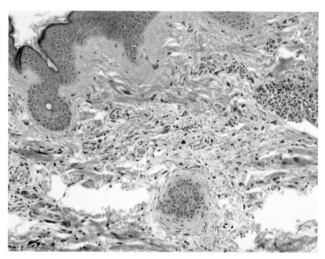

FIGURE 5-18

FIGURE 5-18   Nevus of Ota. Note the subtle population of pigmented, dendritic cell in the dermis.

BLUE NEVUS

This is a common, benign melanocytic lesion that presents as a solitary blue-black macule or papule (1 cm in diameter), most commonly on the dorsal area of hands and feet (360, 361).

PATHOLOGY (FIGURE 5-19A, B)

- The lesion is located in the reticular dermis.
- Occasionally there may be a junctional component or a standard intradermal nevus. Such lesions are combined nevus.
- Population of elongated, finely branching, bipolar dendritic melanocytes in the interstitial dermis
- Mitotic figures are rarely seen, and there is no pleomorphism.
- Interspersed, densely pigmented melanophages
- The melanocytes can be seen around adnexal structures, blood vessels, and nerves.
- Dermal fibrosis

(*text continued on page 290*)

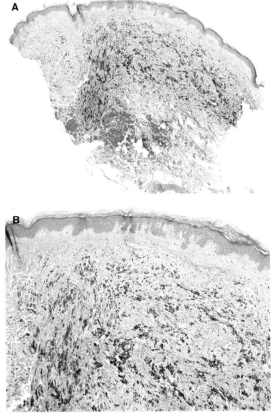

FIGURE 5-19

FIGURE 5-19   (A) Blue nevus. Heavily pigmented spindled cell in the dermis. (B) Note the increased number of dendritic melanocytes in the dermis accompanied by pigmented melanophages.

Dermal Melanocytoses (*continued*)

CELLULAR BLUE NEVUS

Cellular blue nevi are uncommon melanocytic lesions. They show a female predominance most commonly in young adults. Clinically, they present as slowly growing, grayish dome-shaped papules/nodules (1–2 cm in diameter). These lesions can be located in the scalp, face, trunk, and extremities; however, the majority of cases are located in the sacrococcygeal region and buttocks (360, 362).

PATHOLOGY (FIGURE 5-20A–D)

- Well-defined nodular mass that fills the dermis and into the subcutaneous fat (dumbbell architecture)
- The tumors characteristically show a biphasic pattern composed of an admixture of plump, spindle cells with pale cytoplasm and elongated spindle cell dendritic melanocytes with variable pigmentation.
- Commonly densely pigmented melanophages
- Sclerotic stroma
- Very rare mitotic figures
- Some tumors may show nodules of spindle-shaped melanocytes surrounded by dense collagenous septa
- Occasional perineural invasion

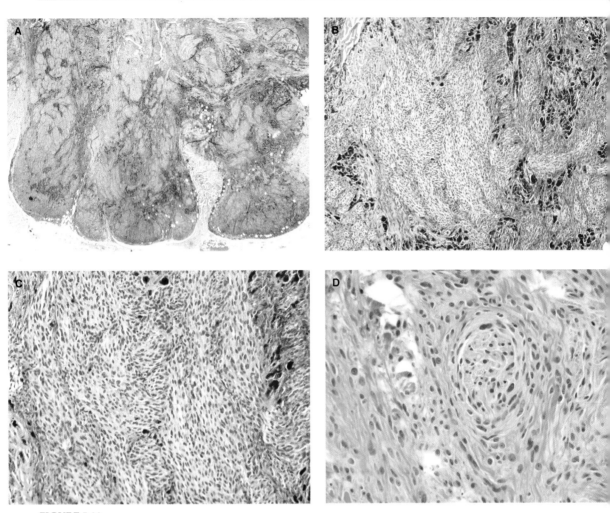

FIGURE 5-20

FIGURE 5-20   (A) Cellular blue nevus. Large nodular mass occupying the entire dermis and focally involving the subcutaneous fat. (B) The tumor is composed of a dual cell population of spindled and epithelioid cells admixed with heavily pigmented melanophages. (C) Elongated spindled cells with large oval vesicular nuclei. (D) Note the perineurial involvement.

Melanoma

Melanoma is one of the most serious forms of skin cancer and the sixth most common cancer in North America. Melanoma is a disease predominantly seen in adults but occasionally may affect children. The development of melanoma is multifactorial and related to multiple risk factors, including excessive exposure to ultraviolet light (the most important risk factor), fair complexion, childhood sunburns, an increased number of dysplastic nevi, family history of melanoma, and older age. Associated risk factors for the development of melanoma include xeroderma pigmentosum, familial dysplastic nevus syndrome, and possibly immunosuppression. Melanoma may develop in precursor melanocytic nevi (acquired or dysplastic nevi); however, >70% of cases arise de novo. In Caucasians, the leg (especially the calf) is the site of predilection in females, whereas the back is in males. In African American and Hispanic individuals, the most common site is the plantar foot. Clinically, worrisome signs for melanoma include a changing mole, variation in color, increase in diameter, asymmetric borders, and ulceration. The prognosis of patients with melanoma is primarily determined by the thickness of the primary tumor (Breslow), presence of ulceration, mitotic rate, and presence and extent of metastatic disease (lymph node involvement). Breslow thickness is the most important single prognostic indicator, and it is measured from the upper portion of the granular cell layer to the deepest point of invasion (in ulcerated tumors, it is measured from the base of the ulcer). Familial melanoma has been associated with *CDKN2A* (9p21) (363–365).

There are four main subtypes of melanoma: superficial spreading, nodular, lentigo maligna, and acral lentiginous.

LENTIGO MALIGNA MELANOMA
Typically it arises in sun-damaged areas of the skin in older individuals, mostly on the head, neck, and arms (chronically sun-damaged skin). The in situ lesion is usually present for 10 to 15 years before invasive tumor develops (364, 365).

PATHOLOGY (FIGURE 5-21A–C)
- The epidermis is usually atrophic, and the dermis shows marked solar elastosis
- It is composed of an asymmetric population of atypical melanocytes located along the dermal epidermal junction.
- Melanocytes usually show a retraction artifact from the surrounding keratinocytes and have pleomorphic, hyperchromatic, angulated nuclei.
- Characteristic involvement of eccrine ducts and the outer root sheath epithelium of hair follicles
- Multinucleated giant melanocytes ("star-burst giant cells") may be present at the basal layer of the epidermis.

(text continued on page 294)

FIGURE 5-21   (A) Lentigo maligna melanoma (in situ). Thin (atrophic) epidermis with an atypical population of intraepidermal melanocytes showing confluent growth, irregularly shaped nests, and involvement of follicles. (B) Intraepidermal confluent growth pattern and the marked melanocytic atypia. Note the extension into skin adnexa (follicles). (C) Higher magnification showing the atypical melanocytes with irregular hyperchromatic nuclei.

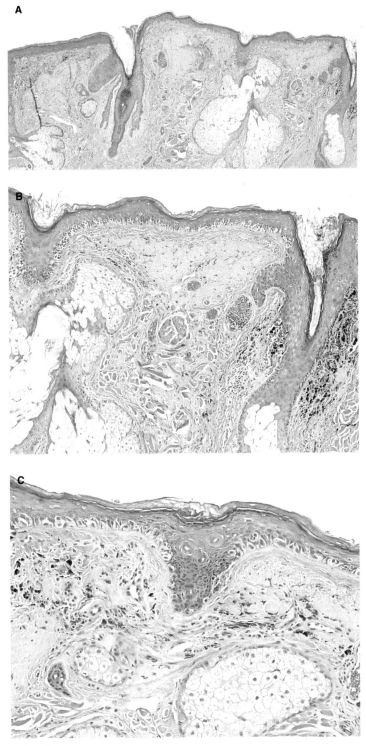

A

B

C

FIGURE 5-21

Melanoma *(continued)*

■ Rarely marked pagetoid spread.
■ Invasive tumor can be multifocal and is usually of the spindle cell type (it may be desmoplastic).

SUPERFICIAL SPREADING MELANOMA

This is the most common subtype of melanoma. It is most common on the trunk in men and on the legs in women. One-fourth of superficial spreading melanomas are found in association with a preexisting nevus. Clinically, it presents as a flat or elevated brown lesion with variegates pigmentation (364).

PATHOLOGY (FIGURE 5-22A–D)

■ The radial growth phase shows an asymmetrical proliferation of atypical melanocytes arranged in single cells and in clusters throughout all levels of the epidermis (pagetoid cells).
■ The melanocytic cells are epithelioid with abundant cytoplasm, often showing dusty melanin pigmentation. These atypical melanocytes often show pleomorphic vesicular nuclei with prominent eosinophilic nucleoli.
■ Invasive tumor is mostly of the epithelioid type with easily encountered atypical mitoses.

(text continued on page 296)

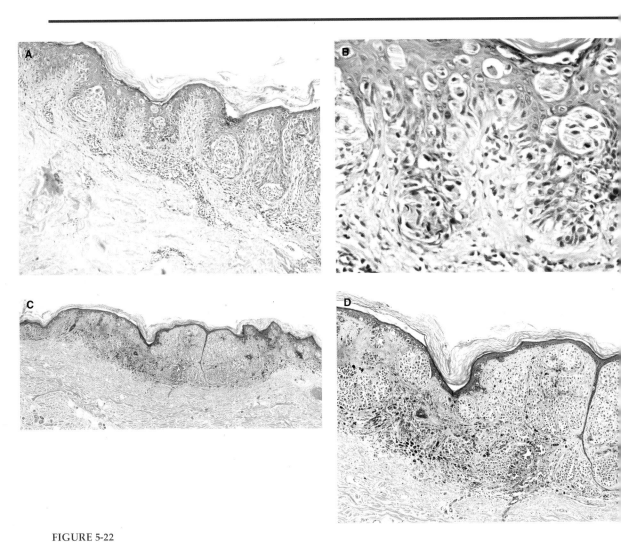

FIGURE 5-22

FIGURE 5-22   (A) Superficial spreading melanoma (in situ). In contrast with lentigo maligna, the
epidermis has preserved rete ridges. Melanocytes are widely scattered throughout the
epidermis and show marked pagetoid upward migration. (B) Higher magnification of
the epithelioid melanocytes with dusky cytoplasm and pleomorphic nuclei. Note the
pagetoid upward migration. (C) Large intraepidermal nests and atypical infiltrate of
melanocytes in dermis. (D) Higher magnification of the atypical nests in the dermis.
Note the lack of maturation toward the base (cells have the same size and shape).

Melanoma (*continued*)

NODULAR MELANOMA

This variant is detected with a vertical growth phase and has no radial growth phase. It shows a relatively poor prognosis (due to the thickness) and affects more males than females (2:1). The trunk and legs are most commonly involved. Clinically, it presents as a dark brown to black papule, which may ulcerate and bleed with minor trauma (366).

PATHOLOGY (FIGURE 5-23A–C)

- This variant has no evidence of radial growth phase (the lesion does not show an intraepidermal component beyond three epidermal ridges).
- Large vertical growth phase.
- The dermal component is composed by epithelioid or spindle cells.
- Mitotic figures are usually frequent and may be of atypical shape.

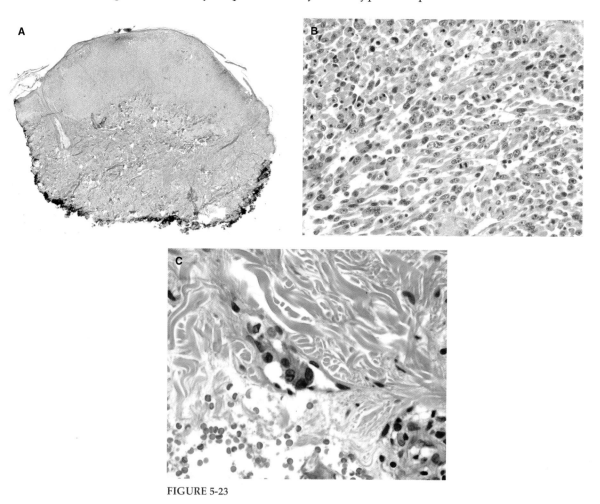

FIGURE 5-23

FIGURE 5-23 (A) Nodular melanoma. Dermal nodule without a radial growth phase. (B) High power showing the atypical epithelioid cells with marked pleomorphism. Note the atypical mitotic figures. (C) Vascular invasion.

ACRAL LENTIGINOUS (MUCOSAL) MELANOMA

This is the least common type of melanoma in White individuals; however, it is the most common type of melanoma in African American, Asian, and Hispanic individuals. They arise most commonly on palmar, plantar, subungual, and occasionally, mucosal surfaces. Not all melanomas arising in acral sites are acral lentiginous melanomas since they should also show the characteristic histologic criteria (see below). This type of melanoma is most commonly seen in older females (367).

PATHOLOGY (FIGURE 5-24A, B)

■ It shows a radial growth phase that can be subtle; it may look misleadingly benign, with a lentiginous pattern of small melanocytes.

■ With progression, the lower levels of the epidermis show large numbers of atypical melanocytes, typically pigmented with dendritic shape, pleomorphic, and usually with marked pagetoid spread.

■ Some of these melanocytes are plump with a surrounding clear halo.

■ Focal junctional nests.

■ Frequent lichenoid infiltrate.

■ The invasive component may consist of epithelioid cells or spindle cells and may display a desmoplastic stromal response.

■ Relatively frequent neurotropism.

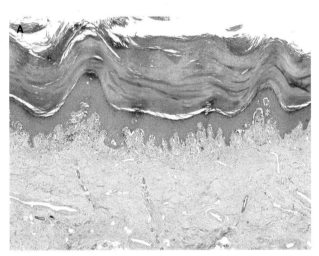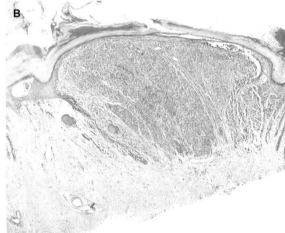

FIGURE 5-24

FIGURE 5-24   (A) Acral lentiginous melanoma. In situ component showing irregular acanthosis and hyperplasia of epidermis. The intraepidermal cells are distributed in a lentiginous pattern (single cells along the dermal–epidermal junction). (B) Acral lentiginous melanoma with prominent dermal invasion.

Desmoplastic Melanoma

Desmoplastic melanoma (DM) is a rare variant. It tends to occur on sun-exposed areas of the head, neck, or upper back, as well as in acral locations, in older individuals. Most cases arise in elderly males. DM is often associated with a lentigo maligna but can develop in the absence of a clinically detectable precursor lesion. When pure (lesions having more than 90% of the invasive component with desmoplastic features), DM appears to behave clinically more like a sarcoma with high local recurrence and low metastatic potential (the lung is the most common site rather than regional lymph nodes). Poor prognostic indicators are high mitotic rate, tumor thickness, and inadequate excision (368, 369).

PATHOLOGY (FIGURE 5-25A–D)

- These tumors are characterized by an infiltrative, paucicellular, spindle cell proliferation with marked fibromyxoid stroma.
- The infiltrate often extends into the subcutaneous fat and even into the skeletal muscle and bone.
- The tumor cells show hyperchromatic, elongated nuclei, and their morphology closely resembles that of fibroblasts seen in a scar.
- The spindle cells form long fascicles that are arranged in acute angles to the horizontal axis of the epidermis; there are also single, dispersed spindle cells.
- Occasional mitotic figures
- Characteristic lymphoid nodular aggregates
- Careful examination of the overlying epidermis shows features of atypical melanocytic hyperplasia or lentigo maligna in at least 50% of cases.
- Common perineural invasion
- IHC: DM usually shows strong positivity for S-100p and NSE. HMB-45 can sometimes be positive in the superficial portion of the tumor cells; however, most of the time it is totally negative. MART-1 shows positivity in 24% to 60% of cases (negativity for MART1 in a spindle-cell melanocytic lesion points to the diagnosis). Antityrosinase is negative in DM. p75, SOX10, and smooth muscle actin are often positive.

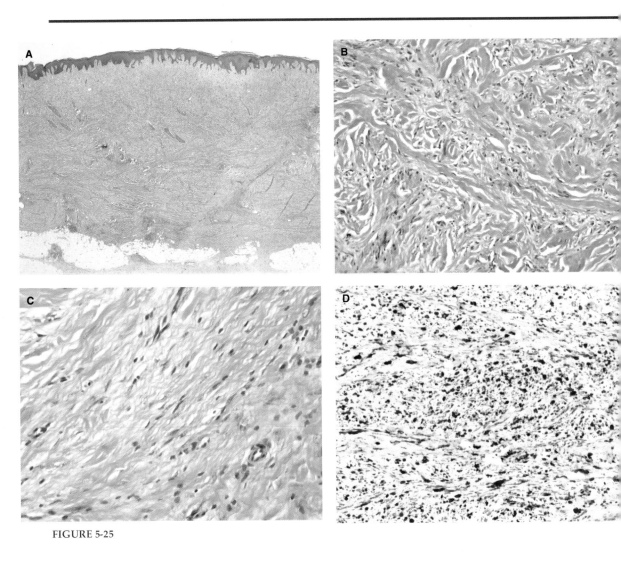

FIGURE 5-25

FIGURE 5-25   (A) Desmoplastic melanoma. Lower magnification showing a subtle spindle cell tumor
in the dermis resembling a dermal scar. Note the characteristic, scattered lymphoid
aggregates. (B) Higher magnification showing spindle cells with only mild cytologic
atypia. (C) Higher magnification of the spindle cells in areas reminiscent of a scar.
(D) S100p expression.

Cutaneous Metastatic Melanoma

Melanoma usually metastasizes first to the regional lymph nodes and then to skin, subcutaneous soft tissue, lung, and brain. Metastatic melanoma involving the skin appears as a dermal nodule or plaque-like lesion, often in close proximity to the primary tumor (370).

PATHOLOGY (FIGURE 5-26A–C)
■ Well-circumscribed, nonencapsulated nodule, in the dermis and subcutaneous tissue.
■ Rarely there may be epidermal involvement (epidermotropic metastasis).
■ Most cells are similar to each one (monomorphous).
■ Usually similar to the cells in the primary lesion.
■ Common well-formed epidermal collarette.
■ Frequent vascular invasion.

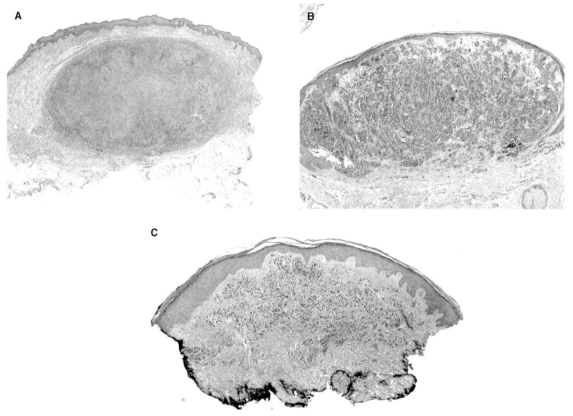

FIGURE 5-26

FIGURE 5-26   (A) Metastatic melanoma. Classic nodular pattern of growth. Note the well-defined neoplasm in the dermis without connection to the overlying epidermis. (B) In this example there is irregular distribution of the melanin pigment, epidermal collarette, and focal intraepidermal component. (C) Note the absence of intraepidermal component but the lesion shows a pattern of pseudomaturation since the deeply located melanocytes disperse among collagen fibers resemble the pattern of an intradermal nevus.

Cutaneous Lymphoproliferative Disorders

6

CUTANEOUS B-CELL LYMPHOMAS

PRIMARY CUTANEOUS FOLLICLE CENTER LYMPHOMA

PRIMARY CUTANEOUS MARGINAL ZONE B-CELL LYMPHOMA

MANTLE CELL LYMPHOMA

DIFFUSE LARGE B-CELL LYMPHOMA, LEG TYPE

PRIMARY CUTANEOUS DIFFUSE LARGE B-CELL LYMPHOMA, OTHER

LYMPHOMATOID GRANULOMATOSIS

INTRAVASCULAR B-CELL LYMPHOMA (ANGIOTROPIC LARGE CELL LYMPHOMA)

CUTANEOUS T-CELL LYMPHOMAS

MYCOSIS FUNGOIDES

SÉZARY SYNDROME

SUBCUTANEOUS PANNICULITIS-LIKE T-CELL LYMPHOMA

PRIMARY CUTANEOUS CD8+ AGGRESSIVE EPIDERMOTROPIC CYTOTOXIC T-CELL LYMPHOMA

PRIMARY CUTANEOUS GAMMA/DELTA T-CELL LYMPHOMA

EXTRANODAL NK/T-CELL LYMPHOMA, NASAL TYPE

HYDROA VACCINIFORME-LIKE LYMPHOMA

LYMPHOMATOID PAPULOSIS

PRIMARY CUTANEOUS ANAPLASTIC LARGE T-CELL LYMPHOMA

PRIMARY CUTANEOUS CD4+ SMALL/MEDIUM T-CELL LYMPHOMA

CUTANEOUS ADULT T-CELL LEUKEMIA/LYMPHOMA

CUTANEOUS B-CELL LYMPHOMAS

Primary Cutaneous Follicle Center Lymphoma

Primary cutaneous follicle center lymphoma (PCFCL) is the most common B-cell lymphoma on the skin, accounting for approximately 55% of cases. Clinically, it presents with red-brown papules or nodules localized on the scalp, forehead, and trunk. Most affected individuals are adults (median age, 51 years) with an equal sex distribution. The majority of "nodal" follicular lymphomas (>90%) have a t(14;18) translocation with *bcl-2* gene rearrangement; in contrast, PCFCL is usually negative for *bcl-2* and lacks the t(14;18) translocation. Patients with PCFCL have an excellent prognosis, with a 5-year disease-specific survival rate of 95%. It is crucial to perform complete staging to distinguish PCFCL from secondary involvement of systemic lymphoma (371–374).

PATHOLOGY (FIGURE 6-1A, B)
- PCFCL lesions can show a nodal, nodal and diffuse, or diffuse pattern consisting of medium to large centrocytes with a variable number of centroblasts.
- Consistent sparing of the epidermis
- Small reactive T-cells admixed with the neoplastic B cells
- IHC: The atypical lymphocytes are positive for CD19, CD20, CD79a, and bcl-6. CD10 is usually expressed in lesions with follicular growth pattern but not in lesions with a diffuse growth pattern. *bcl-2* and MUM-1 are detected in only less than 10% of the cases. As mentioned above, there is no t(14;18) translocation.
- Most cases show monoclonal IgH rearrangement.

FIGURE 6-1   (A) Primary cutaneous follicle center lymphoma. Note the nodular infiltrate with follicular pattern. (B) Primary cutaneous follicle center lymphoma. Diffuse pattern of growth of small lymphocytes with irregular, hyperchromatic nuclei (centrocytes).

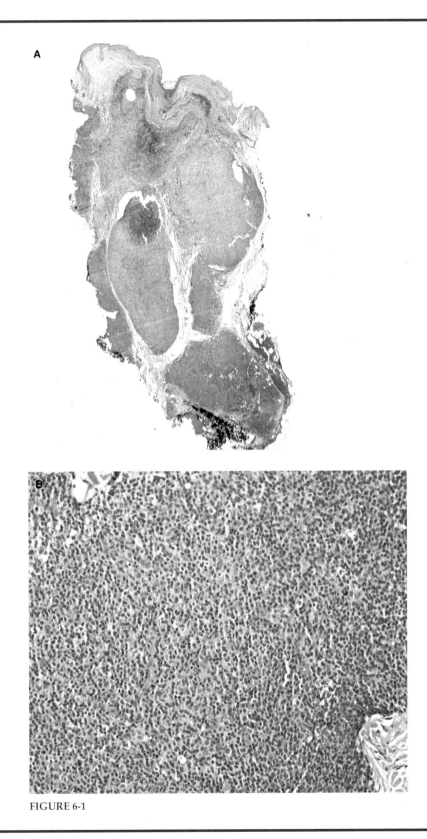

FIGURE 6-1

Primary Cutaneous Marginal Zone B-Cell Lymphoma

Primary cutaneous marginal zone B-cell lymphoma (PCMZL) is the second most common cutaneous B-cell lymphoma (25% of cases). Clinically it presents with red or violaceous papular or nodular lesions on the trunk or arms. A proportion of PCMZL may be related to infection by *Borrelia burgdorferi* in certain geographic locations (Europe). Cytogenetic and molecular analyses have shown that fewer than 25% of PCMZL harbor the t(14;18). The t(11;18) and t(3;14) have been reported in approximately 7% and 10% of PCMZL, respectively. The prognosis is excellent, with a 5-year disease-free survival rate of 98% to 100% despite multiple relapses (375, 376).

PATHOLOGY (FIGURE 6-2A–C)

- Nodular or less commonly diffuse infiltrate in the dermis and subcutaneous tissue (epidermis is spared)
- The infiltrates are composed of a mixed population of small- to medium-sized lymphocytes, marginal zone B-cells, lymphoplasmacytoid cells, and plasma cells, with few centroblasts and reactive T-cells.
- Frequent reactive germinal centers
- Monotypic plasma cells are often located at the periphery of the infiltrates and in the superficial dermis beneath the epidermis.
- IHC: The neoplastic cells express CD19, CD20, CD22, CD79a, and bcl-2. The neoplastic cells are negative for CD23, CD10, cyclin D-1, and bcl-6. CD43 coexpression can be seen in some cases. The B-cells in the reactive follicles are, as expected, CD10+ and bcl-6+, but bcl-2–. There is cytoplasmic expression of immunoglobulin with light chain restriction. Monoclonal rearrangement is seen in 50% to 60% of cases.

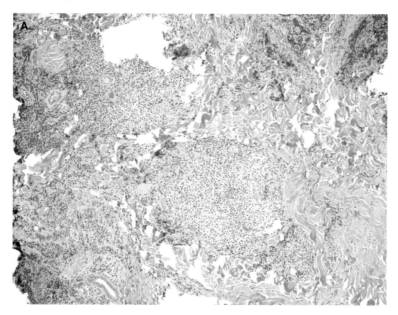

FIGURE 6-2 (A) Primary cutaneous marginal zone B-cell lymphoma. Note the dense and nodular deep dermal lymphoid infiltrate resembling germinal centers.

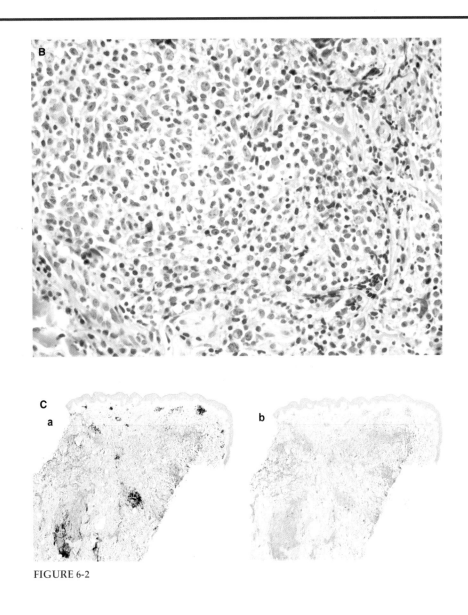

FIGURE 6-2

FIGURE 6-2   (B) Primary cutaneous marginal zone B-cell lymphoma. Note the atypical lymphocytes admixed with scattered plasma cells. (C) Primary cutaneous marginal zone B-cell lymphoma. (a) Kappa (b) Lambda (in situ hybridization). Note the increased kappa to lambda ratio (5:1).

Mantle Cell Lymphoma

Mantle cell lymphoma (MCL) is a rare B-cell lymphoma that derives from the inner mantle zone of follicles that most commonly involves lymph nodes. It is more common in older adults (median 60 years) with predilection for males. MCL uncommonly involves skin, and most cases of cutaneous MCL represent secondary involvement from widespread dissemination. However, rarely skin lesions may represent the first manifestation of the disease. Clinically, it presents as solitary or multiple purple to red nodules. MCL is associated with a t(11;14) in most cases. The prognosis of MCL is poor and the medium survival is approximately 5 years (377–379).

PATHOLOGY (FIGURE 6-3A–C)
- Nodular and diffuse monotonous population of atypical lymphocytes occupying the entire dermis and sometimes the subcutaneous fat.
- Lymphocytes are small to medium size and have irregular hyperchromatic nuclei.
- In the nodular areas there are reactive follicles with a rim of tumor cells.
- IHC: The neoplastic lymphocytes are CD20+, CD79a+ and co-express CD5, CD43, cyclin D1, and bcl-2, while being negative for CD23, bcl-6, and CD10.

A

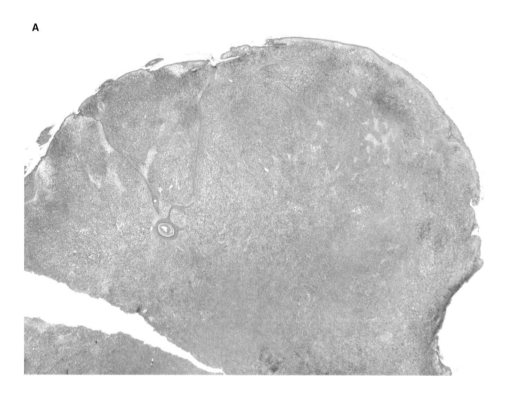

FIGURE 6-3 (A) Mantle cell lymphoma. Low power showing a polypoid lesion in dermis composed of sheets of atypical lymphocytes. (B) There is a dense monomorphic population of lymphoid cells with hyperchromatic nuclei. (C) Strong nuclear expression of bcl-1 (cyclin D-1).

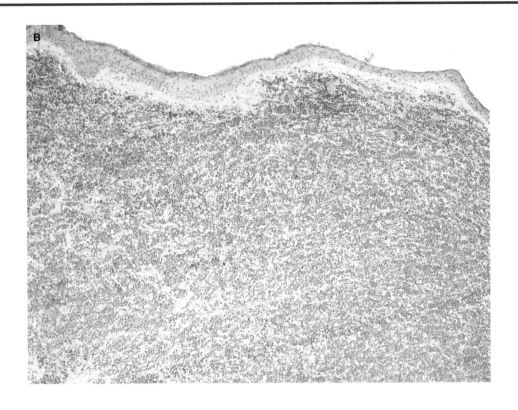

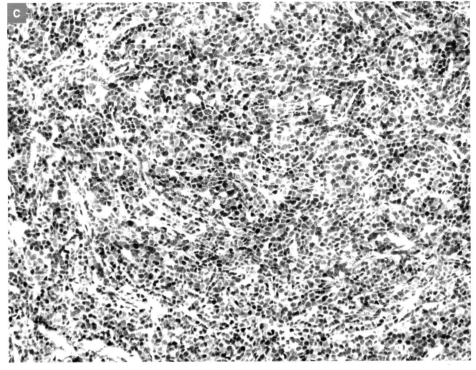

FIGURE 6-3

Diffuse Large B-Cell Lymphoma, Leg Type

Diffuse large B-cell lymphoma, leg type (PCDLBCL-LT) is a B-cell lymphoma of intermediate behavior. These tumors are more commonly seen on the legs of elderly females; however, a small subset of cases (10%–15%) can arise at cutaneous sites different from the leg including the trunk, upper limbs, head and neck, etc. Clinically, it presents as solitary or multiple nodules. Relapses and extracutaneous dissemination are common with relatively frequent central nervous system involvement. The course of disease is characterized with frequent relapses and dissemination into extracutaneous regions. The 5-year disease-specific survival rates ranged from 43% to 63% (377, 380–382).

PATHOLOGY (FIGURE 6-4A–C)

- PCDLBCL-LT shows a diffuse dermal infiltrate in the entire dermis and with frequent invasion into the subcutis.
- Sheets of centroblasts and immunoblasts that efface adnexal structures
- Numerous mitotic figures, some of atypical shape
- Usually there is a Grenz zone (very rare epidermotropism).
- IHC: The neoplastic lymphocytes express CD20 and CD79A and almost always coexpress bcl-2, MUM1, and FOXP1. Up to 10% of cases do not express bcl-2 or MUM-1. The majority of cases express also bcl-6. CD10 is usually negative.

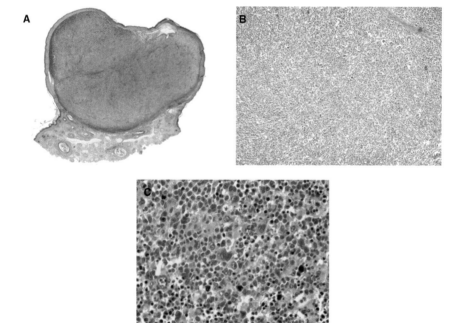

FIGURE 6-4

FIGURE 6-4   Diffuse large B-cell lymphoma, leg type. (A) Diffuse polypoid infiltrate of large atypical lymphocytes. The tumor cells abut into the epidermis. (B) Diffuse population of atypical lymphocytes as a mixture of centroblasts and immunoblasts. (C) High power of the large atypical lymphocytes with marked apoptosis.

Primary Cutaneous Diffuse Large B-Cell Lymphoma, Other

Primary cutaneous diffuse large B-cell lymphoma, other (PCDLBCL-O) is a term used for cases of large B-cell lymphoma arising in the skin that do not fit as PCDLBCL-LT, PCMZL, or PCFCL. The WHO classification of skin tumors (2006) considered these lymphomas to show features typical of PDLBCL-LT but lacking bcl-2 expression; however, recent studies suggest that there are no significant clinical differences between bcl-2+ and bcl-2– PCDLBCL-LT. PCDLBCL-O is not considered a separate entity by many authors, but as of now it represents a category into which some large B-cell lymphomas can be placed until future studies clarify the current classification system (377).

Lymphomatoid Granulomatosis

Lymphomatoid granulomatosis (LyG) is a B-cell, progressive, Epstein–Barr virus (EBV)-driven lymphoproliferative disease. LyG is diagnosed more commonly in men than in women, typically between the fourth and sixth decades of life. The lung is the most frequently involved organ and virtually all patients have pulmonary disease at some point during the course of their illness. Other organs involved include skin, kidneys, central nervous system, upper respiratory tract, and gastrointestinal tract, with a striking sparing of lymphoid tissues. Clinically, the cutaneous lesions are quite heterogeneous but typically appear as scattered subcutaneous or dermal nodules of variable size. In up to 10% of patients, the skin lesions will antedate the lung lesions. The prognosis depends on the grade and extent of the disease; however, it usually follows an aggressive course (383, 384).

PATHOLOGY (FIGURE 6-5A–C)

■ LyG shows a diffuse atypical polymorphous lymphoid infiltrate composed of small lymphocytes (majority of the infiltrate), plasma cells, histiocytes, and large lymphocytes (immunoblasts-like).

■ The malignant B cells usually are medium to large in size with marked pleomorphism.

■ A distinctive morphologic feature is the angiocentric and angiodestructive nature with marked transmural infiltration of the intima of arteries and veins.

■ Common tumor cell necrosis

■ Despite its name there are no granulomas in the infiltrate.

■ IHC: The large cells have a B-cell phenotype expressing CD20 and CD79a. The cells are variably positive for CD30, but CD15, CD56, and CD57 are not expressed. The atypical B cells are EBV positive (EBER). The background population of lymphocytes is composed of CD3+ T-cells predominantly CD4+.

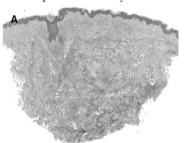
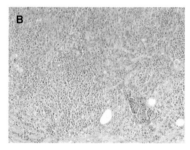
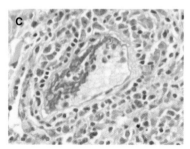

FIGURE 6-5

FIGURE 6-5 Lymphomatoid granulomatosis. (A) Interstitial population of atypical lymphocytes. (B) High power showing the large atypical lymphocytes. (C) Note the angiocentric distribution of atypical lymphocytes.

Intravascular B-Cell Lymphoma (Angiotropic Large Cell Lymphoma)

Intravascular large B-cell lymphoma (IVLBCL) is a rare lymphoma that most commonly affects elderly adults. The tumor cells can invade any systemic organ, but most frequently involve the skin and the central nervous system (less frequently the lung, kidney, and gastrointestinal tract). Lymph nodes are typically spared. Skin manifestations are present at time of diagnosis in 6% to 39% of patients: painful indurated erythema, violaceous plaques, generalized telangiectasia, and ulcerated nodules more commonly located on the trunk and thighs. The prognosis is worse in generalized disease (385–387).

PATHOLOGY (FIGURE 6-6)
- The neoplastic lymphocytes are found within vascular lumina in the dermis and subcutis.
- Perivascular and extravascular arrangement of neoplastic lymphocytes
- The neoplastic lymphocytes are large in size with scanty cytoplasm, round vesicular nuclei, and prominent nucleoli.
- Frequent atypical mitotic figures
- Fibrin thrombi are often observed within vessels, either with or without atypical cells.
- IHC: The neoplastic lymphocytes express CD20, CD79a, CD19, MUM-1, bcl-2, and CD22. CD5 is variably positive (38% of cases). CD10 is expressed in 13% and bcl-6 is expressed in 26% of cases.

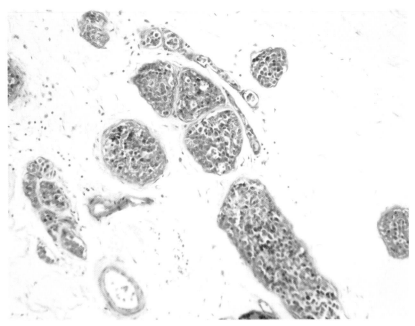

FIGURE 6-6

FIGURE 6-6   Intravascular large B-cell lymphoma. Note the atypical lymphocytes within the lumina of the vessels.

CUTANEOUS T-CELL LYMPHOMAS

Mycosis Fungoides

Mycosis fungoides (MF), although rare, is the most common type of cutaneous T-cell lymphoma (CTCL). There is predilection for males, and it is more common in Black than White patients. The most common age at presentation is 50 years; however, MF can also present in children and adolescents. The course and outcome is variable, ranging from an indolent course with slow progression over years through widespread systemic involvement with high mortality rate. MF is clinically divided into patch, plaque, and tumor stages; however, all stages may be present at the same time in some cases and sometimes the lesions never progress beyond the patch stage (388–390).

Patch stage: It is composed of irregular, slightly scaly, variably sized patches. The lesions have a random distribution but they are more commonly located on the trunk. This stage may persist for many years before progression.

Plaque stage: It is characterized by red scaly plaques with annular arrangement. The plaques may develop de novo or from patches.

Tumor stage: It is usually associated with pre-existing lesions. The tumors are ulcerated and red in color.

PATHOLOGY (FIGURE 6-7A–F)

■ Patch lesion: The histology at this stage can be quite subtle. The epidermis is slightly acanthotic, and mild vacuolar damage with psoriasiform hyperplasia is sometimes present. The neoplastic lymphocytes are seen in a patchy lichenoid distribution in the superficial dermis, with small numbers within the epidermis showing mild cytologic atypia and surrounded by a clear halo. There is palisading and alignment of lymphocytes along the basal layer of the epidermis. Also highly characteristic is the presence of intraepidermal epidermotropic lymphocytes in areas with minimal spongiosis.

■ Plaque lesion: There is a dense band-like lymphocytic infiltrate in the dermis and marked epidermotropism forming Pautrier microabscesses. The cells are small in size and show a characteristic cerebriform appearance. The epidermis is acanthotic with frequent psoriasiform hyperplasia.

(*text continued on page 314*)

FIGURE 6-7   (A) Mycosis fungoides (patch stage). Subtle lichenoid lymphocytic infiltrate in the dermis. Note the epidermotropic lymphocytes with only focal spongiosis, disproportionate to the number of lymphocytes. (B) Mycosis fungoides (patch stage). Epidermotropism with focal spongiosis. Note that the atypical lymphocytes are surrounded by the characteristic clear halo. (C) Mycosis fungoides (plaque stage). Epidermal psoriasiform hyperplasia. Note the subtle infiltrate in the dermis with focal epidermotropism. (D) Mycosis fungoides (plaque stage). Lichenoid infiltrate with marked epidermotropism. (E) Mycosis fungoides (plaque stage). High magnification of the atypical epidermotropic lymphocytes. (F) Mycosis fungoides (tumor stage). Dense atypical lymphocytic infiltrate filling up the entire dermis.

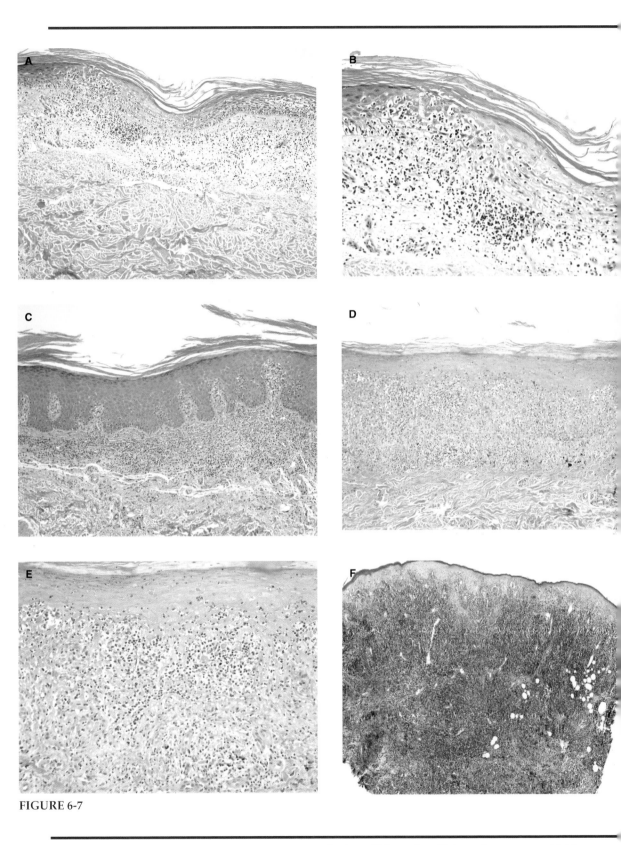

FIGURE 6-7

Mycosis Fungoides *(continued)*

■ Tumor lesion: The biopsy shows a dense nodular infiltrate sometimes involving the subcutaneous fat. The lesions are often ulcerated, and the amount of epidermotropism varies. In addition to showing cerebriform cells, there are increased numbers of large lymphoid cells.

■ IHC: MF is a T-cell lymphoma of alpha/beta T-cell helper lymphocytes; thus, it will express CD3, CD4, BF-1, CD45RO, and CD5. Occasionally the neoplastic cells display CD8+ phenotype. It has been suggested that CD7 expression is mostly lost in MF, in contrast to inflammatory dermatoses; however, its diagnostic value is not specific as its expression can often be lost in some reactive conditions and be present in some MF cases. CD30 expression correlates with large cell transformation.

■ Clonal T-cell receptor (TCR) gene rearrangement may be identified in the majority of cases. However, these results should be interpreted with caution since *TCR* gene rearrangements are present in a variety of inflammatory dermatoses.

VARIANTS

■ Folliculotropic MF: This variant presents in middle-aged to elderly males and clinically shows follicular papules and patchy alopecia, particularly in the head and neck area (face and scalp). This variant has a higher incidence of disease progression with worse prognosis than standard MF. The most important histologic feature of this variant is the presence of medium to large cerebriform lymphoid cells infiltrating the hair follicle (391, 392).

■ Pagetoid reticulosis (Woringer–Kolopp disease): It is a solitary, asymptomatic, well-defined, scaly patch or plaque (psoriasis-like) on the extremities that slowly enlarges. Histologically, the epidermis shows psoriasiform changes and is characteristically infiltrated by medium to large atypical lymphocytes with vacuolated cytoplasm arranged in clusters (mimicking Paget disease or melanoma) (393) (Figure 6-8A, B).

■ Granulomatous slack skin disease/granulomatous MF: Very rare. It is characterized by slow development of pendulous, lax skin, most commonly in the areas of the axillae and groin. Histologically, it shows a dense infiltrate of atypical lymphocytes often involving the dermis and even extending to the subcutis. Characteristically there is a granulomatous infiltrate with many multinucleate giant cells (Langhans type) with elastophagocytosis and focal lymphophagocytosis (394) (Figure 6-9A, B).

■ Hypopigmented MF: This is a rare subtype of MF, more often seen in children and adolescents with dark skin. Clinically, it presents with asymptomatic scaly, hypopigmented patches, most often affecting the trunk and extremities. Histologically, this variant is very similar to classical MF except for the prominent epidermotropism (disproportionate to the number of dermal lymphocytes) and presence of marked pigment incontinence. The immunophenotype of hypopigmented MF is more likely to be CD8+ (395).

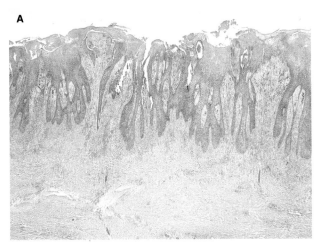
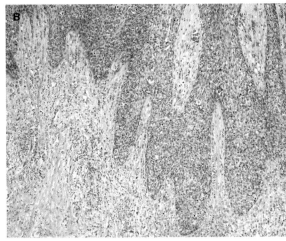

FIGURE 6-8

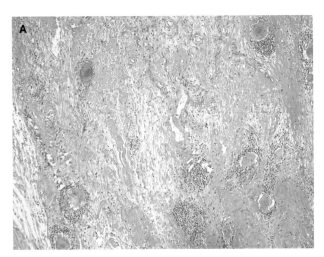
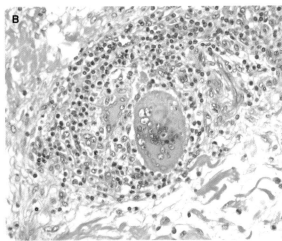

FIGURE 6-9

FIGURE 6-8   (A) Pagetoid reticulosis. Marked epidermal hyperplasia with a diffuse infiltrate of large atypical lymphocytes. (B) Pagetoid reticulosis. Large, atypical lymphocytes diffusely infiltrating the epidermis.

FIGURE 6-9   (A) Granulomatous slack skin. Granulomatous infiltrate with large multinucleated giant cells. (B) Granulomatous slack skin. High magnification of the large multinucleated giant cells.

Sézary Syndrome

Sézary syndrome (SS) is a leukemic variant of CTCL that is characterized by erythroderma, keratoderma, lymphadenopathy, and atypical lymphocytes with cerebriform nuclei in peripheral blood. It is more often seen in Black males in the fifth to seventh decades of life and clinically presents with erythroderma that is intensely pruritic. There is frequent palmoplantar keratoderma. Also common are alopecia, hepatomegaly, nail dystrophy, and lymphadenopathy. These patients tend to have a poor prognosis (396–399).

PATHOLOGY
- Biopsies of SS may show only subtle changes in about 40% of cases, and multiple biopsies sometimes are necessary to obtain a diagnosis.
- Perivascular or a band-like infiltrate involving the papillary dermis and sometimes also the upper reticular dermis.
- Epidermotropism is present in some of cases; however, it can be minimal or even absent.
- Small lymphocytes admixed with some larger cells with cerebriform nuclei.
- Fibrous papillary dermis with thickened collagen bundles and scattered melanophages.
- IHC: The neoplastic lymphocytes in the skin and blood are CD3+, CD4+, CD45RO+, CD8–, CD7–, CD2–, and CD30–.

Subcutaneous Panniculitis-Like T-Cell Lymphoma

Subcutaneous panniculitis-like T-cell lymphoma (SPTCL) is a rare alpha/beta cytotoxic cutaneous lymphoma characterized by primary involvement of subcutaneous tissue mimicking panniculitis. SPTCL is more commonly seen in adults and less commonly in children and young adults. Clinically, it presents with erythematous nodules or deep-seated plaques located most commonly on the extremities and trunk. SPTCL has a relatively favorable clinical course and usually remains confined to the skin with recurrent lesions and rare extracutaneous spread. SPTCL should be separated from other, more aggressive CTCLs by correlation of clinical presentation, morphologic features, and immunophenotype (400–403).

PATHOLOGY (FIGURE 6-10A, B)
- Dense nodular or diffuse infiltrate located in the subcutaneous fat, resembling lobular panniculitis
- Deep reticular dermis may be involved (superficial dermis and epidermis are unaffected).
- The neoplastic lymphocytes vary in size from small to intermediate-sized with only rare large pleomorphic cells.
- The neoplastic lymphocytes are arranged in the subcutis as single cells or small clusters around adipocytes in a wreath-like pattern ("rimming"; this phenomenon can be seen in other T-cell lymphomas and also in reactive conditions).
- Characteristic fat necrosis
- Common histiocytic infiltrate with granulomatous morphology
- Reactive small lymphocytes, plasma cells, and neutrophils in the background
- Rare angioinvasion
- Variable admixture of karyorrhexis and cytophagocytosis
- IHC: The neoplastic lymphoid cells show an alpha/beta, T-cell, cytotoxic phenotype (CD3+, CD4–, CD8+, BF-1+). There is also expression of cytotoxic molecules (granzyme B, TIA-1, and perforin) and CD45RO. Occasionally there is loss of the pan-T-cell antigens CD2, CD5, and CD7. Anti-CD30 and CD56 are negative.
- TCR rearrangement shows a monoclonal population of T cells.

DIFFERENTIAL DIAGNOSIS
The main differential diagnosis of SPTCL is with lupus panniculitis. The two disorders may show overlapping histologic features; however, a diagnosis of lupus panniculitis should be considered when seeing small nodular aggregates of B-cells with reactive germinal centers formation (especially at the periphery of the fat lobule), presence of numerous plasma cells, and epidermal involvement (interface damage) are noted. A cytotoxic phenotype (CD3+, CD8+, and CD4–) is seen in SPTCL, but this can also be seen in lupus panniculitis. A polyclonal pattern (on TCR rearrangement studies) favors a diagnosis of lupus.

(continued)

Subcutaneous Panniculitis-Like T-Cell Lymphoma *(continued)*

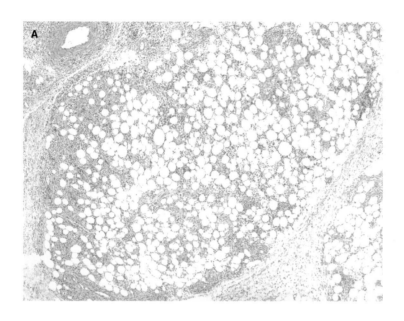

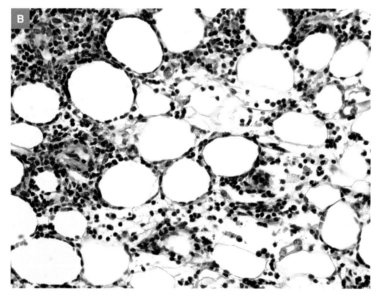

FIGURE 6-10

FIGURE 6-10　Subcutaneous panniculitis-like T-cell lymphoma. (A) Note the dense and atypical nodular lymphocytic infiltrate in subcutaneous tissue (lobular panniculitis-like). (B) Infiltrate of atypical lymphocytes mimicking lobular panniculitis. Note the rimming of atypical lymphocytes around adipocytes.

Primary Cutaneous CD8+ Aggressive Epidermotropic Cytotoxic T-Cell Lymphoma

Primary cutaneous CD8+ aggressive epidermotropic cytotoxic T-cell lymphoma is a rare CTCL characterized by an aggressive behavior. More common in elderly patients, it presents with generalized, rapidly progressing papules, patches, plaques, nodules, and tumors, often with central necrosis or ulceration. Oral involvement is common. There is usually widespread visceral metastasis to testis, lungs, spleen, and the central nervous system and without lymph node involvement. This lymphoma has a high mortality rate (404–406).

PATHOLOGY (FIGURE 6-11A, B)
- The biopsy shows an extensive infiltrate of atypical lymphocytes in a nodular or diffuse growth usually extending deep into the dermis down to the subcutaneous fat.
- There is marked epidermotropism, particularly in the basal cell layer. These features can be seen throughout the different stages of the disease (less pronounced).
- The atypical lymphoid infiltrate is composed of medium to large pleomorphic lymphocytes and immunoblasts.
- Usually with syringotropism and folliculotropism
- Rare angiocentricity and angioinvasion
- IHC: The neoplastic lymphocytes have a cytotoxic phenotype (CD3+, CD8+, BF-1+, CD4–). The cells are usually CD7+ and CD45RA+. Anti-CD45RO, CD30, and CD56 are negative. The tumor cells express the cytotoxic markers (TIA-1, granzyme B, and perforin). The neoplastic lymphocytes may lose pan t-cell markers such as CD2 and CD5. There is clonal rearrangement of the *TCR* gene.

(continued)

Primary Cutaneous CD8+ Aggressive Epidermotropic Cytotoxic T-Cell Lymphoma (*continued*)

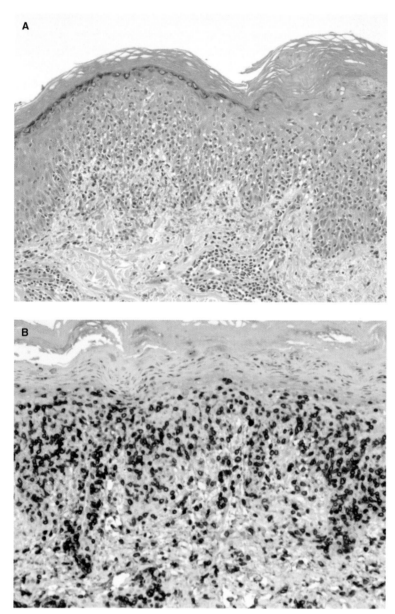

FIGURE 6-11

FIGURE 6-11   (A) Primary cutaneous CD8+, aggressive, epidermotropic cytotoxic T-cell lymphoma. Note the markedly atypical epidermotropic lymphocytes. (B) Primary cutaneous CD8+, aggressive, epidermotropic cytotoxic T-cell lymphoma. CD8 is strongly positive in the epidermotropic T cells.

Primary Cutaneous Gamma/Delta T-Cell Lymphoma

Primary cutaneous gamma/delta T-cell lymphoma (PCGD-TCL) is a rare T-cell lymphoma. Most cases are seen in adult males. Clinically, it presents with generalized deep indurated plaques and patches and ulcerated nodules on the extremities and trunk. Although it may resemble inflammatory panniculitis, PCGD-TCL is usually more extensive with a tendency to ulcerate. Hemophagocytic syndrome is a frequent complication. The prognosis is poor (377, 407–409).

PATHOLOGY (FIGURE 6-12A, B)

- Diffuse proliferation of atypical lymphocytes with marked epidermotropism.
- The infiltrate often affects the subcutis.
- The neoplastic lymphoid cells are small, medium, or large and have coarse, clumped chromatin.
- Occasionally with a lichenoid or vacuolar interface reaction with variable exocytosis
- Common angiocentricity and angioinvasion
- Cases with associated hemagophagocytic syndrome show large macrophages engulfing lymphocytes.
- IHC: The neoplastic lymphocytes express CD2, CD3, and cytotoxic markers (TIA-1, perforin, and granzyme B). CD56 and CD5 are expressed in 40% and 12% of cases, respectively. Most cases are negative for both CD4 and CD8; however, CD8 can be expressed in some cases. CD45RA is expressed in 33% of cases. Some cases show a gamma/delta T-cell phenotype demonstrated by the absence of BF-1 and expression of gamma M-1. There is no evidence of EBV.

(continued)

Primary Cutaneous Gamma/Delta
T-Cell Lymphoma *(continued)*

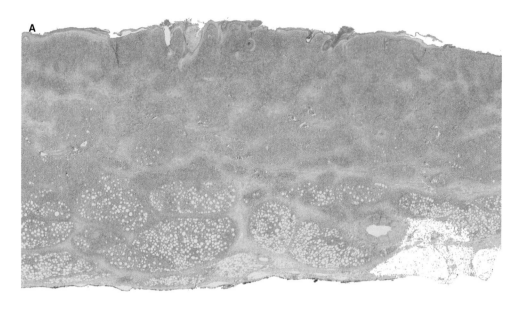

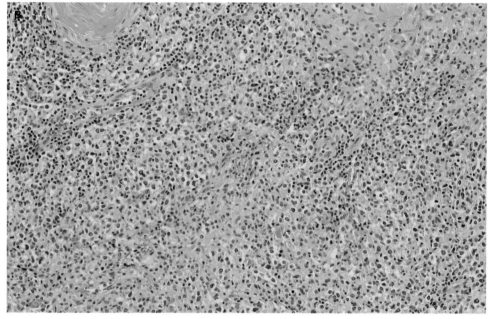

FIGURE 6-12

FIGURE 6-12   (A) Primary cutaneous gamma/delta T-cell lymphoma. Diffuse infiltrate of neoplastic lymphocytes involving the subcutaneous fat. (B) Primary cutaneous gamma/delta T-cell lymphoma. High-power magnification showing large atypical lymphocytes.

Extranodal NK/T-Cell Lymphoma, Nasal Type

Extranodal NK/T-cell lymphoma, nasal type is very rare. Clinically, it is most commonly located on the upper respiratory tract, but extranasal presentation is not uncommon, especially affecting the skin and subcutis. This lymphoma is more prevalent in Asians and in Native Americans of Mexico, Central America, and South America. It is almost always associated with EBV infection. Adult males are more commonly affected (median age is 50 years). Hemophagocytic syndrome is sometimes a complication. This is an aggressive lymphoma with a high mortality rate (410–412).

PATHOLOGY
- Dense diffuse dermal atypical lymphocytic infiltrate, often extending into the subcutaneous fat.
- There is marked angiocentricity with angiodestruction.
- Occasionally with epidermotropism
- The cytomorphology of the tumor cells is variable, ranging from small to medium or large atypical lymphocytes.
- Reactive inflammatory cells are seen in the background.
- Abundant mitotic figures
- Occasional pseudoepitheliomatous hyperplasia
- IHC: The tumor cells are classically positive for CD3 (cytoplasmic), CD2, and CD56, and express cytotoxic molecules (TIA1, perforin, and granzyme B). In the majority of cases the neoplastic lymphocytes are negative for CD4, CD5, CD7, and CD8; however, they can sometimes express either CD4 or CD8. Anti-CD30 may rarely be positive. Almost all cases show evidence of EBV by in situ hybridization (EBER). Majority of cases show no clonal rearrangement of the TCR (germline).

Hydroa Vacciniforme-Like Lymphoma

Hydroa vacciniforme-like lymphoma (HVL) has recently been categorized by the World Health Organization as one of the EBV-related lymphoproliferative disorders of childhood. HVL is a rare lymphoproliferative disorder that clinically resembles hydroa vacciniforme (HV). This neoplastic process is particularly seen in Latin America and Asia. Clinically, the lesions are commonly seen on sun-exposed areas including the face and extremities and are characterized by an edematous papulovesicular eruption (413–416).

PATHOLOGY (FIGURE 6-13A–C)
- Relatively dense and diffuse atypical population of lymphocytes in the dermis and sometimes involving the subcutaneous fat.
- The cytologic atypia in some cases may be minimal.
- Commonly superficial and deep perivascular pattern.
- Angiocentricity, angiodestruction, and infiltration of adnexal structures are common.
- IHC: The neoplastic lymphocytes are positive for CD2, CD3, CD45RO, CD8, and cytotoxic proteins (TIA-1, granzyme B, perforin). Anti-CD4 is negative; however, some cases show a CD4–/CD8– phenotype. Anti-CD30 and CD56 are negative. EBV by in situ hybridization (EBER) is positive.

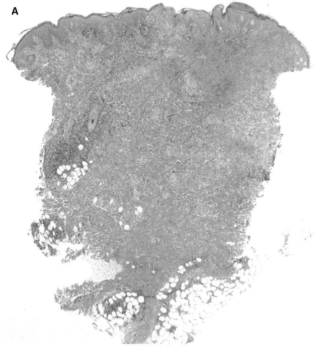

A

FIGURE 6-13

FIGURE 6-13   (A) Hydroa vacciniforme-like lymphoma. Superficial and deep perivascular atypical lymphocytic infiltrate.

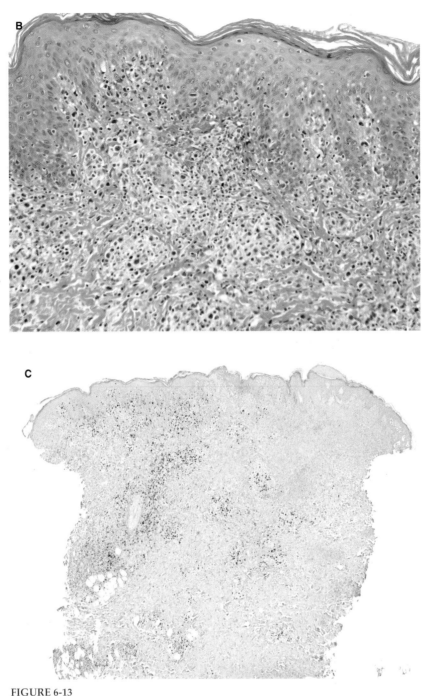

FIGURE 6-13

FIGURE 6-13   (B) Hydroa vacciniforme-like lymphoma. Note the atypical lymphocytic infiltrate surrounding the blood vessels with only focal epidermotropism. (C) Hydroa vacciniforme-like lymphoma. Positive for EBER (in situ hybridization).

Lymphomatoid Papulosis

Lymphomatoid papulosis (LyP) is an indolent CD30+ lymphoproliferative disorder with a chronic clinical course. Clinically, it is characterized by the presence of recurrent pruritic papules and nodules at different stages of development that spontaneously regress (wax and wane) and are predominantly on the trunk and extremities. The disease is usually indolent, occasionally following a short self-limiting course or following a chronic evolution of 5 to 10 years or longer. LyP can be associated with other lymphomas including MF and primary cutaneous anaplastic large cell lymphoma (9% and 20% of cases) (377, 417–419).

PATHOLOGY (FIGURE 6-14A–G)
■ The histology of LyP is variable with five main histologic types so far described.
■ Type A (classic type): It is the conventional type, characterized by a wedge-shaped dermal infiltrate composed of a mixture of large atypical lymphocytes (Reed–Sternberg-like cells), small lymphocytes, eosinophils, neutrophils, and histiocytes. Epidermotropism is variable.
■ Type B (MF-like): This type is rare and is characterized by band-like or superficial perivascular infiltrate with epidermotropism. The lymphoid cells are small to medium in size with cerebriform appearance. The distinction of this type of LyP from MF needs thorough clinical pathologic correlation, as both disorders may show identical histologic changes.

(*text continued on page 328*)

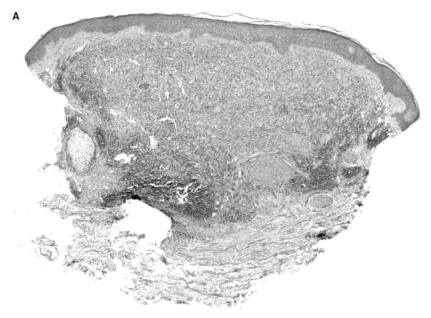

FIGURE 6-14

FIGURE 6-14 (A) Lymphomatoid papulosis type A. Wedge-shaped dermal infiltrate composed by a mixture of large atypical lymphocytes and reactive inflammatory infiltrate.

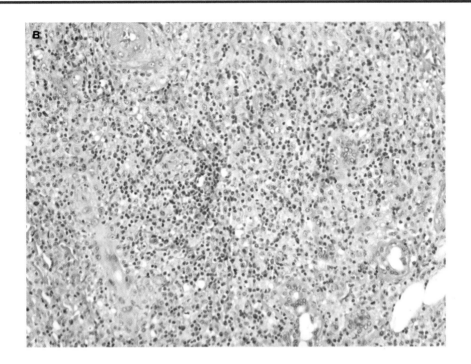

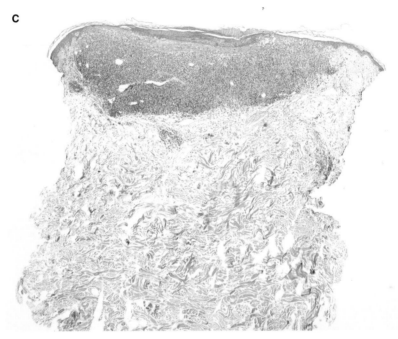

FIGURE 6-14

FIGURE 6-14 (B) Lymphomatoid papulosis. Note the atypical lymphocytic infiltrate admixed with eosinophils, histiocytes, and rare plasma cells. (C) Lymphomatoid papulosis type B. Note the band-like infiltrate with focal epidermotropism mimicking mycosis fungoides.

Chapter 6: Cutaneous Lymphoproliferative Disorders   *327*

Lymphomatoid Papulosis (*continued*)

- Type C (anaplastic large cell lymphoma [ALCL]-like): This type is composed of a dense monotonous population of large atypical lymphoid cells admixed with few small lymphocytes, eosinophils, and neutrophils. The histologic features of this type of LyP are identical to cases of ALCL and thus clinical correlation is necessary.
- Type D: This type is characterized by large numbers of medium-sized, pleomorphic lymphocytes infiltrating the epidermis with a pagetoid reticulosis-like pattern. The lymphoid cells have a cytotoxic (CD8+) phenotype. Thus clinical-pathologic correlation is necessary to distinguish this variant from an epidermotropic aggressive cytotoxic T-cell lymphoma.
- Type E: This recently described variant shows small papules that rapidly ulcerate and subsequently regress within weeks. There are clusters of large, convoluted lymphocytes arranged in an angiocentric and angiodestructive pattern. Thus, it mimics histologically angiocentric T-cell lymphoma and other aggressive lymphomas.
- IHC: The atypical lymphoid cells in LyP express CD30; however, in type B LyP many of the lymphoid cells may be negative for this antigen. LyP usually shows a T-cell helper phenotype (CD4+ and CD8–); however, type B cells usually show a cytotoxic phenotype (CD4–/CD8+). CD56 expression can be seen rarely. ALK-1 is negative. Pan-T-cell antigens, such as CD2, CD3, CD5, and CD7, can be expressed but there is occasional partial loss of these antigens.

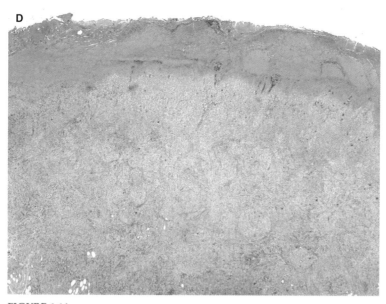

FIGURE 6-14

FIGURE 6-14 (D) Lymphomatoid papulosis type C. Ulcerated lesion with a dense, monomorphic population of large atypical lymphoid cells in the dermis mimicking ALCL. (E) High magnification of Type C LyP showing atypical lymphocytes with anaplastic-like appearance. (F) Lymphomatoid papulosis. CD30 expression in the large, atypical lymphocytes. (G) Lymphomatoid papulosis type D. Epidermotropic atypical lymphocytes. This example was positive for CD8 mimicking an aggressive cytotoxic T-cell lymphoma.

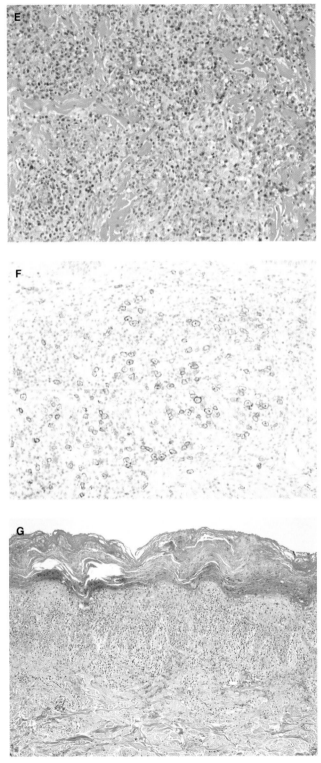

FIGURE 6-14

Primary Cutaneous Anaplastic Large T-Cell Lymphoma

Primary cutaneous anaplastic large T-cell lymphoma (PCALCL) is defined as a CD30+ lymphoproliferative disorder with skin-only involvement and without systemic dissemination at presentation. Clinically, it presents in adults as solitary or localized, ulcerated papules. There may be partial or complete spontaneous regression. PCLACL typically lacks the t(2;5) characteristic of the systemic variant. The prognosis of PCALCL is favorable, with an estimated 5-year survival of 90% (418, 420, 421).

PATHOLOGY (FIGURE 6-15A–C)
- Diffuse and nodular dermal infiltrate
- The neoplastic lymphoid cells have ample cytoplasm and pleomorphic vesicular nuclei with prominent nucleoli.
- Some tumor cells may show bizarre forms including multinucleated giant cells (Reed–Sternberg-like cells).
- Small- to medium-sized neoplastic lymphocytes
- Focal epidermotropism
- Mitotic figures are common, including atypical forms.
- Occasionally prominent pseudoepitheliomatous hyperplasia
- Diverse amounts of reactive lymphocytes, eosinophils, neutrophils, and macrophages and plasma cells
- IHC: This is a T-cell lymphoma and most cases show a T-helper phenotype (CD3+, CD4+, CD8–); however, a small number of cases may show a cytotoxic phenotype (CD8+). More than 75% of the neoplastic cells are CD30+. There is variable loss of various pan-T-cell antigens. Most of the neoplastic cells express cytotoxic molecules (TIA-1, perforin, or granzyme B). Rare cases may express CD56. In contrast to nodal ALCL, EMA and ALK-1 are almost invariably absent in PCALCL. The presence of ALK-1 positivity usually indicates cutaneous spread of primary systemic ALCL; however, there are rare examples of PCALCL showing ALK-1 positivity without the t(2;5) translocation.

FIGURE 6-15 (A) Primary cutaneous anaplastic large T-cell lymphoma. Note the diffuse population of atypical lymphocytes with marked cytologic atypia. (B) Primary cutaneous anaplastic large T-cell lymphoma. Note the increased number of mitotic figures and the anaplastic-appearing cells. (C) Primary cutaneous anaplastic large T-cell lymphoma. Diffuse expression of CD30.

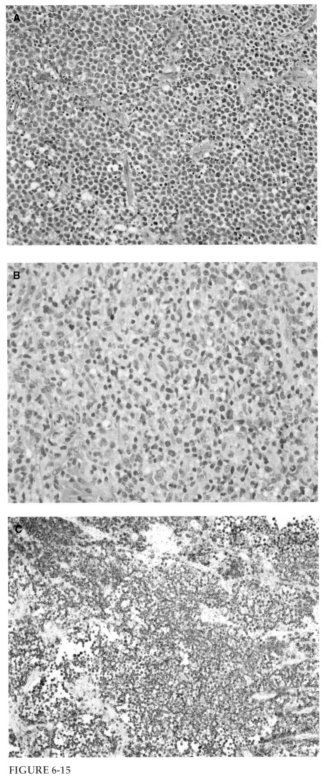

FIGURE 6-15

Primary Cutaneous CD4+ Small/Medium T-Cell Lymphoma

Primary cutaneous CD4+ small/medium T-cell lymphoma is still considered a provisional entity, defined as a neoplasm of small- to medium-sized CD4+ lymphocytes in patients lacking the patches or plaques typical for MF. Most patients are adult or elderly and present with solitary tumors (there may be multiple lesions) commonly on the face, neck or upper trunk. The prognosis is good, with a 5-year survival of around 80% (422, 423).

PATHOLOGY (FIGURE 6-16A–C)

- Nodular or diffuse lymphoid infiltrate often involving the entire dermis and sometimes into the subcutis
- The lymphoid cells are fairly uniform and composed of small- to medium-sized lymphocytes with pale scanty cytoplasm and hyperchromatic noncerebriform nuclei.
- Large lymphoid cells, when present, make up less than 30% of the population.
- Mitotic figures are rare and there is minimal epidermotropism.
- Reactive inflammatory cells in the background including lymphocytes, neutrophils, eosinophils, and plasma cells.
- IHC: The neoplastic lymphoid cells show a T-helper phenotype (CD3+, CD4+, CD8–), and there may be loss of pan T-cell marker such as CD7, CD5, and CD2. Anti-CD30 is negative. There is a large reactive infiltrate of B-cells in the background (CD20+). The neoplastic lymphocytes express follicular T-cell markers, such as PD-1 and CXCL13. Note: Rare cases may show CD8 expression.

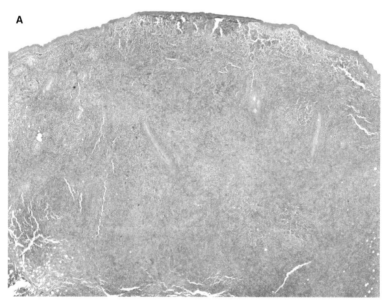

FIGURE 6-16

FIGURE 6-16 (A) Primary cutaneous CD4+ small/medium T-cell lymphoma. Nodular infiltrate of lymphocytes replacing almost the entire dermis.

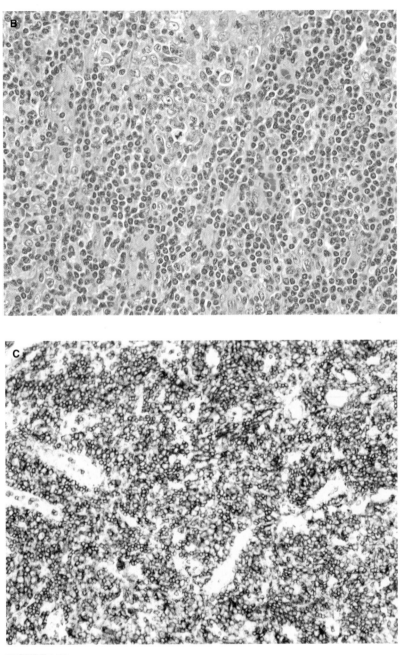

FIGURE 6-16

FIGURE 6-16   (B) Primary cutaneous CD4+ small/medium T-cell lymphoma. Uniform, small- to medium-sized lymphocytes. (C) Primary cutaneous CD4+ small/medium T-cell lymphoma. Strong CD4 expression of the small- and medium-sized atypical T-cells.

Cutaneous Adult T-Cell Leukemia/Lymphoma

Cutaneous adult T-cell leukemia/lymphoma (ATLL) is a systemic lymphoproliferative disorder induced by human T-cell leukemia virus type 1 (HTLV-1) with common skin involvement. This disease is endemic in the Caribbean islands and south of Japan and rare in other regions. Four forms of the disease have been described: aggressive acute, chronic, smoldering, and lymphomatous form. Patients are usually adults with rare cases in young adults. Clinically, skin manifestations can be seen in about half of the patients (especially the indolent form of the disease), showing plaques and patches similar to MF. The prognosis is poor in general but patients with purely cutaneous lesions have better prognosis (424, 425).

PATHOLOGY (FIGURE 6-17A–C)

■ Infiltrate of small to medium/large pleomorphic lymphocytes in upper dermis.
■ Marked epidermotropism.
■ In the nodular and tumor stage the dermal infiltrate is more extensive and can extend into the subcutaneous fat.
■ IHC: The neoplastic lymphoid cells are usually CD2+, CD3+, CD5+, CD4+, and CD7−. The tumor cells are positive for CD25. Rarely, the tumor cells are CD4+/CD8+ or CD4−/CD8−. The large cells may rarely express CD30.

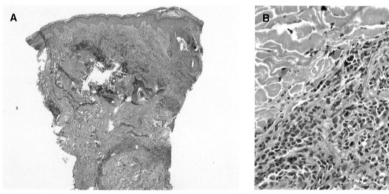

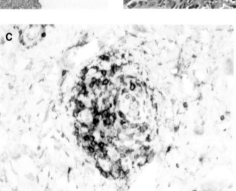

FIGURE 6-17

FIGURE 6-17   Adult T-cell leukemia. (A) Infiltrate of atypical lymphocytes in upper and deep dermis (mainly perivascular). (B) Higher magnification of the atypical lymphocytes. (C) CD25 expression.

References

1. Rogers M, McCrossin I, Commens C. Epidermal nevi and the epidermal nevus syndrome. A review of 131 cases. *J Am Acad Dermatol.* 1989;20(3):476–488. [Epub March 1, 1989].
2. Tay YK, Weston WL, Ganong CA, Klingensmith GJ. Epidermal nevus syndrome: association with central precocious puberty and woolly hair nevus. *J Am Acad Dermatol.* 1996;35(5 Pt 2): 839–842. [Epub November 1, 1996].
3. Happle R, Koch H, Lenz W. The CHILD syndrome. Congenital hemidysplasia with ichthyosiform erythroderma and limb defects. *Eur J Pediatr.* 1980;134(1):27–33. [Epub June 1, 1980].
4. Nabai H, Mehregan AH. Nevus comedonicus. A review of the literature and report of twelve cases. *Acta Derm Venereol.* 1973;53(1):71–74. [Epub January 1, 1973].
5. Lefkowitz A, Schwartz RA, Lambert WC. Nevus comedonicus. *Dermatology.* 1999;199(3):204–207. [Epub December 11, 1999].
6. Mehregan AH, Rahbari H. Benign epithelial tumors of the skin part I: epidermal tumors. *Cutis.* 1977;19(1):43–48. [Epub January 1, 1977].
7. Prieto VG, Casal M, McNutt NS. Lichen planus-like keratosis. A clinical and histological reexamination. *Am J Surg Pathol.* 1993;17(3):259–263. [Epub March 1, 1993].
8. Kaddu S, Dong H, Mayer G, Kerl H, Cerroni L. Warty dyskeratoma—"follicular dyskeratoma": analysis of clinicopathologic features of a distinctive follicular adnexal neoplasm. *J Am Acad Dermatol.* 2002;47(3):423–428. [Epub August 28, 2002].
9. Cohen PR, Ulmer R, Theriault A, Leigh IM, Duvic M. Epidermolytic acanthomas: clinical characteristics and immunohistochemical features. *Am J Dermatopathol.* 1997;19(3):232–241. [Epub June 1, 1997].
10. Brownstein MH. Acantholytic acanthoma. *J Am Acad Dermatol.* 1988;19(5 Pt 1):783–786. [Epub November 1, 1988].
11. DiMaio DJ, Cohen PR. Incidental focal acantholytic dyskeratosis. *J Am Acad Dermatol.* 1998;38(2 Pt 1):243–247. [Epub March 5, 1998].
12. Brownstein MH, Fernando S, Shapiro L. Clear cell acanthoma: clinicopathologic analysis of 37 new cases. *Am J Clin Pathol.* 1973;59(3):306–311. [Epub March 1, 1973].
13. Memon AA, Tomenson JA, Bothwell J, Friedmann PS. Prevalence of solar damage and actinic keratosis in a Merseyside population. *Br J Dermatol.* 2000;142(6):1154–1159. [Epub June 10, 2000].

14. Salasche SJ. Epidemiology of actinic keratoses and squamous cell carcinoma. *J Am Acad Dermatol.* 2000;42(1 Pt 2):4–7. [Epub December 22, 1999].
15. Ragi G, Turner MS, Klein LE, Stoll HL Jr. Pigmented Bowen's disease and review of 420 Bowen's disease lesions. *J Dermatol Surg Oncol.* 1988;14(7):765–769. [Epub July 1, 1988].
16. Kossard S, Rosen R. Cutaneous Bowen's disease. An analysis of 1001 cases according to age, sex, and site. *J Am Acad Dermatol.* 1992;27(3):406–410. [Epub September 1, 1992].
17. Clayman GL, Lee JJ, Holsinger FC, et al. Mortality risk from squamous cell skin cancer. *J Clin Oncol.* 2005;23(4):759–765. [Epub February 1, 2005].
18. Evans HL, Smith JL. Spindle cell squamous carcinomas and sarcoma-like tumors of the skin: a comparative study of 38 cases. *Cancer.* 1980;45(10):2687–2697. [Epub May 15, 1980].
19. Buonaccorsi JN, Plaza JA. Role of CD10, wide-spectrum keratin, p63, and podoplanin in the distinction of epithelioid and spindle cell tumors of the skin: an immunohistochemical study of 81 cases. *Am J Dermatopathol.* 2012. [Epub January 20, 2012].
20. Argenyi ZB. Spindle cell neoplasms of the skin: a comprehensive diagnostic approach. *Semi Dermatol.* 1989;8(4):283–297. [Epub December 1, 1989].
21. Kraus FT, Perezmesa C. Verrucous carcinoma. Clinical and pathologic study of 105 cases involving oral cavity, larynx and genitalia. *Cancer.* 1966;19(1):26–38. [Epub January 1, 1966].
22. Majewski S, Jablonska S. Human papillomavirus-associated tumors of the skin and mucosa. *J Am Acad Dermatol.* 1997;36(5 Pt 1):659–685; quiz 86–88. [Epub May 1, 1997].
23. Swanson SA, Cooper PH, Mills SE, Wick MR. Lymphoepithelioma-like carcinoma of the skin. *Mod Pathol.* 1988;1(5):359–365. [Epub September 1, 1988].
24. Wick MR, Swanson PE, LeBoit PE, Strickler JG, Cooper PH. Lymphoepithelioma-like carcinoma of the skin with adnexal differentiation. *J Cutan Pathol.* 1991;18(2):93–102. [Epub April 1, 1991].
25. Gillum PS, Morgan MB, Naylor MF, Everett MA. Absence of Epstein-Barr virus in lymphoepitheliomalike carcinoma of the skin. Polymerase chain reaction evidence and review of five cases. *Am J Dermatopathol.* 1996;18(5):478–482. [Epub October 1, 1996].
26. Kingman J, Callen JP. Keratoacanthoma. A clinical study. *Arch Dermatol.* 1984;120(6):736–740. [Epub June 1, 1984].
27. Ujiie H, Kato N, Natsuga K, Tomita Y. Keratoacanthoma developing on nevus sebaceous in a child. *J Am Acad Dermatol.* 2007;56(suppl 2):S57–S58. [Epub January 17, 2007].
28. Magee KL, Rapini RP, Duvic M, Adler-Storthz K. Human papillomavirus associated with keratoacanthoma. *Arch Dermatol.* 1989;125(11):1587–1589. [Epub November 1, 1989].
29. Gross G, Hagedorn M, Ikenberg H, et al. Bowenoid papulosis. Presence of human papillomavirus (HPV) structural antigens and of HPV 16-related DNA sequences. *Arch Dermatol.* 1985;121(7):858–863. [Epub July 1, 1985].
30. Lookingbill DP, Kreider JW, Howett MK, Olmstead PM, Conner GH. Human papillomavirus type 16 in bowenoid papulosis, intraoral papillomas, and squamous cell carcinoma of the tongue. *Arch Dermatol.* 1987;123(3):363–368. [Epub March 1, 1987].
31. Plaza JA, Suster S. The Toker tumor: spectrum of morphologic features in primary neuroendocrine carcinomas of the skin (Merkel cell carcinoma). *Ann Diagn Pathol.* 2006;10(6):376–385. [Epub November 28, 2006].
32. Gollard R, Weber R, Kosty MP, Greenway HT, Massullo V, Humberson C. Merkel cell carcinoma: review of 22 cases with surgical, pathologic, and therapeutic considerations. *Cancer.* 2000;88(8):1842–1851. [Epub April 13, 2000].
33. Skelton HG, Smith KJ, Hitchcock CL, McCarthy WF, Lupton GP, Graham JH. Merkel cell carcinoma: analysis of clinical, histologic, and immunohistologic features of 132 cases with relation to survival. *J Am Acad Dermatol.* 1997;37(5 Pt 1):734–739. [Epub November 21, 1997].
34. Heath M, Jaimes N, Lemos B, et al. Clinical characteristics of Merkel cell carcinoma at diagnosis in 195 patients: the AEIOU features. *J Am Acad Dermatol.* 2008;58(3):375–381. [Epub February 19, 2008].
35. Kassem A, Schopflin A, Diaz C, et al. Frequent detection of Merkel cell polyomavirus in human Merkel cell carcinomas and identification of a unique deletion in the VP1 gene. *Cancer Res.* 2008;68(13):5009–5013. [Epub July 3, 2008].

36. Lloyd J, Flanagan AM. Mammary and extramammary Paget's disease. *J Clin Pathol*. 2000;53(10):742–749. [Epub November 7, 2000].

37. Guarner J, Cohen C, DeRose PB. Histogenesis of extramammary and mammary Paget cells. An immunohistochemical study. *Am J Dermatopathol*. 1989;11(4):313–318. [Epub August 1, 1989].

38. Plaza JA, Torres-Cabala C, Ivan D, Prieto VG. HER-2/neu expression in extramammary Paget disease: a clinicopathologic and immunohistochemistry study of 47 cases with and without underlying malignancy. *J Cutan Pathol*. 2009;36(7):729–733. [Epub June 13, 2009].

39. Chanda JJ. Extramammary Paget's disease and occult hypernephroma. *J Am Acad Dermatol*. 1985;13(6):1053–1055. [Epub December 1, 1985].

40. Goldblum JR, Hart WR. Vulvar Paget's disease: a clinicopathologic and immunohistochemical study of 19 cases. *Am J Surg Pathol*. 1997;21(10):1178–1187. [Epub October 23, 1997].

41. Reibold R, Undeutsch W, Fleiner J. [Trichoadenoma of Nikolowski—review of four decades and seven new cases]. *Hautarzt*. 1998;49(12):925–928. [Epub January 23, 1999]. Das Trichoadenom (Nikolowski). Ubersicht von vier Jahrzehnten und sieben eigene Falle.

42. Yamaguchi J, Takino C. A case of trichoadenoma arising in the buttock. *J Dermatol*. 1992;19(8): 503–506. [Epub August 1, 1992].

43. Schulz T, Hartschuh W. The trichofolliculoma undergoes changes corresponding to the regressing normal hair follicle in its cycle. *J Cutan Pathol*. 1998;25(7):341–353. [Epub October 9, 1998].

44. Misago N, Kimura T, Toda S, Mori T, Narisawa Y. A revaluation of trichofolliculoma: the histopathological and immunohistochemical features. *Am J Dermatopathol*. 2010;32(1):35–43. [Epub September 5, 2009].

45. Schulz T, Hartschuh W. Folliculo-sebaceous cystic hamartoma is a trichofolliculoma at its very late stage. *J Cutan Pathol*. 1998;25(7):354–364. [Epub October 9, 1998].

46. Simon RS, de Eusebio E, Alvarez-Vieitez A, Sanchez Yus E. Folliculo-sebaceous cystic hamartoma is but the sebaceous end of tricho-sebo-folliculoma spectrum. *J Cutan Pathol*. 1999;26(2):109. [Epub March 19, 1999].

47. Mehregan AH. Hair follicle tumors of the skin. *J Cutan Pathol*. 1985;12(3–4):189–195. [Epub June 1, 1985].

48. Liang YH, Sun CS, Ye XY, Zhang W, Yang S, Zhang XJ. Novel substitution and frameshift mutations of CYLD in two Chinese families with multiple familial trichoepithelioma. *Br J Dermatol*. 2008;158(5):1156–1158. [Epub March 28, 2008].

49. Heinritz W, Grunewald S, Strenge S, et al. A case of Brooke-Spiegler syndrome with a new mutation in the CYLD gene. *Br J Dermatol*. 2006;154(5):992–994. [Epub April 26, 2006].

50. Bettencourt MS, Prieto VG, Shea CR. Trichoepithelioma: a 19-year clinicopathologic re-evaluation. *J Cutan Pathol*. 1999;26(8):398–404. [Epub November 7, 1999].

51. Dervan PA, O'Hegarty M, O'Loughlin S, Corrigan T. Solitary familial desmoplastic trichoepithelioma. A study by conventional and electron microscopy. *Am J Dermatopathol*. 1985;7(3):277–282. [Epub June 1, 1985].

52. Lazorik FC, Wood MG. Multiple desmoplastic trichoepitheliomas. *Arch Dermatol*. 1982;118(5): 361–362. [Epub May 1, 1982].

53. Brownstein MH. Trichilemmoma. Benign follicular tumor or viral wart? *Am J Dermatopathol*. 1980;2(3):229–231. [Epub January 1, 1980].

54. Reed RJ. Tricholemmoma. A cutaneous hamartoma. *Am J Dermatopathol*. 1980;2(3):227–228. [Epub January 1, 1980].

55. Starink TM. Cowden's disease: analysis of fourteen new cases. *J Am Acad Dermatol*. 1984;11(6):1127–1141. [Epub December, 1, 1984].

56. Mangas C, Hilari JM, Ribera M, et al. Cowden disease in a family: a clinical and genetic diagnosis. *J Am Acad Dermatol*. 2005;53(2):359–360. [Epub July 16, 2005].

57. Roson E, Gomez Centeno P, Sanchez-Aguilar D, Peteiro C, Toribio J. Desmoplastic trichilemmoma arising within a nevus sebaceous. *Am J Dermatopathol*. 1998;20(5):495–497. [Epub October 28, 1998].

58. Lee JY, Tang CK, Leung YS. Clear cell carcinoma of the skin: a tricholemmal carcinoma? *J Cutan Pathol*. 1989;16(1):31–39. [Epub February 1, 1989].

59. Kim JY, Kim YC. Trichoblastoma and syringocystadenoma papilliferum arising in naevus sebaceous in a 4-year-old boy. *Clin Exp Dermatol.* 2007;32(2):218–219. [Epub March 8, 2007].
60. Uzquiano MC, Prieto VG, Nash JW, et al. Metastatic basal cell carcinoma exhibits reduced actin expression. *Mod Pathol.* 2008;21(5):540–543. [Epub January 29, 2008].
61. Santa Cruz DJ, Barr RJ, Headington JT. Cutaneous lymphadenoma. *Am J Surg Pathol.* 1991;15(2):101–110. [Epub February 1, 1991].
62. Pardal-de-Oliveira F, Sanches A. Cutaneous lymphadenoma. *Histopathology.* 1994;25(4):384–387. [Epub October 1, 1994].
63. Cribier B, Grosshans E. Tumor of the follicular infundibulum: a clinicopathologic study. *J Am Acad Dermatol.* 1995;33(6):979–984. [Epub December 1, 1995].
64. Steffen C. Winer's dilated pore: the infundibuloma. *Am J Dermatopathol.* 2001;23(3):246–253. [Epub June 8, 2001].
65. Vakilzadeh F. [Pilar sheath acanthoma]. *Hautarzt.* 1987;38(1):40–42. [Epub January 1, 1987]. Haarscheidenakanthom.
66. Ubogy-Rainey Z, James WD, Lupton GP, Rodman OG. Fibrofolliculomas, trichodiscomas, and acrochordons: the Birt-Hogg-Dube syndrome. *J Am Acad Dermatol.* 1987;16(2 Pt 2):452–457. [Epub February 1, 1987].
67. Fujita WH, Barr RJ, Headley JL. Multiple fibrofolliculomas with trichodiscomas and acrochordons. *Arch Dermatol.* 1981;117(1):32–35. [Epub January 1, 1981].
68. Marrogi AJ, Wick MR, Dehner LP. Pilomatrical neoplasms in children and young adults. *Am J Dermatopathol.* 1992;14(2):87–94. [Epub April 1, 1992].
69. Taaffe A, Wyatt EH, Bury HP. Pilomatricoma (Malherbe). A clinical and histopathologic survey of 78 cases. *Int J Dermatol.* 1988;27(7):477–480. [Epub September 1, 1988].
70. Hardisson D, Linares MD, Cuevas-Santos J, Contreras F. Pilomatrix carcinoma: a clinicopathologic study of six cases and review of the literature. *Am J Dermatopathol.* 2001;23(5):394–401. [Epub January 22, 2002].
71. Ackerman AB, Penneys NS. Montgomery's tubercles. Sebaceous glands. *Obstet Gynecol.* 1971;38(6):924–927. [Epub December 1, 1971].
72. Templeton SF. Folliculosebaceous cystic hamartoma: a clinical pathologic study. *J Am Acad Dermatol.* 1996;34(1):77–81. [Epub January 1, 1996].
73. El-Darouty MA, Marzouk SA, Abdel-Halim MR, El-Komy MH, Mashaly HM. Folliculo-sebaceous cystic hamartoma. *Int J Dermatol.* 2001;40(7):454–457. [Epub October 27, 2001].
74. Morioka S. The natural history of nevus sebaceus. *J Cutan Pathol.* 1985;12(3–4):200–213. [Epub June 1, 1985].
75. Feuerstein RC, Mims LC. Linear nevus sebaceus with convulsions and mental retardation. *Am J Dis Child.* 1962;104:675–679. [Epub December 1, 1962].
76. Ferguson JW, Geary CP, MacAlister AD. Sebaceous cell adenoma. Rare intra-oral occurrence of a tumour which is a frequent marker of Torre's syndrome. *Pathology.* 1987;19(2):204–208. [Epub April 1, 1987].
77. Misago N, Narisawa Y. Sebaceous neoplasms in Muir-Torre syndrome. *Am J Dermatopathol.* 2000;22(2):155–161. [Epub April 19, 2000].
78. Nelson BR, Hamlet KR, Gillard M, Railan D, Johnson TM. Sebaceous carcinoma. *J Am Acad Dermatol.* 1995;33(1):1–15; quiz 6–8. [Epub July 1, 1995].
79. Moreno C, Jacyk WK, Judd MJ, Requena L. Highly aggressive extraocular sebaceous carcinoma. *Am J Dermatopathol.* 2001;23(5):450–455. [Epub January 22, 2002].
80. Kass LG, Hornblass A. Sebaceous carcinoma of the ocular adnexa. *Surv Ophthalmol.* 1989;33(6):477–490. [Epub May 1, 1989].
81. Schwartz RA, Torre DP. The Muir-Torre syndrome: a 25-year retrospect. *J Am Acad Dermatol.* 1995;33(1):90–104. [Epub July 1, 1995].
82. Dores GM, Curtis RE, Toro JR, Devesa SS, Fraumeni JF Jr. Incidence of cutaneous sebaceous carcinoma and risk of associated neoplasms: insight into Muir-Torre syndrome. *Cancer.* 2008;113(12):3372–3381. [Epub October 22, 2008].

83. Burgdorf WH, Pitha J, Fahmy A. Muir-Torre syndrome. Histologic spectrum of sebaceous proliferations. *Am J Dermatopathol.* 1986;8(3):202–208. [Epub June 1, 1986].

84. Fernandez-Flores A. Considerations on the performance of immunohistochemistry for mismatch repair gene proteins in cases of sebaceous neoplasms and keratoacanthomas with reference to Muir-Torre syndrome. *Am J Dermatopathol.* 2012;34(4):416–422. [Epub November 30, 2011].

85. Ponti G, Longo C. Microsatellite instability and mismatch repair protein expression in sebaceous tumors, keratocanthoma, and basal cell carcinomas with sebaceous differentiation in Muir-Torre syndrome. *J Am Acad Dermatol.* 2013;68(3):509–510. [Epub February 12, 2013].

86. Kazakov DV, Mikyskova I, Kutzner H, et al. Hidradenoma papilliferum with oxyphilic metaplasia: a clinicopathological study of 18 cases, including detection of human papillomavirus. *Am J Dermatopathol.* 2005;27(2):102–110. [Epub March 31, 2005].

87. Woodworth H Jr, Dockerty MB, Wilson RB, Pratt JH. Papillary hidradenoma of the vulva: a clinicopathologic study of 69 cases. *Am J Obstet Gynecol.* 1971;110(4):501–508. [Epub June 15, 1971].

88. Mammino JJ, Vidmar DA. Syringocystadenoma papilliferum: report of an unusual case. *Int J Dermatol.* 1991;30(11):828. [Epub November 1, 1991].

89. Cribier B, Scrivener Y, Grosshans E. Tumors arising in nevus sebaceus: a study of 596 cases. *J Am Acad Dermatol.* 2000;42(2 Pt 1):263–268. [Epub January 22, 2000].

90. Umbert P, Winkelmann RK. Tubular apocrine adenoma. *J Cutan Pathol.* 1976;3(2):75–87. [Epub January 1, 1976].

91. Ishiko A, Shimizu H, Inamoto N, Nakmura K. Is tubular apocrine adenoma a distinct clinical entity? *Am J Dermatopathol.* 1993;15(5):482–487. [Epub October 1, 1993].

92. Brownstein MH, Phelps RG, Magnin PH. Papillary adenoma of the nipple: analysis of fifteen new cases. *J Am Acad Dermatol.* 1985;12(4):707–715. [Epub April 1, 1985].

93. Thompson LD, Nelson BL, Barnes EL. Ceruminous adenomas: a clinicopathologic study of 41 cases with a review of the literature. *Am J Surg Pathol.* 2004;28(3):308–318. [Epub April 24, 2004].

94. Maheshwari MB, Hejmadi RK, Stores OP, O'Connell J. Ceruminous gland tumour. *Histopathology.* 2002;41(3):275–276. [Epub September 5, 2002].

95. Fernandez-Figueras MT, Puig L, Trias I, Lorenzo JC, Navas-Palacios JJ. Benign myoepithelioma of the skin. *Am J Dermatopathol.* 1998;20(2):208–212. [Epub April 29, 1998].

96. Kutzner H, Mentzel T, Kaddu S, Soares LM, Sangueza OP, Requena L. Cutaneous myoepithelioma: an under-recognized cutaneous neoplasm composed of myoepithelial cells. *Am J Surg Pathol.* 2001;25(3):348–355. [Epub February 27, 2001].

97. Henner MS, Shapiro PE, Ritter JH, Leffell DJ, Wick MR. Solitary syringoma. Report of five cases and clinicopathologic comparison with microcystic adnexal carcinoma of the skin. *Am J Dermatopathol.* 1995;17(5):465–470. [Epub October 1, 1995].

98. Patrizi A, Neri I, Marzaduri S, Varotti E, Passarini B. Syringoma: a review of twenty-nine cases. *Acta Derm Venereol.* 1998;78(6):460–462. [Epub December 2, 1998].

99. Helwig EB. Eccrine acrospiroma. *J Cutan Pathol.* 1984;11(5):415–420. [Epub October 1, 1984].

100. Gilaberte Y, Grasa MP, Carapeto FJ. Clear cell hidradenoma. *J Am Acad Dermatol.* 2006;54 (suppl 5):248–249. [Epub April 25, 2006].

101. Kazakov DV, Vanecek T, Belousova IE, Mukensnabl P, Kollertova D, Michal M. Skin-type hidradenoma of the breast parenchyma with t(11;19) translocation: hidradenoma of the breast. *Am J Dermatopathol.* 2007;29(5):457–461. [Epub September 25, 2007].

102. Winnes M, Molne L, Suurkula M, et al. Frequent fusion of the CRTC1 and MAML2 genes in clear cell variants of cutaneous hidradenomas. *Genes, Chromosomes Cancer.* 2007;46(6):559–563. [Epub March 6, 2007].

103. Gauerke S, Driscoll JJ. Hidradenocarcinomas: a brief review and future directions. *Arch Pathol Lab Med.* 2010;134(5):781–785. [Epub May 6, 2010].

104. Souvatzidis P, Sbano P, Mandato F, Fimiani M, Castelli A. Malignant nodular hidradenoma of theskin: report of seven cases. *J Eur Acad Dermatol Venereol.* 2008;22(5):549–554. [Epub April 16, 2008].

105. Wong TY, Suster S, Nogita T, Duncan LM, Dickersin RG, Mihm MC Jr. Clear cell eccrine carcinomas of the skin. A clinicopathologic study of nine patients. *Cancer*. 1994;73(6):1631–1643. [Epub March 15, 1994].

106. Rahbari H. Hidroacanthoma simplex—a review of 15 cases. *Br J Dermatol*. 1983;109(2):219–225. [Epub August 1, 1983].

107. Goldman P, Pinkus H, Rogin JR. Eccrine poroma; tumors exhibiting features of the epidermal sweat duct unit. *AMA Arch Dermatol*. 1956;74(5):511–521. [Epub November 1, 1956].

108. Kakinuma H, Miyamoto R, Iwasawa U, Baba S, Suzuki H. Three subtypes of poroid neoplasia in a single lesion: eccrine poroma, hidroacanthoma simplex, and dermal duct tumor. Histologic, histochemical, and ultrastructural findings. *Am J Dermatopathol*. 1994;16(1):66–72. [Epub February 1, 1994].

109. Winkelmann RK, McLeod WA. The dermal duct tumor. *Arch Dermatol*. 1966;94(1):50–55. [Epub July 1, 1966].

110. Shaw M, McKee PH, Lowe D, Black MM. Malignant eccrine poroma: a study of twenty-seven cases. *Br J Dermatol*. 1982;107(6):675–680. [Epub December 1, 1982].

111. Robson A, Greene J, Ansari N, et al. Eccrine porocarcinoma (malignant eccrine poroma): a clinicopathologic study of 69 cases. *Am J Surg Pathol*. 2001;25(6):710–720. [Epub June 8, 2001].

112. Pylyser K, De Wolf-Peeters C, Marien K. The histology of eccrine poromas: a study of 14 cases. *Dermatologica*. 1983;167(5):243–249. [Epub January 1, 1983].

113. Mambo NC. Eccrine spiradenoma: clinical and pathologic study of 49 tumors. *J Cutan Pathol*. 1983;10(5):312–320. [Epub October 1, 1983].

114. Wright S, Ryan J. Multiple familial eccrine spiradenoma with cylindroma. *Acta Derm Venereol*. 1990;70(1):79–82. [Epub January 1, 1990].

115. Granter SR, Seeger K, Calonje E, Busam K, McKee PH. Malignant eccrine spiradenoma (spiradenocarcinoma): a clinicopathologic study of 12 cases. *Am J Dermatopathol*. 2000;22(2): 97–103. [Epub April 19, 2000].

116. Argenyi ZB, Nguyen AV, Balogh K, Sears JK, Whitaker DC. Malignant eccrine spiradenoma. A clinicopathologic study. *Am J Dermatopathol*. 1992;14(5):381–390. [Epub October 1, 1992].

117. Hu G, Onder M, Gill M, et al. A novel missense mutation in CYLD in a family with Brooke-Spiegler syndrome. *J Invest Dermatol*. 2003;121(4):732–734. [Epub November 25, 2003].

118. van der Putte SC. The pathogenesis of familial multiple cylindromas, trichoepitheliomas, milia, and spiradenomas. *Am J Dermatopathol*. 1995;17(3):271–280. [Epub June 1, 1995].

119. Lin PY, Fatteh SM, Lloyd KM. Malignant transformation in a solitary dermal cylindroma. *Arch Pathol Lab Med*. 1987;111(8):765–767. [Epub August 1, 1987].

120. Urbanski SJ, From L, Abramowicz A, Joaquin A, Luk SC. Metamorphosis of dermal cylindroma: possible relation to malignant transformation. Case report of cutaneous cylindroma with direct intracranial invasion. *J Am Acad Dermatol*. 1985;12(1 Pt 2):188–195. [Epub January 1, 1985].

121. Gerretsen AL, van der Putte SC, Deenstra W, van Vloten WA. Cutaneous cylindroma with malignant transformation. *Cancer*. 1993;72(5):1618–1623. [Epub September 1, 1993].

122. Chen AH, Moreano EH, Houston B, Funk GF. Chondroid syringoma of the head and neck: clinical management and literature review. *Ear Nose Throat J*. 1996;75(2):104–108. [Epub February 1, 1996].

123. Kazakov DV, Belousova IE, Bisceglia M, et al. Apocrine mixed tumor of the skin ("mixed tumor of the folliculosebaceous-apocrine complex"). Spectrum of differentiations and metaplastic changes in the epithelial, myoepithelial, and stromal components based on a histopathologic study of 244 cases. *J Am Acad Dermatol*. 2007;57(3):467–483. [Epub August 21, 2007].

124. Redono C, Rocamora A, Villoria F, Garcia M. Malignant mixed tumor of the skin: malignant chondroid syringoma. *Cancer*. 1982;49(8):1690–1696. [Epub April 15, 1982].

125. Ishimura E, Iwamoto H, Kobashi Y, Yamabe H, Ichijima K. Malignant chondroid syringoma. Report of a case with widespread metastasis and review of pertinent literature. *Cancer*. 1983;52(10):1966–1973. [Epub November 15, 1983].

126. Kazakov DV, Suster S, LeBoit PE, et al. Mucinous carcinoma of the skin, primary, and secondary: a clinicopathologic study of 63 cases with emphasis on the morphologic spectrum

of primary cutaneous forms: homologies with mucinous lesions in the breast. *Am J Surg Pathol.* 2005;29(6):764–782. [Epub May 18, 2005].

127. Kalebi A, Hale M. Primary mucinous carcinoma of the skin: usefulness of p63 in excluding metastasis and first report of psammoma bodies. *Am J Dermatopathol.* 2008;30(5):510. [Epub September 23, 2008].

128. Carson HJ, Gattuso P, Raslan WF, Reddy V. Mucinous carcinoma of the eyelid. An immunohistochemical study. *Am J Dermatopathol.* 1995;17(5):494–498. [Epub October 1, 1995].

129. Urso C, Paglierani M, Bondi R. Histologic spectrum of carcinomas with eccrine ductal differentiation (sweat-gland ductal carcinomas). *Am J Dermatopathol.* 1993;15(5):435–440. [Epub October 1, 1993].

130. McLean SR, Shousha S, Francis N, et al. Metastatic ductal eccrine adenocarcinoma masquerading as an invasive ductal carcinoma of the male breast. *J Cutan Pathol.* 2007;34(12):934–938. [Epub November 16, 2007].

131. Plaza JA, Ortega PF, Stockman DL, Suster S. Value of p63 and podoplanin (D2-40) immunoreactivity in the distinction between primary cutaneous tumors and adenocarcinomas metastatic to the skin: a clinicopathologic and immunohistochemical study of 79 cases. *J Cutan Pathol.* 2010;37(4):403–410. [Epub April 10, 2010].

132. Ivan D, Nash JW, Prieto VG, et al. Use of p63 expression in distinguishing primary and metastatic cutaneous adnexal neoplasms from metastatic adenocarcinoma to skin. *J Cutan Pathol.* 2007;34(6):474–480. [Epub May 24, 2007].

133. Goldstein DJ, Barr RJ, Santa Cruz DJ. Microcystic adnexal carcinoma: a distinct clinicopathologic entity. *Cancer.* 1982;50(3):566–572. [Epub August 1, 1982].

134. LeBoit PE, Sexton M. Microcystic adnexal carcinoma of the skin. A reappraisal of the differentiation and differential diagnosis of an underrecognized neoplasm. *J Am Acad Dermatol.* 1993;29(4):609–618. [Epub October 1, 1993].

135. Cooper PH, Mills SE. Microcystic adnexal carcinoma. *J Am Acad Dermatol.* 1984;10(5 Pt 2): 908–914. [Epub May 1, 1984].

136. Ceballos PI, Penneys NS, Acosta R. Aggressive digital papillary adenocarcinoma. *J Am Acad Dermatol.* 1990;23(2 Pt 2):331–334. [Epub August 1, 1990].

137. Duke WH, Sherrod TT, Lupton GP. Aggressive digital papillary adenocarcinoma (aggressive digital papillary adenoma and adenocarcinoma revisited). *Am J Surg Pathol.* 2000;24(6):775–784. [Epub June 8, 2000].

138. Frey J, Shimek C, Woodmansee C, et al. Aggressive digital papillary adenocarcinoma: a report of two diseases and review of the literature. *J Am Acad Dermatol.* 2009;60(2):331–339. [Epub September 30, 2008].

139. McGavran MH, Binnington B. Keratinous cysts of the skin. Identification and differentiation of pilar cysts from epidermal cysts. *Arch Dermatol.* 1966;94(4):499–508. [Epub October 1, 1966].

140. Narisawa Y, Kohda H. Cutaneous cysts of Gardner's syndrome are similar to follicular stem cells. *J Cutan Pathol.* 1995;22(2):115–121. [Epub April 1, 1995].

141. Lopez-Rios F, Rodriguez-Peralto JL, Castano E, Benito A. Squamous cell carcinoma arising in a cutaneous epidermal cyst: case report and literature review. *Am J Dermatopathol.* 1999;21(2): 174–177. [Epub April 28, 1999].

142. Delacretaz J. Keratotic basal-cell carcinoma arising from an epidermoid cyst. *J Dermatol Surg Oncol.* 1977;3(3):310–311. [Epub May 1, 1977].

143. Egawa K, Inaba Y, Honda Y, Johno M, Ono T. 'Cystic papilloma': human papillomavirus in a palmar epidermoid cyst. *Arch Dermatol.* 1992;128(12):1658–1659. [Epub December 1, 1992].

144. Pinkus H. "Sebaceous cysts" are trichilemmal cysts. *Arch Dermatol.* 1969;99(5):544–555. [Epub May 1, 1969].

145. Brownstein MH, Arluk DJ. Proliferating trichilemmal cyst: a simulant of squamous cell carcinoma. *Cancer.* 1981;48(5):1207–1214. [Epub September 1, 1981].

146. Janitz J, Wiedersberg H. Trichilemmal pilar tumors. *Cancer.* 1980;45(7):1594–1597. [Epub April 1, 1980].

147. Chintapatla S, Safarani N, Kumar S, Haboubi N. Sacrococcygeal pilonidal sinus: historical review, pathological insight and surgical options. *Tech Coloproctol.* 2003;7(1):3–8. [Epub May 17, 2003].

148. Hull TL, Wu J. Pilonidal disease. *Surg Clin North Am.* 2002;82(6):1169–1185. [Epub January 9, 2003].

149. Fernandez-Flores A. Morphologic image on infundibular origin of verrucous cyst. *Am J Dermatopathol.* 2008;30(2):199–200. [Epub March 25, 2008].

150. Kim H, Seok JY, Kim SH, et al. Human papillomavirus type 59 identified in a verrucous cyst of the flank. *Eur J Dermatol.* 2006;16(3):254–257. [Epub May 20, 2006].

151. Tomkova H, Fujimoto W, Arata J. Expression of keratins (K10 and K17) in steatocystoma multiplex, eruptive vellus hair cysts, and epidermoid and trichilemmal cysts. *Am J Dermatopathol.* 1997;19(3):250–253. [Epub June 1, 1997].

152. Stiefler RE, Bergfeld WF. Eruptive vellus hair cysts—an inherited disorder. *J Am Acad Dermatol.* 1980;3(4):425–429. [Epub October 1, 1980].

153. Moon SE, Lee YS, Youn JI. Eruptive vellus hair cyst and steatocystoma multiplex in a patient with pachyonychia congenita. *J Am Acad Dermatol.* 1994;30(2 Pt 1):275–276. [Epub February 1, 1994].

154. Cho S, Chang SE, Choi JH, Sung KJ, Moon KC, Koh JK. Clinical and histologic features of 64 cases of steatocystoma multiplex. *J Dermatol.* 2002;29(3):152–156. [Epub May 7, 2002].

155. Bratton C, Suskind DL, Thomas T, Kluka EA. Autosomal dominant familial frontonasal dermoid cysts: a mother and her identical twin daughters. *Int J Pediatr Otorhinolaryngol.* 2001;57(3):249–253. [Epub February 27, 2001].

156. Ogle RF, Jauniaux E. Fetal scalp cysts—dilemmas in diagnosis. *Prenat Diagn.* 1999;19(12):1157–1159. [Epub December 11, 1999].

157. Sperling LC, Sakas EL. Eccrine hidrocystomas. *J Am Acad Dermatol.* 1982;7(6):763–770. [Epub December 1, 1982].

158. Farmer ER, Helwig EB. Cutaneous ciliated cysts. *Arch Dermatol.* 1978;114(1):70–73. [Epub January 1, 1978].

159. al-Nafussi AI, Carder P. Cutaneous ciliated cyst: a case report and immunohistochemical comparison with fallopian tube. *Histopathology.* 1990;16(6):595–598. [Epub June 1, 1990].

160. Kurban RS, Bhawan J. Cutaneous cysts lined by nonsquamous epithelium. *Am J Dermatopathol.* 1991;13(5):509–517. [Epub October 1, 1991].

161. deMello DE, Lima JA, Liapis H. Midline cervical cysts in children. Thyroglossal anomalies. *Arch Otolaryngol Head Neck Surg.* 1987;113(4):418–420. [Epub April 1, 1987].

162. Michalopoulos N, Papavramidis TS, Karayannopoulou G, et al. Cervical thymic cysts in adults. *Thyroid.* 2011;21(9):987–992. [Epub May 21, 2011].

163. Coleman WR, Homer RS, Kaplan RP. Branchial cleft heterotopia of the lower neck. *J Cutan Pathol.* 1989;16(6):353–358. [Epub December 1, 1989].

164. Fraga S, Helwig EB, Rosen SH. Bronchogenic cysts in the skin and subcutaneous tissue. *Am J Clin Pathol.* 1971;56(2):230–238. [Epub August 1, 1971].

165. van der Putte SC, Toonstra J. Cutaneous 'bronchogenic' cyst. *J Cutan Pathol.* 1985;12(5):404–409. [Epub October 1, 1985].

166. Nagore E, Sanchez-Motilla JM, Febrer MI, Aliaga A. Median raphe cysts of the penis: a report of five cases. *Pediatr Dermatol.* 1998;15(3):191–193. [Epub July 9, 1998].

167. Paul AY, Pak HS, Welch ML, Toner CB, Yeager J. Pseudocyst of the auricle: diagnosis and management with a punch biopsy. *J Am Acad Dermatol.* 2001;45(suppl 6):S230–S232. [Epub November 17, 2001].

168. Heim S, Mandahl N, Rydholm A, Willen H, Mitelman F. Different karyotypic features characterize different clinico-pathologic subgroups of benign lipogenic tumors. *Int J Cancer.* 1988;42(6):863–867. [Epub December 15, 1988].

169. Rydholm A, Berg NO. Size, site and clinical incidence of lipoma. Factors in the differential diagnosis of lipoma and sarcoma. *Acta Orthop Scand.* 1983;54(6):929–934. [Epub December 1, 1983].

170. Mandahl N, Heim S, Arheden K, Rydholm A, Willen H, Mitelman F. Three major cytogenetic subgroups can be identified among chromosomally abnormal solitary lipomas. *Hum Genet.* 1988;79(3):203–208. [Epub July 1, 1988].

171. Dixon AY, McGregor DH, Lee SH. Angiolipomas: an ultrastructural and clinicopathological study. *Hum Pathol.* 1981;12(8):739–747. [Epub August 1, 1981].
172. Fletcher CD, Martin-Bates E. Spindle cell lipoma: a clinicopathological study with some original observations. *Histopathology.* 1987;11(8):803–817. [Epub August 1, 1987].
173. Dal Cin P, Sciot R, Polito P, et al. Lesions of 13q may occur independently of deletion of 16q in spindle cell/pleomorphic lipomas. *Histopathology.* 1997;31(3):222–225. [Epub November 14, 1997].
174. Azzopardi JG, Iocco J, Salm R. Pleomorphic lipoma: a tumour simulating liposarcoma. *Histopathology.* 1983;7(4):511–523. [Epub July 1, 1983].
175. Griffin TD, Goldstein J, Johnson WC. Pleomorphic lipoma. Case report and discussion of "atypical" lipomatous tumors. *J Cutan Pathol.* 1992;19(4):330–333. [Epub August 1, 1992].
176. Finley AG, Musso LA. Naevus lipomatosus cutaneus superficialis (Hoffman-Zurhelle). *Br J Dermatol.* 1972;87(6):557–564. [Epub December 1, 1972].
177. Mehregan AH, Tavafoghi V, Ghandchi A. Nevus lipomatosus cutaneus superficialis (Hoffmann-Zurhelle). *J Cutan Pathol.* 1975;2(6):307–313. [Epub January 1, 1975].
178. Raj S, Calonje E, Kraus M, Kavanagh G, Newman PL, Fletcher CD. Cutaneous pilar leiomyoma: clinicopathologic analysis of 53 lesions in 45 patients. *Am J Dermatopathol.* 1997;19(1):2–9. [Epub February 1, 1997].
179. Alam NA, Bevan S, Churchman M, et al. Localization of a gene (MCUL1) for multiple cutaneous leiomyomata and uterine fibroids to chromosome 1q42.3-q43. *Am J Hum Genet.* 2001;68(5): 1264–1269. [Epub April 3, 2001].
180. MacDonald DM, Sanderson KV. Angioleiomyoma of the skin. *Br J Dermatol.* 1974;91(2):161–168. [Epub August 1, 1974].
181. Hachisuga T, Hashimoto H, Enjoji M. Angioleiomyoma. A clinicopathologic reappraisal of 562 cases. *Cancer.* 1984;54(1):126–130. [Epub July 1, 1984].
182. Johnson MD, Jacobs AH. Congenital smooth muscle hamartoma. A report of six cases and a review of the literature. *Arch Dermatol.* 1989;125(6):820–822. [Epub June 1, 1989].
183. Gagne EJ, Su WP. Congenital smooth muscle hamartoma of the skin. *Pediatr Dermatol.* 1993;10(2):142–145. [Epub June 1, 1993].
184. Dahl I, Angervall L. Cutaneous and subcutaneous leiomyosarcoma. A clinicopathologic study of 47 patients. *Pathol Eur.* 1974;9(4):307–315. [Epub January 1, 1974].
185. Kaddu S, Beham A, Cerroni L, et al. Cutaneous leiomyosarcoma. *Am J Surg Pathol.* 1997;21(9):979–987. [Epub September 23, 1997].
186. Massi D, Franchi A, Alos L, et al. Primary cutaneous leiomyosarcoma: clinicopathological analysis of 36 cases. *Histopathology.* 2010;56(2):251–262. [Epub January 28, 2010].
187. Blackburn WR, Cosman B. Histologic basis of keloid and hypertrophic scar differentiation. Clinicopathologic correlation. *Arch Pathol.* 1966;82(1):65–71. [Epub July 1, 1966].
188. Murray JC, Pollack SV, Pinnell SR. Keloids: a review. *J Am Acad Dermatol.* 1981;4(4):461–470. [Epub April 1, 1981].
189. Bernstein KE, Lattes R. Nodular (pseudosarcomatous) fasciitis, a nonrecurrent lesion: clinicopathologic study of 134 cases. *Cancer.* 1982;49(8):1668–1678. [Epub April 15, 1982].
190. Weinreb I, Shaw AJ, Perez-Ordonez B, Goldblum JR, Rubin BP. Nodular fasciitis of the head and neck region: a clinicopathologic description in a series of 30 cases. *J Cutan Pathol.* 2009;36(11):1168–1173. [Epub May 28, 2009].
191. Perez-Montiel MD, Plaza JA, Dominguez-Malagon H, Suster S. Differential expression of smooth muscle myosin, smooth muscle actin, h-caldesmon, and calponin in the diagnosis of myofibroblastic and smooth muscle lesions of skin and soft tissue. *Am J Dermatopathol.* 2006;28(2):105–111. [Epub April 21, 2006].
192. Nagamine N, Nohara Y, Ito E. Elastofibroma in Okinawa. A clinicopathologic study of 170 cases. *Cancer.* 1982;50(9):1794–1805. [Epub November 1, 1982].
193. Balachandran K, Allen PW, MacCormac LB. Nuchal fibroma. A clinicopathological study of nine cases. *Am J Surg Pathol.* 1995;19(3):313–317. [Epub March 1, 1995].
194. Diwan AH, Graves ED, King JA, Horenstein MG. Nuchal-type fibroma in two related patients with Gardner's syndrome. *Am J Surg Pathol.* 2000;24(11):1563–1567. [Epub November 15, 2000].

195. Coffin CM, Hornick JL, Zhou H, Fletcher CD. Gardner fibroma: a clinicopathologic and immunohistochemical analysis of 45 patients with 57 fibromas. *Am J Surg Pathol.* 2007;31(3): 410–416. [Epub February 28, 2007].

196. Banik R, Lubach D. Skin tags: localization and frequencies according to sex and age. *Dermatologica.* 1987;174(4):180–183. [Epub January 1, 1987].

197. Kahana M, Grossman E, Feinstein A, Ronnen M, Cohen M, Millet MS. Skin tags: a cutaneous marker for diabetes mellitus. *Acta Derm Venereol.* 1987;67(2):175–177. [Epub January 1, 1987].

198. Kamino H, Lee JY, Berke A. Pleomorphic fibroma of the skin: a benign neoplasm with cytologic atypia. A clinicopathologic study of eight cases. *Am J Surg Pathol.* 1989;13(2):107–113. [Epub February 1, 1989].

199. Rapini RP, Golitz LE. Sclerotic fibromas of the skin. *J Am Acad Dermatol.* 1989;20(2 Pt 1):266–271. [Epub February 1, 1989].

200. Al-Daraji WI, Ramsay HM, Ali RB. Storiform collagenoma as a clue for Cowden disease or PTEN hamartoma tumour syndrome. *J Clin Pathol.* 2007;60(7):840–842. [Epub May 22, 2007].

201. Fetsch JF, Laskin WB, Miettinen M. Superficial acral fibromyxoma: a clinicopathologic and immunohistochemical analysis of 37 cases of a distinctive soft tissue tumor with a predilection for the fingers and toes. *Hum Pathol.* 2001;32(7):704–714. [Epub August 4, 2001].

202. Luzar B, Calonje E. Superficial acral fibromyxoma: clinicopathological study of 14 cases with emphasis on a cellular variant. *Histopathology.* 2009;54(3):375–377. [Epub February 25, 2009].

203. Calonje E, Guerin D, McCormick D, Fletcher CD. Superficial angiomyxoma: clinicopathologic analysis of a series of distinctive but poorly recognized cutaneous tumors with tendency for recurrence. *Am J Surg Pathol.* 1999;23(8):910–917. [Epub August 6, 1999].

204. Kacerovska D, Sima R, Michal M, et al. Carney complex: a clinicopathologic and molecular biological study of a sporadic case, including extracutaneous and cutaneous lesions and a novel mutation of the PRKAR1A gene. *J Am Acad Dermatol.* 2009;61(1):80–87. [Epub June 23, 2009].

205. Cooper PH, Mackel SE. Acquired fibrokeratoma of the heel. *Arch Dermatol.* 1985;121(3):386–388. [Epub March 1, 1985].

206. Hare PJ, Smith PA. Acquired (digital) fibrokeratoma. *Br J Dermatol.* 1969;81(9):667–670. [Epub September 1, 1969].

207. Dickey GE, Sotelo-Avila C. Fibrous hamartoma of infancy: current review. *Pediatr Dev Pathol.* 1999;2(3):236–243. [Epub April 7, 1999].

208. Fletcher CD, Powell G, van Noorden S, McKee PH. Fibrous hamartoma of infancy: a histochemical and immunohistochemical study. *Histopathology.* 1988;12(1):65–74. [Epub January 1, 1988].

209. Laskin WB, Miettinen M, Fetsch JF. Infantile digital fibroma/fibromatosis: a clinicopathologic and immunohistochemical study of 69 tumors from 57 patients with long-term follow-up. *Am J Surg Pathol.* 2009;33(1):1–13. [Epub October 3, 2008].

210. Bhawan J, Bacchetta C, Joris I, Majno G. A myofibroblastic tumor. Infantile digital fibroma (recurrent digital fibrous tumor of childhood). *Am J Pathol.* 1979;94(1):19–36. [Epub January 1, 1979].

211. Fetsch JF, Laskin WB, Miettinen M. Palmar-plantar fibromatosis in children and preadolescents: a clinicopathologic study of 56 cases with newly recognized demographics and extended follow-up information. *Am J Surg Pathol.* 2005;29(8):1095–1105. [Epub July 12, 2005].

212. Reitamo JJ, Hayry P, Nykyri E, Saxen E. The desmoid tumor. I. Incidence, sex-, age- and anatomical distribution in the Finnish population. *Am J Clin Pathol.* 1982;77(6):665–673. [Epub June 1, 1982].

213. Ayala AG, Ro JY, Goepfert H, Cangir A, Khorsand J, Flake G. Desmoid fibromatosis: a clinicopathologic study of 25 children. *Semin Diagn Pathol.* 1986;3(2):138–150. [Epub May 1, 1986].

214. Schwartz RA, Fernandez G, Kotulska K, Jozwiak S. Tuberous sclerosis complex: advances in diagnosis, genetics, and management. *J Am Acad Dermatol.* 2007;57(2):189–202. [Epub July 20, 2007].

215. Jozwiak J, Galus R. Molecular implications of skin lesions in tuberous sclerosis. *Am J Dermatopathol.* 2008;30(3):256–261. [Epub May 23, 2008].

216. Graham JH, Sanders JB, Johnson WC, Helwig EB. Fibrous papule of the nose: a clinicopathological study. *J Invest Dermatol*. 1965;45(3):194–203. [Epub September 1, 1965].
217. Bansal C, Stewart D, Li A, Cockerell CJ. Histologic variants of fibrous papule. *J Cutan Pathol*. 2005;32(6):424–428. [Epub June 15, 2005].
218. Agrawal SK, Bhattacharya SN, Singh N. Pearly penile papules: a review. *Int J Dermatol*. 2004;43(3):199–201. [Epub March 11, 2004].
219. Smolle J, Auboeck L, Gogg-Retzer I, Soyer HP, Kerl H. Multinucleate cell angiohistiocytoma: a clinicopathological, immunohistochemical and ultrastructural study. *Br J Dermatol*. 1989;121(1):113–121. [Epub July 1, 1989].
220. Shapiro PE, Nova MP, Rosmarin LA, Halperin AJ. Multinucleate cell angiohistiocytoma: a distinct entity diagnosable by clinical and histologic features. *J Am Acad Dermatol*. 1994;30(3): 417–422. [Epub March 1, 1994].
221. Vilanova JR, Flint A. The morphological variations of fibrous histiocytomas. *J Cutan Pathol*. 1974;1(4):155–164. [Epub January 1, 1974].
222. Meister P, Konrad E, Krauss F. Fibrous histiocytoma: a histological and statistical analysis of 155 cases. *Pathol Res Pract*. 1978;162(4):361–379. [Epub August 1, 1978].
223. Fletcher CD, Evans BJ, MacArtney JC, Smith N, Wilson Jones E, McKee PH. Dermatofibrosarcoma protuberans: a clinicopathological and immunohistochemical study with a review of the literature. *Histopathology*. 1985;9(9):921–938. [Epub September 1, 1985].
224. Edelweiss M, Malpica A. Dermatofibrosarcoma protuberans of the vulva: a clinicopathologic and immunohistochemical study of 13 cases. *Am J Surg Pathol*. 2010;34(3):393–400. [Epub February 9, 2010].
225. Maire G, Pedeutour F, Coindre JM. COL1A1-PDGFB gene fusion demonstrates a common histogenetic origin for dermatofibrosarcoma protuberans and its granular cell variant. *Am J Surg Pathol*. 2002;26(7):932–937. [Epub July 20, 2002].
226. Patel KU, Szabo SS, Hernandez VS, et al. Dermatofibrosarcoma protuberans COL1A1-PDGFB fusion is identified in virtually all dermatofibrosarcoma protuberans cases when investigated by newly developed multiplex reverse transcription polymerase chain reaction and fluorescence in situ hybridization assays. *Hum Pathol*. 2008;39(2):184–193. [Epub October 24, 2007].
227. Erdem O, Wyatt AJ, Lin E, Wang X, Prieto VG. Dermatofibrosarcoma protuberans treated with wide local excision and followed at a cancer hospital: prognostic significance of clinicopathologic variables. *Am J Dermatopathol*. 2012;34(1):24–34. [Epub July 26, 2011].
228. Wang WL, Patel KU, Coleman NM, et al. COL1A1:PDGFB chimeric transcripts are not present in indeterminate fibrohistiocytic lesions of the skin. *Am J Dermatopathol*. 2010;32(2):149–153. [Epub November 27, 2009].
229. Horenstein MG, Prieto VG, Nuckols JD, Burchette JL, Shea CR. Indeterminate fibrohistiocytic lesions of the skin: is there a spectrum between dermatofibroma and dermatofibrosarcoma protuberans? *Am J Surg Pathol*. 2000;24(7):996–1003. [Epub July 15, 2000].
230. Ushijima M, Hashimoto H, Tsuneyoshi M, Enjoji M. Giant cell tumor of the tendon sheath (nodular tenosynovitis). A study of 207 cases to compare the large joint group with the common digit group. *Cancer*. 1986;57(4):875–884. [Epub February 15, 1986].
231. Monaghan H, Salter DM, Al-Nafussi A. Giant cell tumour of tendon sheath (localised nodular tenosynovitis): clinicopathological features of 71 cases. *J Clin Pathol*. 2001;54(5):404–407. [Epub May 1, 2001].
232. Costa MJ, Weiss SW. Angiomatoid malignant fibrous histiocytoma. A follow-up study of 108 cases with evaluation of possible histologic predictors of outcome. *Am J Surg Pathol*. 1990;14(12):1126–1132. [Epub December 1, 1990].
233. Raddaoui E, Donner LR, Panagopoulos I. Fusion of the FUS and ATF1 genes in a large, deep-seated angiomatoid fibrous histiocytoma. *Diagn Mol Pathol*. 2002;11(3):157–162. [Epub September 10, 2002].
234. Rossi S, Szuhai K, Ijszenga M, et al. EWSR1-CREB1 and EWSR1-ATF1 fusion genes in angiomatoid fibrous histiocytoma. *Clin Cancer Res*. 2007;13(24):7322–7328. [Epub December 21, 2007].

235. Fretzin DF, Helwig EB. Atypical fibroxanthoma of the skin. A clinicopathologic study of 140 cases. *Cancer.* 1973;31(6):1541–1552. [Epub June 1, 1973].
236. Buonaccorsi JN, Plaza JA. Role of CD10, wide-spectrum keratin, p63, and podoplanin in the distinction of epithelioid and spindle cell tumors of the skin: an immunohistochemical study of 81 cases. *Am J Dermatopathol.* 2012;34(4):404–411. [Epub January 20, 2012].
237. Kanner WA, Brill LB II, Patterson JW, Wick MR. CD10, p63 and CD99 expression in the differential diagnosis of atypical fibroxanthoma, spindle cell squamous cell carcinoma and desmoplastic melanoma. *J Cutan Pathol.* 2010;37(7):744–750. [Epub February 27, 2010].
238. Remstein ED, Arndt CA, Nascimento AG. Plexiform fibrohistiocytic tumor: clinicopathologic analysis of 22 cases. *Am J Surg Pathol.* 1999;23(6):662–670. [Epub June 12, 1999].
239. Luzar B, Calonje E. Cutaneous fibrohistiocytic tumours—an update. *Histopathology.* 2010;56(1):148–165. [Epub January 9, 2010].
240. Taher A, Pushpanathan C. Plexiform fibrohistiocytic tumor: a brief review. *Arc Pathol Lab Med.* 2007;131(7):1135–1138. [Epub July 10, 2007].
241. Gonzalez-Crussi F, Reyes-Mugica M. Cellular hemangiomas ("hemangioendotheliomas") in infants. Light microscopic, immunohistochemical, and ultrastructural observations. *Am J Surg Pathol.* 1991;15(8):769–778. [Epub August 1, 1991].
242. Smoller BR, Apfelberg DB. Infantile (juvenile) capillary hemangioma: a tumor of heterogeneous cellular elements. *J Cutan Pathol.* 1993;20(4):330–336. [Epub August 1, 1993].
243. Mo JQ, Dimashkieh HH, Bove KE. GLUT1 endothelial reactivity distinguishes hepatic infantile hemangioma from congenital hepatic vascular malformation with associated capillary proliferation. *Hum Pathol.* 2004;35(2):200–209. [Epub March 3, 2004].
244. Calduch L, Ortega C, Navarro V, Martinez E, Molina I, Jorda E. Verrucous hemangioma: report of two cases and review of the literature. *Pediatr Dermatol.* 2000;17(3):213–217. [Epub July 8, 2000].
245. Lara-Corrales I, Somers GR, Ho N. Verrucous hemangioma: a challenging vascular lesion. *J Cutan Med Surg.* 2010;14(3):144–146. [Epub May 22, 2010].
246. Clairwood MQ, Bruckner AL, Dadras SS. Verrucous hemangioma: a report of two cases and review of the literature. *J Cutan Pathol.* 2011;38(9):740–746. [Epub June 9, 2011].
247. Cohen AD, Cagnano E, Vardy DA. Cherry angiomas associated with exposure to bromides. *Dermatology.* 2001;202(1):52–53. [Epub March 13, 2001].
248. Mills SE, Cooper PH, Fechner RE. Lobular capillary hemangioma: the underlying lesion of pyogenic granuloma. A study of 73 cases from the oral and nasal mucous membranes. *Am J Surg Pathol.* 1980;4(5):470–479. [Epub October 1, 1980].
249. Demir Y, Demir S, Aktepe F. Cutaneous lobular capillary hemangioma induced by pregnancy. *J Cutan Pathol.* 2004;31(1):77–80. [Epub December 17, 2003].
250. Fortna RR, Junkins-Hopkins JM. A case of lobular capillary hemangioma (pyogenic granuloma), localized to the subcutaneous tissue, and a review of the literature. *Am J Dermatopathol.* 2007;29(4):408–411. [Epub August 2, 2007].
251. Larson BT, Erdman AG, Tsekos NV, Yacoub E, Tsekos PV, Koutlas IG. Design of an MRI-compatible robotic stereotactic device for minimally invasive interventions in the breast. *J Biomech Eng.* 2004;126(4):458–465. [Epub November 17, 2004].
252. Akiyama M, Inamoto N. Arteriovenous haemangioma in chronic liver disease: clinical and histopathological features of four cases. *British J Dermatol.* 2001;144(3):604–609. [Epub March 22, 2001].
253. Aloi F, Tomasini C, Pippione M. Microvenular hemangioma. *Am J Dermatopathol.* 1993;15(6):534–538. [Epub December 1, 1993].
254. Berk DR, Abramova L, Crone KG, Bayliss SJ. Microvenular haemangioma: report of a paediatric case. *Clin Exp Dermatol.* 2009;34(7):e304–e306. [Epub May 22, 2009].
255. Trindade F, Kutzner H, Requena L, Tellechea O, Colmenero I. Microvenular hemangioma—an immunohistochemical study of 9 cases. *Am J Dermatopathol.* 2012;34(8):810–812. [Epub November 22, 2012].
256. Santa Cruz DJ, Aronberg J. Targetoid hemosiderotic hemangioma. *J Am Acad Dermatol.* 1988;19(3):550–558. [Epub September 1, 1988].

257. Rapini RP, Golitz LE. Targetoid hemosiderotic hemangioma. *J Cutan Pathol.* 1990;17(4):233–235. [Epub August 1, 1990].

258. Al Dhaybi R, Lam C, Hatami A, Powell J, McCuaig C, Kokta V. Targetoid hemosiderotic hemangiomas (hobnail hemangiomas) are vascular lymphatic malformations: a study of 12 pediatric cases. *J Am Acad Dermatol.* 2012;66(1):116–120. [Epub July 30, 2011].

259. Requena L, Kutzner H, Mentzel T. Acquired elastotic hemangioma: A clinicopathologic variant of hemangioma. *J Am Acad Dermatol.* 2002;47(3):371–376. [Epub August 28, 2002].

260. Martorell-Calatayud A, Balmer N, Sanmartin O, Diaz-Recuero JL, Sangu> eza OP. Definition of the features of acquired elastotic hemangioma reporting the clinical and histopathological characteristics of 14 patients. *J Cutan Pathol.* 2010;37(4):460–464. [Epub July 21, 2009].

261. Albano LM, Rivitti C, Bertola DR, et al. Angiokeratoma: a cutaneous marker of Fabry's disease. *Clin Exp Dermatol.* 2010;35(5):505–508. [Epub October 22, 2009].

262. Zampetti A, Orteu CH, Antuzzi D, et al. Angiokeratoma: decision-making aid for the diagnosis of Fabry disease. *Br J Dermatol.* 2012;166(4):712–720. [Epub March 29, 2012].

263. Imperial R, Helwig EB. Angiokeratoma of the scrotum (Fordyce type). *J Urol.* 1967;98(3):379–387. [Epub September 1, 1967].

264. Haye KR, Rebello DJ. Angiokeratoma of Mibelli. *Acta Derm Venereol.* 1961;41:56–60. [Epub January 1, 1961].

265. Lynch PJ, Kosanovich M. Angiokeratoma circumscriptum. *Arch Dermatol.* 1967;96(6):665–668. [Epub December 1, 1967].

266. Hunt SJ, Santa Cruz DJ. Vascular tumors of the skin: a selective review. *Semin Diagn Pathol.* 2004;21(3):166–218. [Epub May 26, 2005].

267. Fletcher CD, Beham A, Schmid C. Spindle cell haemangioendothelioma: a clinicopathological and immunohistochemical study indicative of a non-neoplastic lesion. *Histopathology.* 1991;18(4):291–301. [Epub April 1, 1991].

268. Perkins P, Weiss SW. Spindle cell hemangioendothelioma. An analysis of 78 cases with reassessment of its pathogenesis and biologic behavior. *Am J Surg Pathol.* 1996;20(10):1196–1204. [Epub October 1, 1996].

269. Requena L, Kutzner H. Hemangioendothelioma. *Semin Diagn Pathol.* 2013;30(1):29–44. [Epub January 19, 2013].

270. Brenn T, Fletcher CD. Cutaneous epithelioid angiomatous nodule: a distinct lesion in the morphologic spectrum of epithelioid vascular tumors. *Am J Dermatopathol.* 2004;26(1):14–21. [Epub January 17, 2004].

271. Sangueza OP, Walsh SN, Sheehan DJ, Orland AF, Llombart B, Requena L. Cutaneous epithelioid angiomatous nodule: a case series and proposed classification. *Am J Dermatopathol.* 2008;30(1): 16–20. [Epub January 24, 2008].

272. Rosai J. Angiolymphoid hyperplasia with eosinophilia of the skin. Its nosological position in the spectrum of histiocytoid hemangioma. *Am J Dermatopathol.* 1982;4(2):175–184. [Epub April 1, 1982].

273. Olsen TG, Helwig EB. Angiolymphoid hyperplasia with eosinophilia. A clinicopathologic study of 116 patients. *J Am Acad Dermatol.* 1985;12(5 Pt 1):781–796. [Epub May 1, 1985].

274. Fetsch JF, Weiss SW. Observations concerning the pathogenesis of epithelioid hemangioma (angiolymphoid hyperplasia). *Mod Pathol.* 1991;4(4):449–455. [Epub July 1, 1991].

275. Chan JK, Fletcher CD, Hicklin GA, Rosai J. Glomeruloid hemangioma. A distinctive cutaneous lesion of multicentric Castleman's disease associated with POEMS syndrome. *Am J Surg Pathol.* 1990;14(11):1036–1046. [Epub November 1, 1990].

276. Chung WK, Lee DW, Yang JH, Lee MW, Choi JH, Moon KC. Glomeruloid hemangioma as a very early presenting sign of POEMS syndrome. *J Cutan Pathol.* 2009;36(10):1126–1128. [Epub July 21, 2009].

277. Gonzalez-Guerra E, Haro MR, Farina MC, Martin L, Manzarbeitia L, Requena L. Glomeruloid haemangioma is not always associated with POEMS syndrome. *Clin Exp Dermatol.* 2009;34(7):800–803. [Epub December 17, 2008].

278. Jacobson-Dunlop E, Liu H, Simpson EL, White CR Jr, White KP. Glomeruloid hemangiomas in the absence of POEMS syndrome. *J Cutan Pathol*. 2012;39(4):402–403. [Epub March 27, 2012].

279. Requena L, Sangueza OP. Cutaneous vascular anomalies. Part I. Hamartomas, malformations, and dilation of preexisting vessels. *J Am Acad Dermatol*. 1997;37(4):523–549; quiz 49–52. [Epub October 31, 1997].

280. Hashimoto H, Daimaru Y, Enjoji M. Intravascular papillary endothelial hyperplasia. A clinicopathologic study of 91 cases. *Am J Dermatopathol*. 1983;5(6):539–546. [Epub December 1, 1983].

281. Reed CN, Cooper PH, Swerlick RA. Intravascular papillary endothelial hyperplasia. Multiple lesions simulating Kaposi's sarcoma. *J Am Acad Dermatol*. 1984;10(1):110–113. [Epub January 1, 1984].

282. Peachey RD, Lim CC, Whimster IW. Lymphangioma of skin. A review of 65 cases. *Br J Dermatol*. 1970;83(5):519–527. [Epub November 1, 1970].

283. Meunier L, Barneon G, Meynadier J. Acquired progressive lymphangioma. *Br J Dermatol*. 1994;131(5):706–708. [Epub November 1, 1994].

284. Pelle MT, Pride HB, Tyler WB. Eccrine angiomatous hamartoma. *J Am Acad Dermatol*. 2002;47(3):429–435. [Epub August 28, 2002].

285. Sanmartin O, Botella R, Alegre V, Martinez A, Aliaga A. Congenital eccrine angiomatous hamartoma. *Am J Dermatopathol*. 1992;14(2):161–164. [Epub April 1, 1992].

286. Carroll RE, Berman AT. Glomus tumors of the hand: review of the literature and report on twenty-eight cases. *J Bone Joint Surg Am*. 1972;54(4):691–703. [Epub June 1, 1972].

287. Dervan PA, Tobbia IN, Casey M, O'Loughlin J, O'Brien M. Glomus tumours: an immunohistochemical profile of 11 cases. *Histopathology*. 1989;14(5):483–491. [Epub May 1, 1989].

288. Wick MR, Rocamora A. Reactive and malignant "angioendotheliomatosis": a discriminant clinicopathological study. *J Cutan Pathol*. 1988;15(5):260–271. [Epub October 1, 1988].

289. McMenamin ME, Fletcher CD. Reactive angioendotheliomatosis: a study of 15 cases demonstrating a wide clinicopathologic spectrum. *Am J Surg Pathol*. 2002;26(6):685–697. [Epub May 23, 2002].

290. Rieger E, Soyer HP, Leboit PE, Metze D, Slovak R, Kerl H. Reactive angioendotheliomatosis or intravascular histiocytosis? An immunohistochemical and ultrastructural study in two cases of intravascular histiocytic cell proliferation. *Br J Dermatol*. 1999;140(3):497–504. [Epub May 8, 1999].

291. Lazova R, Slater C, Scott G. Reactive angioendotheliomatosis. Case report and review of the literature. *Am J Dermatopathol*. 1996;18(1):63–69. [Epub February 1, 1996].

292. O'Grady JT, Shahidullah H, Doherty VR, al-Nafussi A. Intravascular histiocytosis. *Histopathology*. 1994;24(3):265–268. [Epub March 1, 1994].

293. Nishie W, Sawamura D, Iitoyo M, Shimizu H. Intravascular histiocytosis associated with rheumatoid arthritis. *Dermatology*. 2008;217(2):144–145. [Epub May 30, 2008].

294. Grekin S, Mesfin M, Kang S, Fullen DR. Intralymphatic histiocytosis following placement of a metal implant. *J Cutan Pathol*. 2011;38(4):351–353. [Epub May 25, 2010].

295. Mentzel T, Beham A, Calonje E, Katenkamp D, Fletcher CD. Epithelioid hemangioendothelioma of skin and soft tissues: clinicopathologic and immunohistochemical study of 30 cases. *Am J Surg Pathol*. 1997;21(4):363–374. [Epub April 1, 1997].

296. Resnik KS, Kantor GR, Spielvogel RL, Ryan E. Cutaneous epithelioid hemangioendothelioma without systemic involvement. *Am J Dermatopathol*. 1993;15(3):272–276. [Epub June 1, 1993].

297. Quante M, Patel NK, Hill S, et al. Epithelioid hemangioendothelioma presenting in the skin: a clinicopathologic study of eight cases. *Am J Dermatopathol*. 1998;20(6):541–546. [Epub December 17, 1998].

298. Hodgkinson DJ, Soule EH, Woods JE. Cutaneous angiosarcoma of the head and neck. *Cancer*. 1979;44(3):1106–1113. [Epub September 1, 1979].

299. Billings SD, Folpe AL. Cutaneous and subcutaneous fibrohistiocytic tumors of intermediate malignancy: an update. *Am J Dermatopathol*. 2004;26(2):141–155. [Epub March 17, 2004].

300. Patton KT, Deyrup AT, Weiss SW. Atypical vascular lesions after surgery and radiation of the breast: a clinicopathologic study of 32 cases analyzing histologic heterogeneity and association with angiosarcoma. *Am J Surg Pathol.* 2008;32(6):943–950. [Epub June 14, 2008].

301. Gengler C, Coindre JM, Leroux A, et al. Vascular proliferations of the skin after radiation therapy for breast cancer: clinicopathologic analysis of a series in favor of a benign process: a study from the French Sarcoma Group. *Cancer.* 2007;109(8):1584–1598. [Epub March 16, 2007].

302. Jayalakshmy PS, Sivaram AP, Augustine J, Bindu P. Postmastectomy-postirradiation atypical vascular lesion of the skin: report of 2 cases. *Case Rep Pathol.* 2012;2012:710318. [Epub October 11, 2012].

303. Viejo-Borbolla A, Schulz TF. Kaposi's sarcoma-associated herpesvirus (KSHV/HHV8): key aspects of epidemiology and pathogenesis. *AIDS Rev.* 2003;5(4):222–229. [Epub March 12, 2004].

304. Tappero JW, Conant MA, Wolfe SF, Berger TG. Kaposi's sarcoma. Epidemiology, pathogenesis, histology, clinical spectrum, staging criteria and therapy. *J Am Acad Dermatol.* 1993;28(3):371–395. [Epub March 1, 1993].

305. O'Connell KM. Kaposi's sarcoma: histopathological study of 159 cases from Malawi. *J Clin Pathol.* 1977;30(8):687–695. [Epub August 1, 1977].

306. Zukerberg LR, Nickoloff BJ, Weiss SW. Kaposiform hemangioendothelioma of infancy and childhood. An aggressive neoplasm associated with Kasabach-Merritt syndrome and lymphangiomatosis. *Am J Surg Pathol.* 1993;17(4):321–328. [Epub April 1, 1993].

307. Tsang WY, Chan JK. Kaposi-like infantile hemangioendothelioma. A distinctive vascular neoplasm of the retroperitoneum. *Am J Surg Pathol.* 1991;15(10):982–989. [Epub October 1, 1991].

308. Vin-Christian K, McCalmont TH, Frieden IJ. Kaposiform hemangioendothelioma. An aggressive, locally invasive vascular tumor that can mimic hemangioma of infancy. *Archives of Dermatol.* 1997;133(12):1573–1578. [Epub January 8, 1998].

309. Le Huu AR, Jokinen CH, Rubin BP, et al. Expression of prox1, lymphatic endothelial nuclear transcription factor, in Kaposiform hemangioendothelioma and tufted angioma. *Am J Surg Pathol.* 2010;34(11):1563–1573. [Epub October 27, 2010].

310. Megahed M. Histopathological variants of neurofibroma. A study of 114 lesions. *Am J Dermatopathol.* 1994;16(5):486–495. [Epub October 1, 1994].

311. Riccardi VM. Von Recklinghausen neurofibromatosis. *N Engl J Med.* 1981;305(27):1617–1627. [Epub December 31, 1981].

312. Honda M, Arai E, Sawada S, Ohta A, Niimura M. Neurofibromatosis 2 and neurilemmomatosis gene are identical. *J Invest Dermatol.* 1995;104(1):74–77. [Epub January 1, 1995].

313. Kurtkaya-Yapicier O, Scheithauer B, Woodruff JM. The pathobiologic spectrum of Schwannomas. *Histol Histopathol.* 2003;18(3):925–934. [Epub June 7, 2003].

314. Reed RJ, Fine RM, Meltzer HD. Palisaded, encapsulated neuromas of the skin. *Arch Dermatol.* 1972;106(6):865–870. [Epub December 1, 1972].

315. Fletcher CD. Solitary circumscribed neuroma of the skin (so-called palisaded, encapsulated neuroma). A clinicopathologic and immunohistochemical study. *Am J Surg Pathol.* 1989;13(7):574–580. [Epub July 1, 1989].

316. Robson AM, Calonje E. Cutaneous perineurioma: a poorly recognized tumour often misdiagnosed as epithelioid histiocytoma. *Histopathology.* 2000;37(4):332–339. [Epub September 30, 2000].

317. Skelton HG, Williams J, Smith KJ. The clinical and histologic spectrum of cutaneous fibrous perineuriomas. *Am J Dermatopathol.* 2001;23(3):190–196. [Epub June 8, 2001].

318. Buley ID, Gatter KC, Kelly PM, Heryet A, Millard PR. Granular cell tumours revisited. An immunohistological and ultrastructural study. *Histopathology.* 1988;12(3):263–274. [Epub March 1, 1988].

319. Ordonez NG. Granular cell tumor: a review and update. *Adv Anat Pathol.* 1999;6(4):186–203. [Epub July 20, 1999].

320. Angervall L, Kindblom LG, Haglid K. Dermal nerve sheath myxoma. A light and electron microscopic, histochemical and immunohistochemical study. *Cancer.* 1984;53(8):1752–1759. [Epub April 15, 1984].

321. Fetsch JF, Laskin WB, Miettinen M. Nerve sheath myxoma: a clinicopathologic and immunohistochemical analysis of 57 morphologically distinctive, S-100 protein- and GFAP-positive, myxoid peripheral nerve sheath tumors with a predilection for the extremities and a high local recurrence rate. *Am J Surg Pathol.* 2005;29(12):1615–1624. [Epub December 6, 2005].

322. Misago N, Inoue T, Narisawa Y. Unusual benign myxoid nerve sheath lesion: myxoid palisaded encapsulated neuroma (PEN) or nerve sheath myxoma with PEN/PEN-like features? *Am J Dermatopathol.* 2007;29(2):160–164. [Epub April 7, 2007].

323. Barnhill RL, Mihm MC Jr. Cellular neurothekeoma. A distinctive variant of neurothekeoma mimicking nevomelanocytic tumors. *Am J Surg Pathol.* 1990;14(2):113–120. [Epub February 1, 1990].

324. Fetsch JF, Laskin WB, Hallman JR, Lupton GP, Miettinen M. Neurothekeoma: an analysis of 178 tumors with detailed immunohistochemical data and long-term patient follow-up information. *Am J Surg Pathol.* 2007;31(7):1103–1114. [Epub June 27, 2007].

325. Plaza JA, Torres-Cabala C, Evans H, Diwan AH, Prieto VG. Immunohistochemical expression of S100A6 in cellular neurothekeoma: clinicopathologic and immunohistochemical analysis of 31 cases. *Am J Dermatopathol.* 2009;31(5):419–422. [Epub June 23, 2009].

326. Uhle P, Norvell SS Jr. Generalized lentiginosis. *J Am Acad Dermatol.* 1988;18(2 Pt 2):444–447. [Epub February 1, 1988].

327. Andersen WK, Labadie RR, Bhawan J. Histopathology of solar lentigines of the face: a quantitative study. *J Am Acad Dermatol.* 1997;36(3 Pt 1):444–447. [Epub March 1, 1997].

328. Buchner A, Hansen LS. Melanotic macule of the oral mucosa. A clinicopathologic study of 105 cases. *Oral Surg Oral Med Oral Pathol.* 1979;48(3):244–249. [Epub September 1, 1979].

329. Ho KK, Dervan P, O'Loughlin S, Powell FC. Labial melanotic macule: a clinical, histopathologic, and ultrastructural study. *J Am Acad Dermatol.* 1993;28(1):33–39. [Epub January 1, 1993].

330. Haneke E. The dermal component in melanosis naeviformis Becker. *J Cutan Pathol.* 1979;6(1): 53–58. [Epub February 1, 1979].

331. Patrizi A, Medri M, Neri I, Fanti PA. Becker naevus associated with basal cell carcinoma, melanocytic naevus and smooth-muscle hamartoma. *J Eur Acad Dermatol Venereol.* 2007;21(1): 130–132. [Epub January 9, 2007].

332. Swerdlow AJ, English J, MacKie RM, et al. Benign melanocytic naevi as a risk factor for malignant melanoma. *Br Med J (Clin Res Ed).* 1986;292(6535):1555–1559. [Epub June 14, 1986].

333. Cochran AJ, Bailly C, Paul E, Dolbeau D. Nevi, other than dysplastic and Spitz nevi. *Semin Diagn Pathol.* 1993;10(1):3–17. [Epub February 1, 1993].

334. Weedon D. Unusual features of nevocellular nevi. *J Cutan Pathol.* 1982;9(5):284–292. [Epub October 1, 1982].

335. Cramer SF. The origin of epidermal melanocytes. Implications for the histogenesis of nevi and melanomas. *Arch Pathol Lab Med.* 1991;115(2):115–119. [Epub February 1, 1991].

336. Horenstein MG, Prieto VG, Burchette JL Jr., Shea CR. Keratotic melanocytic nevus: a clinicopathologic and immunohistochemical study. *J Cutan Pathol.* 2000;27(7):344–350. [Epub August 5, 2000].

337. Adeniran AJ, Prieto VG, Chon S, Duvic M, Diwan AH. Atypical histologic and immunohistochemical findings in melanocytic nevi after liquid nitrogen cryotherapy. *J Am Acad Dermatol.* 2009;61(2):341–345. [Epub April 14, 2009].

338. Boyd AS, Rapini RP. Acral melanocytic neoplasms: a histologic analysis of 158 lesions. *J Am Acad Dermatol.* 1994;31(5 Pt 1):740–745. [Epub November 1, 1994].

339. Blessing K. Benign atypical naevi: diagnostic difficulties and continued controversy. *Histopathology.* 1999;34(3):189–198. [Epub April 27, 1999].

340. Bravo Puccio F, Chian C. Acral junctional nevus versus acral lentiginous melanoma in situ: a differential diagnosis that should be based on clinicopathologic correlation. *Arch Pathol Lab Med.* 2011;135(7):847–852. [Epub July 8, 2011].

341. Seab JA Jr, Graham JH, Helwig EB. Deep penetrating nevus. *Am J Surg Pathol.* 1989;13(1):39–44. [Epub January 1, 1989].

342. Cooper PH. Deep penetrating (plexiform spindle cell) nevus. A frequent participant in combined nevus. *J Cutan Pathol*. 1992;19(3):172–180. [Epub June 1, 1992].

343. Robson A, Morley-Quante M, Hempel H, McKee PH, Calonje E. Deep penetrating naevus: clinicopathological study of 31 cases with further delineation of histological features allowing distinction from other pigmented benign melanocytic lesions and melanoma. *Histopathology*. 2003;43(6):529–537. [Epub November 26, 2003].

344. Luzar B, Calonje E. Deep penetrating nevus: a review. *Arch Pathol Lab Med*. 2011;135(3):321–326. [Epub March 4, 2011].

345. Roth ME, Grant-Kels JM, Ackerman AB, et al. The histopathology of dysplastic nevi. Continued controversy. *Am J Dermatopathol*. 1991;13(1):38–51. [Epub February 1, 1991].

346. Ahmed I, Piepkorn MW, Rabkin MS, et al. Histopathologic characteristics of dysplastic nevi. Limited association of conventional histologic criteria with melanoma risk group. *J Am Acad Dermatol*. 1990;22(5 Pt 1):727–733. [Epub May 1, 1990].

347. Elder DE. Dysplastic naevi: an update. *Histopathology*. 2010;56(1):112–120. [Epub January 9, 2010].

348. Shea CR, Vollmer RT, Prieto VG. Correlating architectural disorder and cytologic atypia in Clark (dysplastic) melanocytic nevi. *Hum Pathol*. 1999;30(5):500–505. [Epub May 20, 1999].

349. Walker GJ, Hussussian CJ, Flores JF, et al. Mutations of the CDKN2/p16INK4 gene in Australian melanoma kindreds. *Hum Mol Genet*. 1995;4(10):1845–1852. [Epub October 1, 1995].

350. Rivers JK, Kopf AW, Vinokur AF, et al. Clinical characteristics of malignant melanomas developing in persons with dysplastic nevi. *Cancer*. 1990;65(5):1232–1236. [Epub March 1, 1990].

351. Spitz S. Melanomas of childhood. *Am J Pathol*. 1948;24(3):591–609. [Epub May 1, 1948].

352. Casso EM, Grin-Jorgensen CM, Grant-Kels JM. Spitz nevi. *J Am Acad Dermatol*. 1992;27 (6 Pt 1):901–913. [Epub December 1, 1992].

353. Requena C, Requena L, Kutzner H, Sanchez Yus E. Spitz nevus: a clinicopathological study of 349 cases. *Am J Dermatopathol*. 2009;31(2):107–116. [Epub March 26, 2009].

354. Zedek DC, McCalmont TH. Spitz nevi, atypical spitzoid neoplasms, and spitzoid melanoma. *Clin Lab Med*. 2011;31(2):311–320. [Epub May 10, 2011].

355. Miteva M, Lazova R. Spitz nevus and atypical spitzoid neoplasm. *Semin Cutan Med Surg*. 2010;29(3):165–173. [Epub November 6, 2010].

356. Rybojad M, Moraillon I, Ogier de Baulny H, Prigent F, Morel P. [Extensive Mongolian spot related to Hurler disease]. *Ann Dermatol Venereol*. 1999;126(1):35–37. [Epub March 30, 1999]. Tache mongolique etendue revelant une maladie de Hurler.

357. Kikuchi I, Inoue S. Natural history of the Mongolian spot. *J Dermatol*. 1980;7(6):449–450. [Epub December 1, 1980].

358. Hidano A, Kajima H, Ikeda S, Mizutani H, Miyasato H, Niimura M. Natural history of nevus of Ota. *Arch Dermatol*. 1967;95(2):187–195. [Epub February 1, 1967].

359. Mishima Y, Mevorah B. Nevus Ota and nevus Ito in American Negroes. *J Invest Dermatol*. 1961;36:133–154. [Epub February 1, 1961].

360. Temple-Camp CR, Saxe N, King H. Benign and malignant cellular blue nevus. A clinicopathological study of 30 cases. *Am J Dermatopathol*. 1988;10(4):289–296. [Epub August 1, 1988].

361. Leopold JG, Richards DB. The interrelationship of blue and common naevi. *J Pathol Bacteriol*. 1968;95(1):37–46. [Epub January 1, 1968].

362. Rodriguez HA, Ackerman LV. Cellular blue nevus. Clinicopathologic study of forty-five cases. *Cancer*. 1968;21(3):393–405. [Epub March 1, 1968].

363. Weyers W, Euler M, Diaz-Cascajo C, Schill WB, Bonczkowitz M. Classification of cutaneous malignant melanoma: a reassessment of histopathologic criteria for the distinction of different types. *Cancer*. 1999;86(2):288–299. [Epub July 27, 1999].

364. Duncan LM. The classification of cutaneous melanoma. *Hematol Oncol Clin North Am*. 2009;23(3):501–513, ix. [Epub May 26, 2009].

365. Elder DE. Pathology of melanoma. *Clin Cancer Res*. 2006;12(7 Pt 2):2308s–23011s. [Epub April 13, 2006].

366. Baumert J, Schmidt M, Giehl KA, et al. Time trends in tumour thickness vary in subgroups: analysis of 6475 patients by age, tumour site and melanoma subtype. *Melanoma Res.* 2009;19(1):24–30. [Epub May 12, 2009].

367. Feibleman CE, Stoll H, Maize JC. Melanomas of the palm, sole, and nailbed: a clinicopathologic study. *Cancer.* 1980;46(11):2492–2504. [Epub December 1, 1980].

368. McCarthy SW, Scolyer RA, Palmer AA. Desmoplastic melanoma: a diagnostic trap for the unwary. *Pathology.* 2004;36(5):445–451. [Epub September 17, 2004].

369. de Almeida LS, Requena L, Rutten A, et al. Desmoplastic malignant melanoma: a clinicopathologic analysis of 113 cases. *Am J Dermatopathol.* 2008;30(3):207–215. [Epub May 23, 2008].

370. Plaza JA, Torres-Cabala C, Evans H, Diwan HA, Suster S, Prieto VG. Cutaneous metastases of malignant melanoma: a clinicopathologic study of 192 cases with emphasis on the morphologic spectrum. *Am J Dermatopathol.* 2010;32(2):129–136. [Epub December 17, 2009].

371. Bergman R, Kurtin PJ, Gibson LE, Hull PR, Kimlinger TK, Schroeter AL. Clinicopathologic, immunophenotypic, and molecular characterization of primary cutaneous follicular B-cell lymphoma. *Arch Dermatol.* 2001;137(4):432–439. [Epub May 1, 2001].

372. Lawnicki LC, Weisenburger DD, Aoun P, Chan WC, Wickert RS, Greiner TC. The t(14;18) and bcl-2 expression are present in a subset of primary cutaneous follicular lymphoma: association with lower grade. *Am J Clin Pathol.* 2002;118(5):765–772. [Epub November 14, 2002].

373. de Leval L, Harris NL, Longtine J, Ferry JA, Duncan LM. Cutaneous b-cell lymphomas of follicular and marginal zone types: use of Bcl-6, CD10, Bcl-2, and CD21 in differential diagnosis and classification. *Am J Surg Pathol.* 2001;25(6):732–741. [Epub June 8, 2001].

374. Santucci M, Pimpinelli N. Primary cutaneous B-cell lymphomas. Current concepts. I. *Haematologica.* 2004;89(11):1360–1371. [Epub November 9, 2004].

375. Bailey EM, Ferry JA, Harris NL, Mihm MC Jr., Jacobson JO, Duncan LM. Marginal zone lymphoma (low-grade B-cell lymphoma of mucosa-associated lymphoid tissue type) of skin and subcutaneous tissue: a study of 15 patients. *Am J Surg Pathol.* 1996;20(8):1011–1023. [Epub August 1, 1996].

376. Cerroni L, Signoretti S, Hofler G, et al. Primary cutaneous marginal zone B-cell lymphoma: a recently described entity of low-grade malignant cutaneous B-cell lymphoma. *Am J Surg Pathol.* 1997;21(11):1307–1315. [Epub November 14, 1997].

377. Willemze R, Jaffe ES, Burg G, et al. WHO-EORTC classification for cutaneous lymphomas. *Blood.* 2005;105(10):3768–3785. [Epub February 5, 2005].

378. Argatoff LH, Connors JM, Klasa RJ, Horsman DE, Gascoyne RD. Mantle cell lymphoma: a clinicopathologic study of 80 cases. *Blood.* 1997;89(6):2067–2078. [Epub March 15, 1997].

379. Sen F, Medeiros LJ, Lu D, et al. Mantle cell lymphoma involving skin: cutaneous lesions may be the first manifestation of disease and tumors often have blastoid cytologic features. *Am J Surg Pathol.* 2002;26(10):1312–1318. [Epub October 3, 2002].

380. Vermeer MH, Geelen FA, van Haselen CW, et al. Primary cutaneous large B-cell lymphomas of the legs. A distinct type of cutaneous B-cell lymphoma with an intermediate prognosis. Dutch Cutaneous Lymphoma Working Group. *Arch Dermatol.* 1996;132(11):1304–1308. [Epub November 1, 1996].

381. Grange F, Beylot-Barry M, Courville P, et al. Primary cutaneous diffuse large B-cell lymphoma, leg type: clinicopathologic features and prognostic analysis in 60 cases. *Arch Dermatol.* 2007;143(9):1144–1150. [Epub September 19, 2007].

382. Plaza JA, Kacerovska D, Stockman DL, et al. The histomorphologic spectrum of primary cutaneous diffuse large B-cell lymphoma: a study of 79 cases. *Am J Dermatopathol.* 2011;33(7): 649–655; quiz 56–58. [Epub September 23, 2011].

383. James WD, Odom RB, Katzenstein AL. Cutaneous manifestations of lymphomatoid granulomatosis. Report of 44 cases and a review of the literature. *Arch Dermatol.* 1981;117(4): 196–202. [Epub April 1, 1981].

384. Beaty MW, Toro J, Sorbara L, et al. Cutaneous lymphomatoid granulomatosis: correlation of clinical and biologic features. *Am J Surg Pathol.* 2001;25(9):1111–1120. [Epub November 2, 2001].

385. Ferreri AJ, Campo E, Seymour JF, et al. Intravascular lymphoma: clinical presentation, natural history, management and prognostic factors in a series of 38 cases, with special emphasis on the 'cutaneous variant'. *Br J Haematol.* 2004;127(2):173–183. [Epub October 6, 2004].

386. Murase T, Yamaguchi M, Suzuki R, et al. Intravascular large B-cell lymphoma (IVLBCL): a clinicopathologic study of 96 cases with special reference to the immunophenotypic heterogeneity of CD5. *Blood.* 2007;109(2):478–485. [Epub September 21, 2006].

387. Orwat DE, Batalis NI. Intravascular large B-cell lymphoma. *Arch Pathol Lab Med.* 2012;136(3): 333–338. [Epub March 1, 2012].

388. Plaza JA, Morrison C, Magro CM. Assessment of TCR-beta clonality in a diverse group of cutaneous T-cell infiltrates. *J Cutan Pathol.* 2008;35(4):358–365. [Epub November 3, 2007].

389. Massone C, Kodama K, Kerl H, Cerroni L. Histopathologic features of early (patch) lesions of mycosis fungoides: a morphologic study on 745 biopsy specimens from 427 patients. *Am J Surg Pathol.* 2005;29(4):550–560. [Epub March 16, 2005].

390. Shapiro PE, Pinto FJ. The histologic spectrum of mycosis fungoides/Sezary syndrome (cutaneous T-cell lymphoma). A review of 222 biopsies, including newly described patterns and the earliest pathologic changes. *Am J Surg Pathol.* 1994;18(7):645–667. [Epub July 1, 1994].

391. Gerami P, Guitart J. The spectrum of histopathologic and immunohistochemical findings in folliculotropic mycosis fungoides. *Am J Surg Pathol.* 2007;31(9):1430–1438. [Epub August 28, 2007].

392. Pereyo NG, Requena L, Galloway J, Sangueza OP. Follicular mycosis fungoides: a clinicohistopathologic study. *J Am Acad Dermatol.* 1997;36(4):563–568. [Epub April 1, 1997].

393. Haghighi B, Smoller BR, LeBoit PE, Warnke RA, Sander CA, Kohler S. Pagetoid reticulosis (Woringer-Kolopp disease): an immunophenotypic, molecular, and clinicopathologic study. *Mod Pathol.* 2000;13(5):502–510. [Epub May 29, 2000].

394. LeBoit PE, Zackheim HS, White CR Jr. Granulomatous variants of cutaneous T-cell lymphoma. The histopathology of granulomatous mycosis fungoides and granulomatous slack skin. *Am J Surg Pathol.* 1988;12(2):83–95. [Epub February 1, 1988].

395. El-Shabrawi-Caelen L, Cerroni L, Medeiros LJ, McCalmont TH. Hypopigmented mycosis fungoides: frequent expression of a CD8+ T-cell phenotype. *Am J Surg Pathol.* 2002;26(4):450–457. [Epub March 27, 2002].

396. Buechner SA, Winkelmann RK. Sezary syndrome. A clinicopathologic study of 39 cases. *Arch Dermatol.* 1983;119(12):979–986. [Epub December 1, 1983].

397. Marti RM, Pujol RM, Servitje O, et al. Sezary syndrome and related variants of classic cutaneous T-cell lymphoma. A descriptive and prognostic clinicopathologic study of 29 cases. *Leuk Lymphoma.* 2003;44(1):59–69. [Epub April 15, 2003].

398. Vonderheid EC, Bernengo MG, Burg G, et al. Update on erythrodermic cutaneous T-cell lymphoma: report of the International Society for Cutaneous Lymphomas. *J Am Acad Dermatol.* 2002;46(1):95–106. [Epub January 5, 2002].

399. Diwan AH, Prieto VG, Herling M, Duvic M, Jone D. Primary Sezary syndrome commonly shows low-grade cytologic atypia and an absence of epidermotropism. *Am J Clin Pathol.* 2005;123(4):510–515. [Epub March 4, 2005].

400. Gonzalez CL, Medeiros LJ, Braziel RM, Jaffe ES. T-cell lymphoma involving subcutaneous tissue. A clinicopathologic entity commonly associated with hemophagocytic syndrome. *Am J Surg Pathol.* 1991;15(1):17–27. [Epub January 1, 1991].

401. Salhany KE, Macon WR, Choi JK, et al. Subcutaneous panniculitis-like T-cell lymphoma: clinicopathologic, immunophenotypic, and genotypic analysis of alpha/beta and gamma/delta subtypes. *Am J Surg Pathol.* 1998;22(7):881–893. [Epub July 21, 1998].

402. Hoque SR, Child FJ, Whittaker SJ, et al. Subcutaneous panniculitis-like T-cell lymphoma: a clinicopathological, immunophenotypic and molecular analysis of six patients. *Br J Dermatol.* 2003;148(3):516–525. [Epub March 26, 2003].

403. Kong YY, Dai B, Kong JC, et al. Subcutaneous panniculitis-like T-cell lymphoma: a clinicopathologic, immunophenotypic, and molecular study of 22 Asian cases according to WHO-EORTC classification. *Am J Surg Pathol.* 2008;32(10):1495–1502. [Epub August 19, 2008].

404. Berti E, Tomasini D, Vermeer MH, Meijer CJ, Alessi E, Willemze R. Primary cutaneous CD8-positive epidermotropic cytotoxic T cell lymphomas. A distinct clinicopathological entity with an aggressive clinical behavior. *Am J Pathol.* 1999;155(2):483–492. [Epub August 6, 1999].

405. Diwan H, Ivan D. CD8-positive mycosis fungoides and primary cutaneous aggressive epidermotropic CD8-positive cytotoxic T-cell lymphoma. *J Cutan Pathol.* 2009;36(3):390–392. [Epub February 18, 2009].

406. Nofal A, Abdel-Mawla MY, Assaf M, Salah E. Primary cutaneous aggressive epidermotropic CD8+ T-cell lymphoma: proposed diagnostic criteria and therapeutic evaluation. *J Am Acad Dermatol.* 2012;67(4):748–759. [Epub January 10, 2012].

407. de Wolf-Peeters C, Achten R. gammadelta T-cell lymphomas: a homogeneous entity? *Histopathology.* 2000;36(4):294–305. [Epub April 12, 2000].

408. Toro JR, Beaty M, Sorbara L, et al. gamma delta T-cell lymphoma of the skin: a clinical, microscopic, and molecular study. *Arch Dermatol.* 2000;136(8):1024–1032. [Epub August 5, 2000].

409. Guitart J, Weisenburger DD, Subtil A, et al. Cutaneous gammadelta T-cell lymphomas: a spectrum of presentations with overlap with other cytotoxic lymphomas. *Am J Surg Pathol.* 2012;36(11):1656–1665. [Epub October 18, 2012].

410. Choi YL, Park JH, Namkung JH, et al. Extranodal NK/T-cell lymphoma with cutaneous involvement: 'nasal' vs. 'nasal-type' subgroups--a retrospective study of 18 patients. *Br J Dermatol.* 2009;160(2):333–337. [Epub November 19, 2008].

411. Ng SB, Lai KW, Murugaya S, et al. Nasal-type extranodal natural killer/T-cell lymphomas: a clinicopathologic and genotypic study of 42 cases in Singapore. *Mod Pathol.* 2004;17(9):1097–1107. [Epub June 15, 2004].

412. Li S, Feng X, Li T, et al. Extranodal NK/T-cell lymphoma, nasal type: a report of 73 cases at MD Anderson Cancer Center. *Am J Surg Pathol.* 2013;37(1):14–23. [Epub December 13, 2012].

413. Iwatsuki K, Satoh M, Yamamoto T, et al. Pathogenic link between hydroa vacciniforme and Epstein-Barr virus-associated hematologic disorders. *Arch Dermatol.* 2006;142(5):587–595. [Epub May 17, 2006].

414. Barrionuevo C, Anderson VM, Zevallos-Giampietri E, et al. Hydroa-like cutaneous T-cell lymphoma: a clinicopathologic and molecular genetic study of 16 pediatric cases from Peru. *Appl Immunohistochem Mol Morphol.* 2002;10(1):7–14. [Epub March 15, 2002].

415. Magana M, Sangueza P, Gil-Beristain J, et al. Angiocentric cutaneous T-cell lymphoma of childhood (hydroa-like lymphoma): a distinctive type of cutaneous T-cell lymphoma. *J Am Acad Dermatol.* 1998;38(4):574–579. [Epub May 15, 1998].

416. Doeden K, Molina-Kirsch H, Perez E, Warnke R, Sundram U. Hydroa-like lymphoma with CD56 expression. *J Cutan Pathol.* 2008;35(5):488–494. [Epub November 3, 2007].

417. Saggini A, Gulia A, Argenyi Z, et al. A variant of lymphomatoid papulosis simulating primary cutaneous aggressive epidermotropic CD8+ cytotoxic T-cell lymphoma. Description of 9 cases. *Am J Surg Pathol.* 2010;34(8):1168–1175. [Epub July 28, 2010].

418. Kempf W. CD30+ lymphoproliferative disorders: histopathology, differential diagnosis, new variants, and simulators. *J Cutan Pathol.* 2006;33(suppl 1):58–70. [Epub January 18, 2006].

419. Plaza JA, Feldman AL, Magro C. Cutaneous CD30-positive lymphoproliferative disorders with CD8 expression: a clinicopathologic study of 21 cases. *J Cutan Pathol.* 2013;40(2):236–247. [Epub November 30, 2012].

420. Bekkenk MW, Geelen FA, van Voorst Vader PC, et al. Primary and secondary cutaneous CD30(+) lymphoproliferative disorders: a report from the Dutch Cutaneous Lymphoma Group on the long-term follow-up data of 219 patients and guidelines for diagnosis and treatment. *Blood.* 2000;95(12):3653–3661. [Epub June 14, 2000].

421. Plaza JA, Ortega P, Lynott J, Mullane M, Kroft S, Olteanu H. CD8-positive primary cutaneous anaplastic large T-cell lymphoma (PCALCL): case report and review of this unusual variant of PCALCL. *Am J Dermatopathol.* 2010;32(5):489–491. [Epub May 6, 2010].

422. Rodriguez Pinilla SM, Roncador G, Rodriguez-Peralto JL, et al. Primary cutaneous CD4+ small/medium-sized pleomorphic T-cell lymphoma expresses follicular T-cell markers. *Am J Surg Pathol.* 2009;33(1):81–90. [Epub November 7, 2008].

423. Grogg KL, Jung S, Erickson LA, McClure RF, Dogan A. Primary cutaneous CD4-positive small/medium-sized pleomorphic T-cell lymphoma: a clonal T-cell lymphoproliferative disorder with indolent behavior. *Mod Pathol.* 2008;21(6):708–715. [Epub March 4, 2008].
424. Uchiyama T, Yodoi J, Sagawa K, Takatsuki K, Uchino H. Adult T-cell leukemia: clinical and hematologic features of 16 cases. *Blood.* 1977;50(3):481–492. [Epub September 1, 1977].
425. Yamaguchi T, Ohshima K, Karube K, et al. Clinicopathological features of cutaneous lesions of adult T-cell leukaemia/lymphoma. *Br J Dermatol.* 2005;152(1):76–81. [Epub January 20, 2005].
426. Sellheyer K, et al. Follicular stem cell marker PHLDA1 (TDAG51) is superior to cytokeratin-20 in differentiating between trichoepithelioma and basal cell carcinoma in small biopsy specimens. *J Cutan Pathol.* 2011; 38(7):542-550.

Index